FACTS AND THEORIES OF
PSYCHOANALYSIS

Founded by C. K. Ogden

The International Library of Psychology

PSYCHOANALYSIS
In 28 Volumes

FACTS AND THEORIES OF PSYCHOANALYSIS

IVES HENDRICK

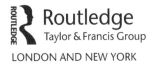

Routledge
Taylor & Francis Group
LONDON AND NEW YORK

First published in 1934 by
Routledge
2 Park Square, Milton Park, Abingdon, Oxfordshire OX14 4RN
711 Third Avenue, New York, NY 10017

First issued in paperback 2014

Routledge is an imprint of the Taylor and Francis Group, an informa business

The publishers have made every effort to contact authors/copyright holders
of the works reprinted in the *International Library of Psychology*.
This has not been possible in every case, however, and we would
welcome correspondence from those individuals/companies
we have been unable to trace.

These reprints are taken from original copies of each book. In many cases
the condition of these originals is not perfect. The publisher has gone to
great lengths to ensure the quality of these reprints, but wishes to point
out that certain characteristics of the original copies will, of necessity, be
apparent in reprints thereof.

British Library Cataloguing in Publication Data
A CIP catalogue record for this book
is available from the British Library

Facts and Theories of Psychoanalysis
ISBN 0415-21093-3
Psychoanalysis: 28 Volumes
ISBN 0415-21132-8
The International Library of Psychology: 204 Volumes
ISBN 0415-19132-7

ISBN 13: 978-1-138-87559-3 (pbk)
ISBN 13: 978-0-415-21093-5 (hbk)

AFFECTIONATELY DEDICATED

T O

MY MOTHER AND FATHER

PREFACE TO

THIRD EDITION

WHEN the summit of a lifetime has been achieved, it becomes
natural for most people to take a backward glance and take note
of what they had already understood in younger days, and what
wisdom (or seeming wisdom) they have since acquired.

The author has had a like experience in preparing this third
edition. In retrospect, it is obvious that twenty-three years ago
there could have been no final judgment as to the truth and validity
of the convictions of that small number of psychiatrists who had
made psychoanalysis their chief life work; there were indeed only
sixty-five members of the American Psychoanalytic Association in
1930. Not only the extraordinary increase within a generation of
the numbers of these practicing analysts, but also the widespread
acceptance of the value of their science in some medical centers
and by a number of other professions seem today full confirmation
of the convictions of the pioneers.

From this perspective, the usefulness of this book to readers
and students over a period of twenty-three years since its first publication would seem partly a result of the original selection of those
facts and theories for emphasis in 1934 which are still in 1957 the
foundation of psychoanalytic science. The decisive role of the unconscious in determining human experience, the facts of repression
and of infantile psychosexuality, the significance of these in normal
development and in the causation of neurotic suffering, the basic
principles of Freud's new method for exploring these regions of the
mind, as well as the invention of the instinct theory, and especially
the libido theory, are all even more certainly recognized as funda-

mental in 1957 than in 1934. In addition, there were a few topics, treated incidentally in the first edition, whose full importance was at that time not fully recognized, but has been in the intervening years. Thus "ego potentiality" was formulated in the first edition, and only extensively discussed and studied as "ego strength" in later years. Similarly, the basic identity of Freud's "Pleasure Principle" and Walter Cannon's concept of "homeostasis" was mentioned in the 1934 edition, and in recent years has received much attention. Some definite aspects of ego psychology which are of primary importance for the comprehension of psychoses and early development were also mentioned in the first edition and have been the basis of much productive work in this later period.

For these reasons it has been found unnecessary to recast the substance or form of presentation of these fundamental subjects for this third edition, though there have been thorough editing and some changes and additions. Chapter II, "Psychosexuality," has been made two chapters (II and III of this new edition), and one section has been somewhat expanded. This has also been the fate of former Chapter V, "Theory of Psychosexuality and Aggression" (Chapters VI and VII in this edition). In keeping with the extensive development of facts and theories of ego psychology during these latter decades, a portion of Chapter VIII (this edition), "The Structure of the Total Personality," already expanded in the second edition, has been rewritten and amplified.

But though these foundations of psychoanalysis have survived the controversies of the years, a new professional structure has arisen, especially in America, with many anterooms and chambers. Part IV of all editions, "The Psychoanalytic Movement," has therefore in large part been rewritten. Thus, though dynamic psychiatry was not new in 1934, its extraordinary development and expansion, and its unanticipated utilization of psychoanalysis, are reflected in this author's development of six pages of the second edition into Chapter XII, "Psychoanalysis and Dynamic Psychiatry," dealing particularly with applications of psychoanalysis to the study of the psychoses and to the techniques of modern psychotherapy. The growth of child psychiatry and the contributions of child analysis to this field have also been phenomenal, and the six pages of the previous edition have therefore become Chapter XIII, "Child Analysis and Child Psychiatry." The establishment of Psychosomatic Medicine as a major specialty has entirely occurred since the first printing of this book; in consequence, the two pages in the first edition and the new chapter on this subject in the second edition have also been in part rewritten: Chapter XIV, "Psychoanalysis and Diseases of the Body." Psychoanalysis has also had a fundamental effect upon basic ideas in the social sciences and non-medical clinical professions, such as clinical psychology, social work, education, and nursing. Former Chapter XI, "Professional and Cultural Applications," has therefore been rewritten as Chapter XV, "Applied Psychoanalysis."

Besides the intrinsic growth of psychoanalysis as a science and therapy, drastic world events have affected its organizational, educational, and practical problems. The shattering of European democracies by the Nazis and the War all but exterminated most centers of analysis in Europe, except England and Holland, and this cataclysm was followed by the emigration of most European analysts to other countries, especially to the United States. Before these events, the basic structure of institutes for psychoanalytic training in this country had been created, but no one had foreseen the extraordinary development of these institutes, either in numbers of students or in their contemporary influence on psychiatry. These new events required expansion of a chapter, in large part newly written, now Chapter XVI, "Psychoanalysis: A New Profession."

The Glossary has been carefully revised and amplified. The "Suggestions for Further Reading," intended as a helpful guide rather than a bibliography of sources, has been brought up to date, with some deletions and some additions. The Index is new.

IVES HENDRICK, M.D.

Boston, Massachusetts
November 1, 1957

SECOND EDITION

FIVE years have passed since this book was published. Psychoanalysis is still a youthful member of the scientific family, the creation of one man still living, and three generations of his followers. Not only has it added its specific discoveries to human knowledge, but it has proved to be a basic science whose principles are applicable to every field of study which involves the mental, emotional, and social functions of the human being. The developments of so youthful a science within a five years' span are more remarkable than those of older disciplines, and their extension to new fields more rapid. Besides this natural progress, the personnel of psychoanalysis and its professional organization have been profoundly affected by the political chaos of Europe. In America, however, the flowering of a closer relationship between psychoanalysis, organic medicine, and general psychiatry than has ever been possible in Europe, as well as the rapid development here of specialized training in this profession, has become more and more manifest.

This revision of the first edition aims to bring this volume up to date. Because its purpose was originally informative, rather than technical or controversial, and there have been no recent discoveries refuting the basic principles of psychoanalysis, many chapters have required no alteration. A discussion of the analytic controversy about the differentiation of female sexuality has been added to Chapter II; the section on identification has been rewritten, and a short discussion of the modern study of character defences has been included in the chapter on the anxiety theory of neurosis; the recent data of therapeutic results at the Institutes in Chicago and London have been included; and the brief discussion of child analysis has been amplified. Two new chapters have been added: one on the psychological study of organic disease, and one on the extra-medical applications of psychoanalysis. The final chapter on professional organizations and education has been rewritten. A new appendix has been added to facilitate cross-reference to cases, suggestions for further reading and glossary have been amplified, and the second edition has been re-indexed.

I. H.

Boston, Massachusetts
September 1, 1939

THE PRESENT volume attempts to give, as completely as brevity allows, an epitome of psychoanalysis, a survey of the whole science as it is understood by the specialist practising it today. No contribution which is not thoroughly discussed in the technical literature is attempted. And in only a few places, such as in emphasizing the concept of "instinct-representatives" and the relationship of unconscious psychology and physiology, in commenting on the therapy and prognosis of schizophrenia, and in formulating the nature of "Ego potentiality" (inevitably recognized by every practitioner, but too little discussed), has the author emphasized special individual interests of his own. The effort is made throughout to help the reader to distinguish consistently those facts and principles which are generally accepted by psychoanalysts at the present time from those which are decidedly controversial.

The book is oriented especially by the desire to make clear the distinction between the facts which are observed by all who practise psychoanalysis, and the theories. Clarity is sought by adequate illustrations from practice or everyday life.

The discussion of education in Chapter XII will show why this book is not designed for technical instruction in the practice of psychoanalysis. Nor does it attempt to convince the reader of what is proved only by direct observation. Its purpose is *informative,* to assist those with an intelligent interest to understand how the analyst himself regards his own work, and why. If it succeeds in this, it fulfils its purpose.

I. H.

Boston, Massachusetts
March 17, 1934

ACKNOWLEDGMENTS

EDITIONS I, II, AND III

THE FIRST acknowledgment of any contributor to psychoanalysis is almost superfluous—an expression of his appreciation of the genius of Sigmund Freud. My more individual indebtedness is to those teachers of the Berlin Institute of Psychoanalysis who enabled me to understand his work: Drs. Franz Alexander, Sandor Rado, Karen Horney, Max Eitingon, and Hanns Sachs—to name only those to whom I owe the most; and to those two men to whom I chiefly owe my scientific and psychiatric preparation for psychoanalytic study, Dr. Milton C. Winternitz, Dean of Yale Medical School (1920–35), and Dr. Charles Macfie Campbell, Professor of Psychiatry, Harvard Medical School (1920–43).

Whatever value this book may have is largely due to the detailed criticisms and suggestions of friends and colleagues who carefully studied my manuscript. Drs. Bertram Lewin, William J. Healy, Augusta Bronner, Franz Alexander, Henry A. Murray, Jr., John Whitehorn, Earl Bond, Miss Betsey Libbey, and Mr. Karl de Schweinitz.

I am indebted to Dr. Otto Fenichel for his preparation of the therapeutic results of the Berlin Institute, and to the Internationaler Psychoanalytischer Verlag for permission to abstract them; to Dr. Isador Coriat for his abstract of the proceedings of the Committee on Psychoanalysis of the British Medical Association (published in *The Psychoanalytic Review*, Vol. XVII, No. 1, January 1930); to Mr. Erik Erikson for revising and drawing the diagrams and criticizing the section on child analysis; and to Drs. Martin Peck, Isador Coriat, and John Murray for assistance in preparing the glossary and reading the proof.

Most of all I am indebted to my patients and students, not only for teaching me the facts of their unconscious minds (and now and then items that had been overlooked in the analysis of my own), but for the privilege of quoting their associations. The formulation of psychoanalysis without the clinical background is worth no printer's ink, but I have carefully tried in the selection and presentation of clinical fragments to avoid the possibility of personal embarrassment.

In the preparation of the second edition, I am indebted especially to Drs. John Abbott, Edgerton Howard, Leon Saul, and Miss Annette Garrett for their suggestions and assistance; to Mrs. Leslie Keay for secretarial collaboration of exceptional merit; and to Drs. Franz Alexander of the Chicago Institute for Psychoanalysis and Ernest Jones of the London Psychoanalytic Institute for permission to publish their statistical studies.

For the third edition, acknowledgment is due first to the authors of two major additions to early psychoanalytic history, the information they brought together, and their scholarship: Ernest Jones's definitive *Life of Sigmund Freud* (New York: Basic Books, Inc.); and Sigmund Freud's *The Origins of Psychoanalysis*, edited by Marie Bonaparte, Anna Freud, and Ernst Kris (New York: Basic Books, Inc.). The author is indebted to these books for several facts mentioned in this edition.

I am indebted to the following among many colleagues and friends who have helped by providing data, checking details, by suggestions, criticisms, editorial corrections, and unstinted encouragement: Drs. Marian Putnam (Chairman, The Children's Center, Boston), Gregory Rochlin (Director, The Children's Unit, Boston Psychopathic Hospital), Lucie Jessner (Professor of Child Psychiatry, University of North Carolina), Eveoleen Rexford (Director, Douglas Thom Clinic, Boston), Miss Helen Ross (Administrative Director, The Chicago Psychoanalytic Institute), Dr. Marion Kenworthy (President-elect, American Psychoanalytic Association), Dr. Richard M. Silberstein, Medical Director, Staten Island Mental Health Center, and Mrs. Margaret M. Otto (Librarian, The New York School of Social Work), for help with the chapter on

Child Analysis and Child Psychiatry; Dr. Ruth Eissler (Honorary Secretary of the International Psychoanalytic Association), for facts concerning psychoanalytic organizations in foreign countries; Dr. Ernest Kahn (Harvard Medical School), Dr. Karl Menninger (Editor, with the collaboration of George Devereux, Ph.D., *A Guide to Psychiatric Books with a Suggested Basic Reading List*), Mrs. Loretta Smith (Librarian, Boston Psychopathic Hospital), and Miss Miriam Putlack (Librarian, Boston Psychoanalytic Institute), for assistance with "Suggestions for Further Reading"; Dr. David Young (Professor, University of North Carolina, Department of Psychiatry) for assistance with several chapters; Dr. Robert Gardner (the Harvard Teaching Unit, Boston Psychopathic Hospital), for reading the chapter on Dynamic Psychiatry; Jerome Bruner, Ph.D. (Professor of Psychology, Harvard University), and Mr. Michael Maccoby (Research Assistant in Psychology, Harvard University) for their illuminating criticism of the chapter on Applied Psychoanalysis; and for the many scholarly corrections and suggestions of Dr. Carl Binger (Harvard University) regarding the chapter on Diseases of the Body and the Glossary; Drs. Alexander Martin, Harold Kelman, and Nathan Freeman of the American Association for the Advancement of Psychoanalysis for kindly helping me to clarify the views of Karen Horney (they take no responsibility for my summary in the text); Dr. George Daniels (Professor of Psychiatry, Columbia Medical School), for historical data in the chapter on Diseases of the Body; Dr. Bertram Lewin (Director, Survey of Psychoanalytic Education) for being the first to examine the Third, as he had been the first to examine the First Edition, *in toto,* and Mr. John McVeigh (Executive Secretary, American Psychoanalytic Association), for statistical data. Most of all I am grateful to my secretary, Mrs. Leslie Keay, for surpassing even the competence and spirit of her assistance with the second edition.

I. H.

CONTENTS

PART III. THERAPY BY PSYCHOANALYSIS

PART ONE

THE FACTS OF
PSYCHOANALYSIS

CHAPTER

I

THE UNCONSCIOUS

P S Y C H O A N A L Y S I S is the science of the unconscious functions of the mind and personality, developed by Sigmund Freud and three generations of his students. The term "psychoanalysis" is properly used in the following ways:

1. to designate *empirical observations* on those mental and emotional determinants of human personality and behavior which are not disclosed by the investigation of rational thought and motivation (either by introspection or by direct study of another);

2. to describe the special *technique* of Freud for the demonstration and study of these unconscious mental events and for the treatment of personality problems, neurotic symptoms, and diseases which are caused or influenced by them; and

3. to signify that *theoretical* system of psychology which consists in the abstraction of these observations and the inductive inferences made from them.

In a broader and less scientific sense, "psychoanalysis" may properly be used to include the application of knowledge of the individual derived from such studies to many allied subjects—to sociology, anthropology, economics, to the arts and literature, to comparative religion and ethics, to such professions as social work, nursing, psychology, pedagogy, and criminology—indeed, to all

branches of learning which deal with human nature and its derivatives. Psychoanalysis has also, especially during the last twenty
years, made significant contributions to medical research and the
therapy of many diseases long known to medicine by the symptoms
of damaged organs or abnormality of function.

"Psychoanalysis" is a word much misused (though far less often than it used to be). Sometimes it is dilettantishly used as a synonym for "psychotherapy," rather than as a special method of psychotherapy—indeed the most thorough method yet devised for
affecting fundamental processes of personality development. Frequently patients without technical knowledge speak of their "psychoanalysis" when they have had some other type of psychiatric
help. At other times "psychoanalysis" is misused in a less compli-
mentary way, usually by those who have studied it seriously but
have no clinical experience, as though the conclusions of psychoanalysts had no more empirical basis than a speculative philosophy
or fanatical dogma. Not infrequently, older physicians, of distinction in their own branch of medicine, are unable to think of psychoanalysis as a branch of science because the possibilities of new
knowledge of human processes derived from the study of psychological data are beyond their own field of experience and comprehension. Most commonly, perhaps, "psychoanalysis" is misused by
intellectuals who argue its validity as though it were a philosophy,
an ethical system, or a set of theories; such discussion, whether it
be heated or dispassionate, seems alien and unproductive to the
analyst himself, whose primary convictions originate in what his patients have told him.

THE UNCONSCIOUS

Though psychoanalysis is concerned with many aspects of
conscious thought, it is the development of a special technique for
exploring unconscious ideas which defines it as a specialized field
of mental science. "Unconscious" is a word which Freud uses in
two senses: as a simple *adjective,* to describe mental phenomena of

which the person is unaware; or, secondly, as a *substantive,* to designate the aggregate of observations of such mental activity. In this substantive and more theoretical sense, Freud refers to "*the* Unconscious," as though it were a special region of the mind. This does not imply any special knowledge of actual anatomical segregation in a definite portion of the brain; it is merely a convenient means of thinking of the totality of those psychological processes which differ from other mental phenomena chiefly in the inability of the subject to recognize or recall them by a simple effort of attention. *The* Unconscious, therefore, is the source of unconsciously motivated thoughts and acts, taken in the aggregate.

It is the particular task of psychoanalytic technique to investigate systematically the details of unconscious thoughts, memories, and wishes. When the objectionable idea or memory occurs to a patient, we say that this idea had been unconscious whenever the patient was previously unaware of it, though it had exerted a causal influence on his symptoms and actions. These unconscious thoughts cannot be discovered by the everyday intellectual processes of rational thought; for, indeed, it is a fact that consciousness of a certain thought can be so painful it evokes the need to keep such ideas in an unconscious state.

Most arguments against the existence of an "Unconscious" are of a philosophical nature, advanced by those who ignore the basic empiricism of Freud. It is this which distinguishes Freud's scientific contribution from that of philosophers, such as Spinoza, Schopenhauer, and Hartmann, who had previously surmised an unconscious type of thinking. Freud's achievement was to prove the validity of many of the intuitive conclusions of these gifted but unscientific men by laborious observations.

Other arguments against the concept of the Unconscious are occasionally advanced by scientists who have applied Freud's technique either inexpertly or not at all.

The Unconscious, like the chemical concept of atoms, is *theoretical* in so far as it is never observed directly; and *empirical* in that it is an essential inference if we are to explain logically and systematically a large mass of isolated observations which may be consistently confirmed. Otherwise the phenomena studied by analysts appear inexplicable and chaotic. These phenomena must be closely related to all vital manifestations of the organs the study of whose functions comprises normal and abnormal physiology. Certainly this is true of the brain. And, indeed, since the modern study of the anatomy of the brain and its network of nerves to other portions of the body was established, specialists in the field have striven to define thought and its pathological effects in terms of structural knowledge. Thrilling as were their achievements in elucidating some diseases in terms of brain anatomy, their efforts to explain those phenomena which Freud has elucidated were unavailing. For, practically, our knowledge of the more subtle and complex physiological functions and neurological pathways is wholly inadequate to describe the Unconscious in a useful way by its unknown chemico-physical properties or anatomical localization. If, however, in accordance with our observations, we formulate our inductions and generalizations in *psychological* terms, we succeed in describing certain properties and general laws of the Unconscious which are of substantial value.

For example, a hysterical paralysis (in which no disease of the tissues can be demonstrated) is obviously the result of some alteration of function in certain muscles and nerves; yet neither normal nor abnormal physiology gives a useful explanation of the process. Neurologists succeed only in diagnosing it as "functional," and many internists as a "general nuisance." On the other hand, psychoanalysis successfully describes this type of symptom in terms of unconscious mental processes which have general validity, not only for the specific case, but for all other symptoms of hysteria in other cases which manifest them. It can also show that some of these same laws are decisive for a large variety of other phenomena (for example, obsessions and dreams), the description of whose obvious properties discloses no resemblance to hysteria. And it can show how the etiology of the hysterical symptom differs from that of these other phenomena, and why an individual patient suffers from paralysis rather than some other abnormal function, and why the paralysis affects that particular part of the body in that particular case.

Freud originally called each impulse which motivates a specific act, phantasy, or symptom a *wish,* as it represents a certain insistent need of the individual, even though it is consciously denied.

Many examples of human behavior could be cited where the effectiveness of a wish which is unconscious is obvious to anybody except the subject. The girl who vehemently criticizes the taste in clothes of a friend often cannot consciously admit the real motive: "I wish I looked like her, and hate her because that man admires her." The mother who consciously maligns a school-teacher who justly punishes her son cannot endure the conscious thought: "My son was bad, not so good as the other children." The real motives of the "reformer" who consciously believes he is protecting others' morality and unconsciously enjoys a mass of obscene literature in the role of public censor are commonly recognized. In Eugene O'Neill's play *Mourning Becomes Electra*, Lavinia contrives the death of Captain Brant, her mother's lover, apparently to defend her father and avenge her mother's turpitude. At the height of angry passion, she suddenly cries: "Brant" to her own lover. Every member of the audience realizes the mistake is not pure chance, but discloses her love of Brant, even though she has so persistently concealed it from herself. The significance of a similar "slip of the tongue" in real life was immediately apparent when a man said to his childless wife: "When you're sewing, I think of Penelope weaving at her *womb*."

These are all examples of the unconscious but effective wishes which are the primary object of psychoanalytic study. The girl does not know her jealousy; the mother cannot think of her child's fault; the reformer may be unaware of his hypocrisy; Lavinia could not endure the thought of a hopeless and guilty love; the husband conceals his thwarted wish for a child. The reason for these people's blindness to their own motives is in every case the same: awareness of the emotion associated with the unconscious thought is too excruciating to be endured, and the painful thought must therefore be excluded from conscious meditation. Nevertheless, though unconscious, the emotional tension associated with each of these ideas impels the individual to some form of expression which has the dual purpose of satisfying indirectly the emotion and of disguising its real source. Thus hatred of a rival is expressed by condemning the rival's taste instead of her success in love; the censor explains his obscenity as an act of social beneficence; Lavinia's life is consumed, not by thoughts of love for Brant, but by thoughts of how bad her mother is and how wronged is her father; the husband affectionately praises his wife's sewing and does not condemn her childlessness.

The technical term for such exclusion of painful thoughts from consciousness is *repression*. The intellectual distortion by which the individual explains an unconsciously motivated act or symptom is termed *rationalization*.

Psychoanalysis has shown that *rationalization* is a secondary process, and that unconscious wishes are more vital factors in the motivation of human conduct. Every mental and social act can be shown by the study of its unconscious motive to have a definite cause, to be purposeful and "emotionally logical," however unreasonable it may appear biologically or intellectually. Rationalizations of such primary wishes do not in themselves constitute abnormality. It is only when unconscious motives produce acts or symptoms which lead to suffering or are detrimental to happiness and success, as is conspicuously the case in all psychoneurotic manifestations, that the repressed, unconscious wishes become of prime medical importance.

Unconscious wishes are generally less obvious than the simple cases cited above and are apparent neither to the subject nor to another person. The special technique of psychoanalysis must then be utilized in order to discover them.

For example, can a more adequate reason than "pure accident" be found why a man loses one of two theater tickets? No other explanation than "pure accident" is apparent to the patient or to his friends. Psychoanalysis discloses a series of memories which had been forgotten, and were "unconscious." On the reverse side of the lost ticket he had scribbled the address of a man with whom he had an appointment. The appointment was of considerable practical importance. Although their relationship was cordial, on one occasion the man had made a casual remark which severely wounded the patient's feelings. This he had forgotten until the memory returned in analysis. He, therefore, had two attitudes concerning his friend: *conscious* friendship and a practical need of his help, and the *unconscious* wish: "I hate the man who said that about me, and don't want to see him again." Those were incompatible attitudes. Yet, though the conscious feeling of friendship was not only more pleasant but advantageous, the wish to avoid a person he at the same time unconsciously hated had determined the "accidental" loss of a card bearing his address and thus fulfilled the wish not to see him again.

The relationship of the unconscious wish to behavior is somewhat more complex in the following example. A man could not remember the name of a recent acquaintance, Mrs. Barney. He was sure his moderate feeling for the lady was pleasant and there was no latent antagonism. By use of psychoanalysis it was demonstrated that her general personality and social position, as well as a similarity of names, had suggested that of another woman, Mrs. Barnet. This woman he scarcely knew, but her name had been frequently mentioned in association with a man whose hostility had greatly injured his business. One sees here how unconscious events may be indirectly associated with an otherwise "innocent" detail of experience and cause forgetfulness. Memory of the lady's name threatened him with the pain of recalling a similar person and consequently a very unpleasant episode of his life. Even though his emotions in regard to neither of the two ladies necessitated repression, a chance association with a repressed and pain-provoking memory affected his mental attitude to them. His forgetfulness is similar to forgetting the name of a town where one once had one's suitcase stolen.

Another patient was much distressed in life by an excessive meekness and lack of self-confidence. For a long time he had been laughed at for a sudden, tic-like movement of his flexed arm across the front of his body. Eventually he recalled that this was a repeated abbreviation of a pose he had occasionally assumed consciously, when much younger, before a mirror, imitating pictures of Napoleon with hand in waistcoat. These phantasies of being world-conqueror had long been forgotten. When they became conscious, the tic disappeared and the patient could no longer argue that his over-modesty and lack of aggression, which were in fact a denial of excessive, childish ambition, were special virtues.

Another man one day saw an overcoat hanging from the doorknob of his older brother's house. Thereafter he had to go home a roundabout way, so that he should not see this door. Such behavior was completely inexplicable until, in the course of analysis, he recalled that the instant he had seen the coat he had thought it was crepe, and then recounted a series of occasions for violently hating his older brother. The illusion that the coat had been crepe had expressed a deep, repressed wish that his brother might be dead. The avoidance of his brother's house was, therefore, a purposeful precaution against the chance of again stimulating the recognition of a hatred which had long been "repressed" and denied by a conscious feeling of special solicitude for his brother's well-being.

Freud's discovery that decisive motives in human thought and conduct are very often unconscious was the outcome of his investigation of the psychoneuroses, at first hysteria, and later the compulsion and obsessional neuroses.[1]

INVESTIGATIONS BY HYPNOSIS

As a young physician, Freud had gained recognition for researches in physiology and neurophysiology in the laboratories of Brücke and Meynert. In his clinical work, he became interested in hysteria, and left Vienna for Paris in 1885, at the age of twenty-nine, to spend a year in Charcot's clinic at the Salpetrière. This

[1] In this book I shall generally follow informal analytic usage, using "neurosis" and "psychoneurosis" as though synonymous, although the existence of organic "neuroses" is fully recognized. Similarly, I shall refer to "sexuality," where the more cumbersome "psychosexuality" would be more exact, and use "analysis" for "psychoanalysis."

world-famous master was demonstrating that symptoms of hysteria could be produced and allayed by hypnotic suggestion. Though Charcot himself attempted to explain the remarkable effectiveness of hypnosis by a physiological theory doomed to early obsolescence, his actual work had fully established the fact that psychological influences could definitely affect bodily mechanisms.

After a visit to the famous Bernheim in 1889 had convinced him of the limitations of hypnotic suggestion, Freud returned to Vienna and became the collaborator of his former teacher, Dr. Josef Breuer. This eminent physician had already, between 1880 and 1882, discovered that hysterical patients could recall experiences of which they had no memory when in a normal waking state.

For example, among other hysterical symptoms a German girl presented paralysis of an arm and inability to converse in her mother tongue, so that generally she understood only English. Under hypnosis a forgotten and tremendously emotional experience was recalled. This was a scene of nursing her dying father, when her arm was pressed against the chair exactly where her paralysis developed, and she spoke an English prayer. Another woman developed a tongue-tic, making a clucking noise every time she became excited; under hypnosis she recalled that this involuntary act began when striving to make no noise which might awaken her child, who was ill. A man who had a severe hysterical pain in his hip recalled under hypnosis that it was first experienced when witnessing the forcible extension of an ankylosed hip-joint of his brother.

Freud now collaborated with Breuer, adopted his technique, and confirmed and amplified his observations. In 1893 they published together their observations and inferences, their conclusive demonstration of significant unconscious mental processes, and their *traumatic theory* of hysteria. They had shown: first, that an event of great subjective emotional significance, if sufficiently painful to the individual, may be excluded from consciousness and cannot be recalled in the normal waking state. Secondly, that under hypnosis this event may be recalled, and it can then be shown that some detail of the traumatic experience, whether it be a single occasion or a series, is identical with details of the hysterical symptom. For example, the patient's emotional experience at the bedside of her father, quoted above, had been forgotten, but the subsequent loss of sensation was in that portion of her arm which had been pressed against the chair. Therefore, they concluded, the experience, though unconscious and not under ordinary circumstances accessible to memory, can exert a lasting effect and cause hysterical symptoms years afterward. This transformation of an emotional impulse into an abnormal physiological function they termed *conversion.*

To explain these observations they formulated the *traumatic theory of hysteria,* concluding that a hysterical symptom is caused by a traumatic psychological event, of whose conscious recollection and voluntary management the patient had been incapable in consequence of regression.

Finally, they showed that if this recollection of the traumatic experience under hypnosis was accompanied by an intense reproduction of the original emotion, often with a hallucinatory reproduction of the trauma, it no longer exerted an unconscious etiologic influence, and the symptom disappeared. This therapeutic event they called *abreaction,* and the method emotional *catharsis.*

Their work had been a conclusive demonstration of unconscious, repressed mental processes which exert dynamic effects long after the original stimulus, and of the possibility of an *etiologic* type of therapy for functional symptoms. A basic principle of psychoanalysis in later years, the role of unconscious ideas in the production of neurotic symptoms, had been fully established. But subsequent work was to show how inadequate was the original traumatic theory as an explanation of psychoneurosis, and of how little permanent value was therapy by hypnotic abreaction. These results of the experiments of Breuer and Freud with hypnosis were the cornerstones on which the edifice of modern psychoanalysis was to be built, but a new method had to be devised, investigated, and extensively elaborated through years of experience to produce psychoanalysis as we know it today.

THE FREE-ASSOCIATION METHOD

With this work Breuer's role in the history of psychoanalysis ends. Freud had already, soon after 1890, become dissatisfied with hypnosis as his instrument of investigation and therapy, for the following reasons: first, not all patients could be hypnotized; secondly, though a specific symptom was cured by emotional "catharsis" during hypnosis, the cure was temporary; and, thirdly, hypnosis influenced only those unconscious factors which were striving for expression and did not affect the prohibiting forces which were responsible for their exclusion from consciousness.

Moreover, hypnosis placed none of the mental functions peculiar to waking life at the disposal of the physician; its effectiveness was dependent on the patient's infantile submission to the suggestive power of the hypnotist, and, though it often cured the symptoms, it circumvented, instead of developed, the patient's own capacity to combat his illness. The cure was symptomatic; it was not a cure of the neurotic illness, and it was soon found to be an ephemeral cure and dependent on a perpetuation of the personal relationship of the patient with his physician.

While working with hypnosis, Freud had already made a discovery of a technical principle whose very naïveté is no less startling because silk-hatted neurologists of that day had overlooked it. He discovered that a great many important communications, which at first he had believed only hypnosis would reveal, would be told by the patient while awake if the physician listened sympathetically. These pertinent references to the intimate feelings could in no way be correlated with the medical learning of the day. For such an attitude toward the patient was the opposite to that of the physician, whose treatment is dependent upon impressing the patient with a knowledge he does or does not possess. Freud had admitted to himself the palpable truth that medicine still knew nothing at all about the causes of hysteria; that major neurologic advances of that day in the study of the nervous system had not resolved this ignorance of the nature of psychoneurosis, and that therefore the exploration of these problems by a psychologic method could be more rewarding.

True, physicians of all time, in their role as humanists, have listened to their patients' troubles; but none had thought to study those revelations systematically, to use them as the raw material of a scientific inquiry. Freud's genius for observing, not only organic symptoms, but human nature, soon led him to appreciate that it was not the most carefully reasoned utterances of his patients that were most helpful in his studies, but those which came spontaneously and with increased emotion. Merely listening to all that some of his patients knew of their own problems, duplicating in some ways the role of the Roman Catholic confessor, would not, of course, have led to psychoanalysis; for it was necessary to learn also what patients did not and could not know of their own unconscious selves. But it was the clue which led to the development of the new free-association technique for the study of human problems, the method which became the keystone of psychoanalytic technique in later years, and is today widely used in dynamic psychiatry and allied professions.

"Free association" is based upon the principle that there are two distinct ways in which ideas are associated with one another in the human mind. That of ordinary waking life is, so to speak, "horizontal"; a series of ideas are associated because of their logical or realistic relationships. To maintain this, the most conscious type of thought in most adults, there is a constant exclusion of ideas which threaten to intrude and break the logical continuity of this "horizontal thinking." The intruders are consciously discarded, or "repressed," from the focus of attention because they are illogical, embarrassing, disgusting, repugnant to ideals, or painful to self-esteem.

The second type of association of ideas may be thought of as "vertical," in the sense of a more immediate relationship to the "deeper," more primitive and imaginative components of the mind. In this type of association, thoughts succeed each other, not because they are rationally related, but because they are *emotionally* related. This occurs to some extent in everyday life—for example, when a girl likes a boy because he has the name of her favorite movie star; or a soldier dislikes an order because the officer has a nose like an older brother's. In normal reverie, such as that which commonly occurs after retiring and before deep sleep, day-dreams and memories may succeed each other in a haphazard way which defies an intellectual appraisal.

A few individuals often think in this associative manner quite naturally; they have an amazing understanding of motivations to which others are usually blinded by their need to rationalize emotion; they understand more easily than other people illogically related events, or what makes two people interact the way they do. Such individuals, more commonly women than men, more commonly artists than lawyers, are usually recognized as especially "intuitive" or "artistic." Most creative minds, at least those whose work is great, possess this gift. And certainly little children all demonstrate it constantly; they do not merely "outgrow" this early talent, but are trained to think consciously in more realistic terms, and educated to esteem the logical, and above all are required in the little segment of any civilization in which they live and think and fraternize to honor and obey the cultural limits on what it is proper to think and know and say. Many fine people are compelled by cultural convention to believe with conscious sincerity that a parent *always* loves a child, or that he loves each son and daughter equally, as though real love were dished out with a measuring cup, though others may observe this is basically an ideal and not always a valid fact. Few normal adults could react without horror, experiencing the news as something which could not really happen, on learning that a three-year-old child, left in her stateroom on a ship alone with her baby brother, got rid of the infant rival by throwing him out the porthole into the sea; yet many little children would immediately recognize this child's feeling of jealousy as natural, as a "fact of life" more fundamental than those which adults insist upon.

The most over-civilized of adults have never lost completely, or truly "outgrown," this capacity for understanding some things without benefit of logical connections. This fact is clearly apparent in group reactions, such as panic or riots or evangelism, where ideas will lead to acts of whose contemplation individuals would have ordinarily been incapable. Moreover, every adult mind is occasionally absorbed by a wish-fulfilling day-dream, or momentarily understands with certainty a secret emotional motive. All adults have some awareness of irrational association, especially when inflamed by passion or when laughing, reading, talking loquaciously, or playing. But few, until they have specially studied these processes, realize to what extent our daily conscious thoughts, those communicated to others and those uncommunicated, are edited, and how much of our conscious mentation is rejected by an unknown but scrupulous censor.

Freud made this second type of thinking, to which scientists had previously paid scant attention, the basis of the "free-association" method. The patient was asked to relax his attention and to report as well as he could each thought which came into his mind. He was specially instructed to try his very best to ignore all self-criticism, intellectual and moral, which might dictate that an exception be made of this or that spontaneous association. These ideas, especially phantasies and painful memories of emotional experience, together with the analyst's observations of the illogical interrelations of these ideas with each other and observations of accompanying gestures, mannerisms, changing voice and respiration, and especially of those occasions when the patient's effort to free associate becomes especially difficult or impossible, constitute the raw data of psychoanalysis. And the science of psychoanalysis is the intellectual organization of these facts of mental processes and emotional experiences revealed by expert use of the free-association method.

The contrast of logical association and free association in mental processes was neatly illustrated in the following incident of a psychoanalysis. The patient criticized the logic of a remark by the analyst and, to prove his point, suggested this illustration: "If two women have brown eyes, it is illogical to say they are the same woman; if one man is run over by a train, and another by an automobile, it is illogical to say it is the same man that was run over."

The patient was asked to give his free associations to "brown eyes," and at random spoke about his mother and sister, who both had brown eyes. His associations to "run over" dealt with a trip his father had made by auto, and a trip the analyst had made by train, and his phantasies that each would be injured. The patient's principle of deductive logic was sound. At the same time, free association disclosed that, in his unconscious, mother and sister *are* the same—that is, they are unconsciously the objects of identical emotions. Further analysis established in many ways that an outstanding feature of his whole development was his need in very early life to escape the position of strong love and resentment for his mother, and the chief method had been to derive from his sister the various pleasures he originally wished from his mother, while rejecting his mother to an extreme degree. Analysis also disclosed that the two men whom he had phantasied as run over were the same man, so far as his unconscious emotions concerning them were identical; for father and analyst were hated for the same reasons at that time. Thus logical contradiction does not necessarily mean emotional contradiction, and it is the special function of "free-association" technique to show relationships which are emotionally decisive even though illogical. Moreover, analysis discloses that not only may two people be felt to be the same, but the same person may be both loved and hated at the same instant. This incident illustrates, not only the difference between logical and emotional identities, but the use of the intellect itself to maintain repressions; for logical argument prevents emotional associations from emerging from the unconscious over and over again.

By this new "free-association" method Freud not only circumvented the disadvantages of hypnotic technique, but very greatly extended his previous knowledge of psychoneurotic etiology. He demonstrated, first, that when free association was consistently used, a patient, while fully conscious, could eventually discover significant wishes and memories which had previously been repressed and unconscious. Secondly, he was able to show that the adult traumata, which he and Breuer had investigated by hypnosis a few years before, were precipitating, and not primary, causes;

that, though they frequently determined the specific features of the individual symptom, the original psychic factors which predisposed an adult to a psychoneurosis and made him especially incapable of recovering normally from such adult traumata were events of the earliest years of life, infantile emotional experiences which still acted with dynamic effectiveness in the unconscious of the neurotic adult. Thirdly, he discovered the relationship of certain sexual impulses and experiences of infancy to psychoneuroses and to other phenomena of adult life. This discovery soon led to intensive investigation of other aspects of childhood development, especially the child's phantasies, his emotional reactions to parents and siblings, and his anxiety reactions to discipline. And, fourthly, he learned that unconscious ideas produced not only hysterical symptoms, but other mental manifestations as well, such as obsessions, weeping, temper fits, typical character traits, dreams, hallucinations, and errors of speech and act in everyday life. We shall now consider briefly his early investigations of dreams, and later return to his studies of the psychoneuroses.

DREAMS

Freud had noticed that when patients associated freely, not infrequently dreams of the night before, or of years past, would occur to them. Thus, quite by accident, while investigating psychoneuroses, Freud discovered that dreams have a definite meaning, even though it is disguised. Free associations to each fragment of a dream often led more quickly to the disclosure of unconscious memories and phantasies than associations to other topics. Applying the technique of free association to the dreams of his patients, and to his own dreams as well, Freud gathered a large amount of data, some of which he published in 1900. He had proved that a dream, like a psychoneurotic symptom, is the conscious expression of an unconscious phantasy which cannot be thought of in waking life unless the technique of free association is skillfully used. This unexpected discovery has subsequently played an important, but not indispensable, role in the technique of analysing the Unconscious. Dreams a.e one of the normal manifestations of unconscious activity, and were shown later to be very similar to the pathological waking thoughts of insane people with delusions.

The dream image regularly represents an unconscious *wish*, but this significance of the image is at the same time disguised from waking recognition.

Ocasionally a dream is so simple—as when a little child dreams of ice cream, or of his mother's face, when she is away from home—that the fulfillment of a wish by the dream is obvious. Far more often the dream appears absurd or unintelligible to the dreamer after he has awakened. But Freud, using the free-association method, showed not only why the mind of the sleeping person selects certain thoughts which produce a dream, but he also unraveled the process by which the original meaning of the dream is disguised from the waking mind. The most common of many devices by which the psychic apparatus effects this disguise is to represent a significant image by one which seems conspicuously absurd or irrelevant, yet is unconsciously associated with the wish.

For example, a patient recalls dreaming of a dog with red eyes. The real unconscious wish of the dream, free association discloses, concerns his grandfather; but his grandfather is disguised from consciousness as a dog, until the patient recalls that throughout childhood he had feared the redness of his grandfather's eyes when he was in a temper. There is no logical connection between dog and grandfather; but over and over analysis shows how unconsciously a single factor which two different objects have in common is utilized to represent both, when the emotional attitude to both is the same. Because of this linking idea, the emotions toward a grandfather could be represented in a dream by the emotions toward a dog, and, after the dreamer awakened, the associated thought of the grandfather remained unconscious, and the "dog" seemed a bizarre and meaningless product of a sleeping mind.

Another patient dreams of a stranger sitting in a chair. Analysis by free association shows the unconscious wish concerns the analyst, whose identity is only discovered when the patient recalls that, of all the people of whom he thinks, only the analyst is visualized sitting as in the dream. Analysis by free association of the posture has led to the unconscious image of a person whose identity is disguised in the conscious dream. Freud termed the dream image itself, that which we recall on awakening as our dream, the *manifest content,* and those images which are the real motive of the dream but have been disguised, the *latent content.* Thus, "dog with red eyes" is manifest content, and "grandfather's eyes" and "grandfather's temper" latent content; "stranger in a chair" is manifest content, "the analyst" is latent content. Psychoanalysis labors to discover the latent content of the dream which is remembered, yet the critics of Freud's dream psychology, as well as inexpert practitioners of dream analysis, persistently overlook that Freud's conclusions are not derived from study of the manifest content alone, but from psychoanalysis of the disguised, unconscious, latent content which is unknown without this work.

Of thousands of observations which confirm Freud's original conclusions, we can cite only one here. A man who is chiefly preoccupied with mental devices for consciously denying and concealing from himself any erotic interest in women reports the following "manifest content" of a dream: "Two Negro boys were wrestling." In analysis the latent content—the phantasies and memories represented by this "harmless" image and previously not admitted in his waking life—is mainly erotic. This becomes known when he recalls a series of experiences which had been immediately excluded by repression from his waking thoughts. "Negroes" remind him of several things: of a Negro couple he had seen the preceding day, when he had observed the woman's figure; of a Negro woman seen with a white man a week before, and the obscene remarks of his companions; of white couples, and erotic adventures which his friends recounted; of youthful experiences of his own; of his zealous curiosity in the accounts of miscegenation which relatives from a southern state had discussed. "Boys wrestling" recalled to him a tussle of childhood, when he had been punished coincidentally for wrestling and for erotic mischief with a little girl, and voluptuous sensations experienced when watching the coaching of wrestling teams at college accompanied by thoughts that some of the wrestlers' holds were like those of amorous couples. In this dream, therefore, was represented in a "harmless" and disguised fashion a series of past erotic thoughts and experiences, each of which had one detail in common with either "Negro," "boys," or "wrestling." This kind of ideas this patient had for a long time consciously regarded as foreign to his nature, and when they did erupt spontaneously, he immediately and involuntarily had excluded them from further conscious thought. The unconscious wish, or "latent" thought of the dream, was: "I want to satisfy my erotic needs like these other people [Negroes, white couples, obscene companions, wrestlers, himself in childhood]." But this had been disguised by a platonic image which was related only by the association of individual details of "Negroes" and "wrestling" with forgotten, unconscious, erotic incidents of his life. In this way the psychic apparatus during sleep had made use of a device which represented the unconscious need but coincidentally made it unrecognizable by his hypermoral waking consciousness.

Thus unconscious past experience is utilized in the psychological construction of the manifest content of dreams. Another mechanism in the formation of dream images is *symbolism*. This had been recognized by Scherner and other students even before Freud's investigations. It was finally proved by him, and especially studied by Wilhelm Stekel. Symbols are elements of dream images (occasionally the whole dream) which are derived not from the experience of the individual, but from a universal propensity of all people to represent certain unconscious thoughts, especially sexual ones, by certain symbols. Thus the male genital is frequently represented by snakes, swords, or trees. The female genital is represented by boxes or by ravines. Experience with the free associations of many individuals has enabled analysts to learn of a large number of such symbols which recur over and over and have for many individuals identical latent meanings. They are conspicuous not only in dreams, but in ritual, in poetry, in art, and in everyday life. For example, a man leaves his key in the automobile switch by chance; in his associations he recalls that at the moment of leaving the car he was thinking of a prospective visit to his sweetheart. Analysts know that repeatedly a genital wish is also symbolically represented in dreams by keys and locks. A large part of the abnormal speech of schizophrenics consists of such symbols, so that at times one who is familiar with them can converse with such a patient in a sort of "dream language" consisting of the prolific use of symbols; this sounds as absurd as Chinese to an Englishman, but is sometimes quite intelligible to the psychotic patient and even the analyst.

UNCONSCIOUS PHANTASIES AND PSYCHONEUROSES

After the discovery, during his early work with Breuer in hypnosis, that adult traumata were precipitating and not primary causes, Freud turned to the investigation of the factors which predispose certain individuals to react to such acute emotional situations with neurotic illness, while others suffer only temporary and normal distress.

Psychoanalysis now became the detailed review of the patient's whole personality and social, vocational, and sexual adaptation, rather than the elucidation and cure of individual symptoms. This involved a survey of the patient's entire development, especially of those earliest experiences which, free association disclosed, were most persistently combated by the conscious mind.

Freud found that unconscious wishes not only produced symptoms, but affected, less obviously but not less vitally, the whole success and happiness of the individual. A hysterical symptom, for example, was often found to be only one expression of a total problem which had prevented a woman from accepting her opportunities for marriage and children.[2] An obsession proved to be a superficial indication of an unconscious problem which had kept a man from doing efficient work and realizing his professional potentialities. If these fundamental problems were relieved, the presenting symptoms automatically disappeared; if only the symptom was helped,

[2] See "Case History," pages 80–1.

of what importance was that to the total life of the patient? Less, the psychoanalyst's experience taught, than the value of an icebag to abdominal pain when an etiological process in the appendix is neglected. It is for this reason that the interest of modern psychoanalysts in the presenting symptom is chiefly that it indicates the presence of a fundamental unconscious problem. Though they concede that hypnosis and other suggestive methods of psychotherapy are often the best expedients for quick and temporary effects, they prefer this laborious and time-consuming method of psychoanalysis for obtaining a lasting amelioration of the neurosis itself.

At first Freud was disposed to revise the conclusions he had reached in his work with Breuer by saying that adult traumata were secondary, and infantile traumata were primary causes of psychoneurosis. Patients had reported to him during psychoanalysis the occurrence of vivid, hitherto unrecalled "memories" from the first three and four years of life, especially incidents of seduction by adults, usually nursemaids. The tremendous emotion which accompanied those unexpected statements of patients during analysis, together with many details which showed a relationship of these events to adult experience, and their consistent occurrence during analysis of psychoneuroses, seemed at first to justify the unanticipated conclusion that these early seductions were the primary cause of most adult neurosis. But as he proceeded, Freud discovered that so large a number of patients reported the same convincing early and apparently traumatic "memories" that it was highly improbable that so many individuals could all have had very similar sexual experiences. When confronted with this dilemma, Freud for a time was strongly inclined to renounce all his previous conclusions and give up investigation by psychoanalysis. On the other hand, the positive evidence of some etiologic relationship of his patient's statements to the neurosis was too overwhelming to be discarded.

Finally Freud hit upon an explanation of this apparent paradox which all subsequent work has confirmed. Even though the external events reported as memories had not actually occurred, the occurrence of the patient's pseudo-memory was a fact in itself. Though it was highly improbable that certain external situations could recur with the frequency with which they were reported, it was not more improbable that all children might be disposed to imagine similar events than that widely separated races should have many similarities in their myths. As psychotic adults have delusions possessing the full value of reality for themselves, so the little child's imagery is possessed of a convincing similitude to actual experience which the normal adult has lost except in dreams. It is not always the image of an event, but may be a phantasy that is repressed; and when such a phantasy is recovered from the unconscious in psychoanalysis, it again manifests that convincing similarity to actual experience it had originally had in childhood. This, however, does not imply that infantile traumata have not in many cases played an important role, and that none of the reported infantile events actually occurred. There is conclusive evidence to the contrary, especially from the analysis of children. But the point is that phantasies of infants when repressed may exert the same dynamic and continued effect on the adult personality as actual experience.

This conception is a landmark second only to the recognition of the unconscious, not only in psychoanalysis but in all departments of clinical psychiatry. It is the point where today psychologically minded scientists part company with those who insist there is no objective validity when statements have no external or logical justification. For the principle applies not only to infantile repression, but to all details of psychological experience which are subjectively distorted. A patient who must wash her hands fifty times a day; a person who believes he is Christ; a man who constantly complains that an amiable wife is a fiend; a pauper who enjoys posing as a millionaire—all such acts and statements may have no rational validity, yet, whether or not evidence (in the legal sense) shows they are representations of fact, it is always a fact that they represent what the individual thinks, feels, or must do. The belief that a witch flew over the house is as authentic an item in the psychology of the believer as the hanging of supposed witches is authentic history. Some psychiatrists who have not accepted this orientation will, for example, spend many hours confirming or refuting a patient's statements that he is illegitimate, and no time at all in investigating the feelings and emotions which motivated or resulted from the belief in a phantasy.

Psychoanalytic study of the relation of unconscious wishes to psychoneurosis shows that, in addition to hereditary predispositions which cannot be appraised exactly, and current environmental problems, which are generally secondary to the fundamental maladaptations of the personality, the following groups of etiological factors are of primary importance in the production of a neurotic problem: (1) adult emotional traumata (acute or chronic); (2) infantile traumata (acute or chronic); (3) certain infantile phantasies. These are the sources of dynamic mental processes, unknown to the individual and therefore unconscious; they motivate many of his life activities, his psychoneurotic symptoms, his traits of character, his relations with other people, and his dreams. They are often rationally incongruous, unknown to the student of organic processes, and unknown to psychiatrists who study only conscious and rational phenomena.

And, finally, Freud discovered that all factors contributing to a neurotic reaction are intimately associated with the sexual life of the patient, and the sexual life of his childhood as well as his adult experiences. Unresolved sexual needs in the adult, often unrecognized by the patient, are potent factors in the production of his neurotic problems, and are usually unresolved in consequence of sexual phantasies and experiences from an early period of life which our culture tends to regard as lacking in lustful interests. Study of the psychoneuroses by psychoanalysis therefore led Freud to understand the importance of childhood sexuality, and conversely the study of the residuals of childhood sexuality in the adult unconscious was essential to an adequate comprehension of unsolved problems of adult life.

PSYCHOSEXUALITY

T H E word "psychosexuality" (colloquially "sexuality"), as used by analysts, comprises a wider group of phenomena than the emotions and acts obviously related to union of the genital organs. "Sexuality" includes "genitality" (the term used by analysts for impulses to normal adult intercourse), but *also* all other aspects of life to which the term "love" is commonly applied—friendship, ideals, parent-child affection, love of abstractions, self-love, etc., and all pleasant bodily sensations. The broadest customary usage of "love" also implies that we *love* what gives us pleasure, or what is essential for our pleasure, and the universal characteristic of "sexuality," as used in psychoanalysis, is also the *pleasure* afforded the subject.

Early in his investigations of psychoneuroses, Freud observed that unconscious wishes and memories which were causal factors in neurotic problems were always closely related to some frustration of either a sexual wish or a hostile wish, and that love and hate are so closely united as to defy separate consideration. For one hates either the rival, actual or imaginary, of an object of love, or the loved one who withholds what is desired.

Though their basic etiology may require months to discover, the concurrence of neurotic problems and sexual dysfunction can usually be established even without analytic technique. Most psychoneurotic patients, if encouraged by sympathetic listening, will themselves describe the travail of the *conscious* sexual life. If it is not worry over masturbation, it is impotence, frigidity, imperfect orgasm, lack of confidence with the other sex, excessive shame, inability to find or woo a mate, or failure to satisfy both sensual and tender needs with the same permanent mate. One therapist who, after receiving psychoanalytic training, continued the treatment of a former patient was told: "I tried to tell you these things for two years, and you would not let me!" Psychoneurosis without conscious sexual problems [1] apparently does not exist. Occasionally a patient may at first minimize them, declaring "those are unimportant things," or diffidently withhold communication of them for some weeks. Eventually their existence is always revealed to the therapist.

Freud's contributions to unconscious sexuality concern both adult and childhood phenomena. Before discussing the latter we shall mention four phenomena which are characteristic of unconscious sexuality at any life epoch, and for both normal and abnormal people: bisexuality, ambivalence, sublimation, and displacement.

BISEXUALITY

Freud showed that the sexual impulses of human beings are notably "bisexual." [2] No man is devoid of some strong wishes of a feminine nature, and there is no woman who has not some masculine tendencies, some wishes to be a man, though such latent "homosexual" inclinations are very generally repudiated by consciousness.

Thus Freud, as so frequently in his work, demonstrated that

---

[1] Possibly "traumatic neurosis," such as some neuroses of combat soldiers, is an exception; but some observations by psychiatrists during the war made this doubtful.

[2] Recent documents indicate that the existence of "bisexuality" was actually recognized by Wilhelm Fliess, who wrote Freud about it, and that Freud suffered an amnesia and forgot his indebtedness to this source. (Ernest Jones, *The Life and Work of Sigmund Freud*, Vol. I., p. 314 ff.)

psychologic forces are reflections of basic elements characteristic of the organic life of the species. For students of the development of the human body have long had knowledge that in the early life of an embryo anatomical progenitors of both male and female reproductive organs are present. As bodily characteristics which distinguish the sex eventually appear, the potential organs of the other sex regress instead of growing; but they do not disappear completely. The mature male still possesses a vestigial remnant of the uterus ("uterus masculinus"), though so far as is known it is functionless, just as his body retains vestiges of the gills of the fish he resembled at one stage of embryonic life. And in the human female, anatomical bisexuality is still more obvious. The woman not only possesses a vagina and a uterus, the primary organs of her biological role in reproduction, but also a *clitoris,* an organ which is literally a little penis, made of the same tissues, provided with the same sensory nerves, and identical in its erectile characteristics with the male's genital. But the clitoris, in contrast to the vestigial uterus of the male, is essential for the full development of female sexual excitement and psychological preparation for the completion of the mating act.

Furthermore, modern biochemistry has demonstrated that the production of female hormones is an essential function of the healthy male, and male hormones are indispensable to normal menstruation and other physiological functions of the woman.

Thus Freud's discovery of the importance of the psychological manifestations of bisexuality in both man and woman illustrates again the fundamental identity of the psychological, anatomic, and physiologic manifestations of the determinants of human life. A little boy who has observed or learned about his mother's pregnancy will frequently play that he can make a baby too; and many of the most cherished traits of a satisfactory husband, his tenderness for wife and child, are expressions of such phantasies of motherhood. One of the most consistent features of a girl's development, her "tomboy" years preceding puberty, when she plays as if she were a boy and resents implications that she is feminine, show equally well the normalcy of male phantasies in a woman. Many creative artists are fully conscious of an intensely pleasurable phantasy of "giving birth" and "reproducing" in their hours of greatest productivity. It is not unlikely indeed that the intensity of the wish of certain men to reproduce is largely responsible for the historical fact that men have created more great works of art and science than women.

But students of conscious psychology alone could scarcely have appreciated the pervasive role of bisexuality in human experience, especially experience determined by the reactions of people to each other. Far more important than these conscious manifestations of bisexuality are the unconscious phantasies revealed during psychoanalysis. As happened so often in Freud's work, his demonstration of unknown or under-emphasized aspects of the normal life and development was a consequence of his deep investigation of neurotic problems. The wish, especially if repressed, to be both male and female, is one of the most important determinants of the conflict of opposed wishes which cannot be resolved without symptoms, maladjustment, and suffering. Unconscious bisexuality is often directly responsible for both symptomatic disturbances of the sexual act and of the love relations of a man and woman. Analyses of many women who have no orgasm show that this is the result of the unconscious thought: "Though I love my husband, I hate him because he has an organ I do not possess." Some cases of impotence in men are cured when adequate conscious expression is given to the unconscious envy of the female function of maternity.

During the analysis of one man for obsessions, he mentioned that he had always been perplexed by two incidents which occurred at fifteen and seventeen years of age respectively. Both times he had suddenly thrown a woman down and examined her sexual organs, and he could not understand it because the attacks had been unpremeditated and were not the sequel of intense sexual desire. Though superficially this appeared a manifestation of an abnormally urgent virility, analysis disclosed that the motive of these attacks was not a pathological failure to control erotic lust, but a reaction to his inability to endure consciousness of the thought: "'This woman has no penis." When, under certain circumstances,

such as seeing nude paintings during a European tour, this idea
could scarcely be excluded from his conscious thoughts, he had
been uncontrollably driven by the phantasy of disproving it by ex-
amining some woman's organs. This motive was revealed by analysis of dreams in which he saw naked women with penises. Though
at three and six he had played with little girls and observed the reality of anatomical differences, he truly believed women had a
penis until his tenth year; and even in his twentieth year he still
insisted "cock" was the word of schoolboys for the *female* genitalia. Months after these unconscious phantasies had been disclosed during an analytic hour, it was learned that this irrational
anxiety was the result of an unconscious wish to be a woman; for if
he consciously thought of himself as the woman he wished to be,
he must think of himself as without that organ which he naturally
prized as a source of sensory pleasure. For some time he had
adopted a ritual during masturbation, wrapping towels about his
chest and buttocks. Eventually he recalled during analysis that he
had originally done this in imitation of the shawl of a movie actress,
whose exposed breasts he had wished were his own. Later he reported a phantasy of himself and the analyst disciplining the elevator boy, and then said: "It was as though I were your secretary,
or, better still, your wife." His assaults were, therefore, attempts to
disprove the biologic fact he had observed in early childhood, that
women have no penis; and the fear of being like them was due to
the strong unconscious urge to be a woman himself. Similar unconscious wishes of this man to be a woman were revealed in numerous other ways and shown to be fundamental in behavior which,
without analysis of the *unconscious* phantasies, could only be rationally ascribed to an abnormally excessive heterosexual urge. Its
special significance was due to the fact that the phantasies derived
from this wish, as well as the early experience which had made it
strong, had been entirely unconscious. Even in cases where "bisexuality" is not the decisive problem, its presence in the unconscious is always revealed in analysis, and plays an important role
in the life of the individual.

AMBIVALENCE

The second contribution of Freud to sexuality is the discovery that impulses of love and hate for the same person often coexist in the unconscious, even when one or the other is consciously denied. For this (as well as bisexuality and some other types of psychological "bipolarity") Freud used the term "ambivalence," as suggested by the Swiss psychiatrist Eugen Bleuler. An example of ambivalence is that of a woman whose conscious affections for her own sex had seemed greater than normal. During analysis it was disclosed that repeatedly in early childhood, adolescence, and adult life she had for brief periods experienced intense hatred of women; this had always been repressed and consequently forgotten until recovered in analysis. Her consciously excessive affection for women was due to her natural love of them *plus* the need of proving she did not also hate them.

Other women are deeply troubled by the inability to fulfill their sexuality except when they have a pair of lovers, and this is often shown to be an adaptation to an otherwise insoluble ambivalence of feelings for men who are emotionally important. Such a woman is always threatened by the return of this unhappy conflict of love and hate, except when the hatred can be directed at one of the pair while the other is then freely loved. If then the hated one is rejected or retires, the former situation of both loving and hating one man recurs, with a repetition of the former events. Freud pointed out how frequently such fundamental ambivalence explains the lives of women who cannot endure life with the first husband, but, after quarreling constantly with him and procuring a divorce, become contented wives without excessive hatred in their second marriages. Some other immature women who quarrel excessively with a child, in spite of ample conscious evidence of a happy family situation, owe their difficulties to an unconscious desire to be as helpless as the babe, with a resulting unconscious ambivalence of love and hatred and reactions to the child which seem incomprehensible. Miscarriages, and probably even sterility, are sometimes physiologic consequences of a similar problem.

Among men ambivalence is equally decisive. Often an adolescent youth must express this repressed desire to hurt a father, or another older man whom he consciously loves and strives to please, by rebellious behavior beyond his conscious control; he may express it by smoking forbidden cigarettes, by failure in his work, by delinquency and crime, and yet be quite unconscious of why he needs to cause such trouble.

One young man, twenty-two years of age, with the symptom of dangerously severe and painful rectal bleeding, was especially difficult to analyze at first. His consciously imperturbable and placid character was maintained by an excessive need for logical reasonableness because all strong feelings were so repressed that he could not know he was aggressive. Eventually, to his great surprise, he discovered charged phantasies that he could be like an older brother, who had become, in the patient's eyes, a "hero" in the Navy, sailed the seven seas, and—most important—won high rating as a radio technician. The patient himself, in spite of his disease, had been doing highly competent work as an electrician in the Navy Yard; he had been conscious of feeling admiration for his brother, but had not been conscious of envy for his career. The patient's symptom, however, was not relieved until its immediate cause became conscious through analysis of a dream; he then learned that the pain and bleeding had begun when he had repressed strong fear that a fellow worker, whose skill did not in fact exceed his own, would be made a foreman. In the dream the feared co-worker wore a uniform like the one his brother wore, and later analytic work showed how this unconscious ambivalence for his brother, and men who reminded him of his brother, had been the chief determinant of the patient's life, dating from the age of five when his parents had kept his brother with them at home while sending him for an otherwise happy summer with his uncle in the country.

Freud regarded the ambivalence of love and hate as deeply rooted in the human constitution, and showed that the development of means to resolve such inevitable conflicts happily is one of the fundamental problems of all human lives.

SUBLIMATION

A third important contribution is Freud's exposition of the unconscious relationship of obviously sexual needs to many other activities of life. Repeatedly he observed how drives to accomplish, to create, and to enjoy experiences of an artistic, playful, or useful sort were transformations of erotic impulses. The same unconscious phantasies would be associated with both a love relationship and an artistic or intellectual activity. For example, analysis of the domestic irritability of a man whose hobby was devising electrical apparatus disclosed the unconscious wish to have his genital regarded by his wife as admiringly as his exhibitionistic urination had been by certain other women and girls in his childhood, and the repression of the pain felt because she did not gratify this vanity. During a period when this was the outstanding emotional feature of his life, there was a marked increment in his interest in the productive elaboration and invention of an ingenious and valuable scientific apparatus. In the analysis of dreams in which this apparatus appeared, the associations showed that it not only had a real rational value in his work, but was also unconsciously associated with tubes which spouted, symbolizing his penis. He often had thought that with his inventions he would "win glory," and the world would be made to acclaim his work. After the disclosure of many hitherto unconscious phantasies of this kind, the intensity of his work became less without diminished productivity, and his domestic irritability was markedly attenuated. Another man whose unconscious had retained the desire to repeat similar experiences of exhibiting the act of urination to little girls in early childhood earned his living by extolling the high pressure of the fire-extinguishers which he sold.

The relationship of many such activities to erotic emotion is often apparent without analysis of the unconscious phantasies. Thus it is with the pleasure in social dancing, the rejected lover who writes poetry, the words which vividly describe a great deal of music—passionate, tender, climactic, etc. At other times, especially when the "virtue" of an activity is very much stressed, the relationship is not apparent except when it is psychoanalyzed. For example, a woman dreamed she was undressing herself before many spectators, and the analyst asked if she would like to be seen unclothed by anyone while awake. For weeks she upbraided the therapist for his "filthy mind," protested the entire absence of any sexual wishes in her own nature, and sermonized about the purity of her own pleasure in "nature." One day she reported her wonderful ecstasy while on a walk. She had experienced such intense happiness in nature that she wanted to run and leap, and she had snatched at an apple on a branch. Then in great confusion she said her pleasure had been inexplicable, it had been something driving her on, until, reaching for the apple, she had very suddenly known that it was to be like Eve and experience the carnal pleasures of Eden that she had craved. Subsequently she told the analyst that prior to her dream of undressing, she had been much troubled by the obsessive thought that it would be fun to observe a man's reaction if she adjusted her skirts less modestly than was her custom. She had experienced without conscious sexual thoughts her feeling of joy in nature and with no knowledge of their sexuality until analysis revealed her repressed phantasies.

Another woman, rejected by a lover, developed strong impulses for æsthetic dancing and, while enthusiastically reporting her pleasure, had the unexpected associations: "It is constantly to have the male organ; I feel like its strength and power and joy when I dance!"

Such "coincidences" are so abundant in analysis as to preclude, except by the most arbitrary pedantry, the supposition that making love and doing other pleasant things are unrelated cubicles of human activity. The other alternative is the hypothesis that a certain amount of sexual energy which originally gives rise to the phantasy of a love relationship may be directed into abstract activities from which either an "æsthetic" or a "useful" but definite pleasure is derived. This gratification by activities which yield pleasure, but do not require another human being (in fact or conscious phantasy) has been called *sublimation*.[3] The actual psychological mechanisms by which an unconscious wish which originally requires an erotic act for its gratification becomes one in which "beauty" or "usefulness" are satisfying in themselves are as unknown as those which produce "conversion" of a mental wish to a physical hysterical symptom. There is not even a satisfactory theory to explain the phenomenon. Nor, for that matter, is there a good hypothesis to explain why the pleasure of two individuals with very similar associated phantasies may be the same, and yet one finds it in chopping firewood and the other in creating a beautiful cabinet.[4] It is somewhat clearer, but insufficiently so, in what way the unconscious phantasy of both these individuals is productive of pleasure, and that of a third leads to a neurotic symptom and suffering. Sublimation, whether as an individual avocation or an artistic act enjoyed by other people, not only yields pleasure, but pleasure which is a consequence of success in resolving a conflict, whereas a neurotic solution is only at best a compromise involving pain. And psychoanalysis leaves no doubt that all art is an expression of unconscious phantasies which the artist and other human beings have in common. But as yet it has found no clue to the difference between those conscious representations of these common impulses which have emotional significance only to the individual who is activated to create, and those of genius which satisfy the æsthetic cravings of all mankind.

[3] The layman often misuses "sublimation" to refer not only to these phenomena, but also to love between human beings from which the sensual element is excluded. Freud called the latter "aim-inhibited love."

[4] Some years after this was written, this author proposed the hypothesis of the *work principle,* that there is a pleasure-yield in the use of organized mental and physical skills in addition to the pleasure from either direct or sublimated gratification of a wish (*Psychoanalytic Quarterly*, Vol. XII, pp. 311–29, 1943). According to this hypothesis, the pleasure of either the wood-chopper or the cabinet-maker would partly depend on the successful use of a skill he had developed.

DISPLACEMENT

Displacement is the representation in consciousness of a part or whole of the original unconscious phantasy by some associated substitute. It is, therefore, one of the main mechanisms by which an unconscious wish attains representation in consciousness, while the integrity of the unconscious, the preservation of the repression of the original idea, is maintained. When displacement has occurred, we may consciously "wish" for something in phantasy, but may not be aware of what was the original nature of the wish.

Displacement was first discovered in the investigation of manifest dreams, in whose development from the recollected "latent content" of the sleeping dreamer it plays an outstanding part. For example, in the dreams of Negro boys wrestling,[5] the unconscious phantasy of coitus was "displaced" by the game of wrestling. In the illustrations above of sublimation, the penis was "displaced" in the man's consciousness by scientific apparatus, and the woman's repressed phantasy of a penis by the movement of the dance. Very soon Freud discovered that displacement also occurs in regard to the portion of the body where a potential pleasure is originally desired. In the analysis of a case of hysteria he found that the origin of a woman's vomiting had been pleasant genital sensations produced by an embrace; this scene had been immediately repressed and replaced in consciousness by unpleasant sensations in the mouth. This phenomenon of unpleasant oral reactions to sexuality is a commonplace in moral "disgust," even in normal, modest people who refer to some reactions to genital stimulation as "leaving a bad taste in the mouth." The source of their sensations has been displaced from the genital to an organ not sexually taboo. Conversely, some cases of genital frigidity are produced by the repression of the consciously distasteful phantasy of taking the penis in the mouth.

Another type of displacement of very great significance is *displacement of object*. This occurs when the partial or complete love

[5] See page 20.

or hatred for a certain individual is denied by consciousness, and though the source of the feeling remains unconscious, the emotions are felt and referred to another person as stimulus "by proxy." In the quoted dream of Negro boys wrestling, white girls were displaced in consciousness by Negro boys. In the man who could not pass his brother's door, the brother was replaced by his door, which then became the "displaced object" of his irrational avoidance. The most complete demonstration of object-displacement is Freud's study of a five-year-old boy who suffered acute terror whenever he encountered a horse. Freud showed that originally the child had feared his father (though without common-sense occasion), but this had become unconscious, and the emotion had been consciously experienced instead for horses, and only for horses.

In other words, one may seem to love or hate a person, an animal, or a thing not only for what he or it is, but also because he or it is a "surrogate" for another whom he unconsciously represents. Object displacement may be partial or complete; or it may be divided among several, one person becoming the object of sensual love, another of tenderness, another the ideal, and still another the object of displaced hatred. Such cases illustrate the importance of the mechanism of displacement in solving the problems of ambivalence. Analysis will also often disclose that an inexplicable conscious love is due to the fact that the beloved unconsciously represents another because of some consciously insignificant association, such as the possession of a common physical feature or name or mannerism. This is often to be observed in such phenomena as "spite marriages," where a rejected suitor very quickly loves another, and in "infatuations" where there appears to be no adequate reason for the irresistible emotional bond.

Displacement is also to be seen in the frequency of very tender feelings of patients for their physician. Analysis discloses this very real affection is not always due to the "nobility" of the doctor or his profession, in whatever degree the individual may or may not realistically justify devotion, but to the peculiar predilections of people to find in physicians, priests, employers, and school-teachers unconscious "surrogates" for those who had given affection, often years before, in childhood. Object displacement in a patient by a psycho-therapist is called *transference,* and is one of the most conspicuous and constant observations of psychoanalysis. Inevitably, if a patient continues to recount his intimate wishes and feelings, he develops an emotional reaction to the physician (or anyone else), regardless of how impersonal and detached the latter's attitude may be.[6]

Thus, by the psychoanalytic study of the unconscious corre-lates of conscious thoughts, erotic and non-erotic, Freud proved the fundamental role of bisexuality, ambivalence, displacement, and sublimation. These are basic attributes of psychosexuality, deter-mining the love relationships of individuals, the pattern of their social lives and pleasure goals. Clear recognition and formulation of their attributes has become indispensable to the understanding of normal personality development and of emotional conflicts which cannot be resolved by conscious decisions and impel the develop-ment of neurotic symptoms.

[6] See "Tranference," pages 192–202.

III

❖–❖–❖–❖

INFANTILE
PSYCHOSEXUALITY

A further contribution to psychosexuality and to the etiology of psychoneuroses, and one of the most fundamental of all Freud's discoveries, is his elucidation of the sexual impulses of the first five years of life. He showed that the sexual wishes of the adult unconscious which give rise to psychoneurosis, as well as to many normal and desirable but emotionally immature aspects of adult life—such as wit, play, superstition, dreams, and religion—are directly related to associated sexual wishes of what Freud called the "infantile period," the first five years of a child's life. In other words, those infantile wishes which were not fully gratified or transformed, in the process of development, into wishes capable of some adult form of conscious gratification, persist in the unconscious of the adult and motivate many features of his life. What the little child had sought to gratify consciously though secretly by masturbation, phantasy, and play, the adult neurotic gratifies unconsciously by symptom or character trait, and the normal adult by such mental processes as dreams, art, and wit. This is Freud's conclusion from the study of unconscious phantasies and memories of childhood, and the manifold correlations of these with other details of the adult's life.

A few examples of infantile sexuality have already been

given. The associations of the man who demonstrated the unconscious relationship of his interest in electrical apparatus and irritability at his wife to the childhood exhibition of his urination are a single illustration of the extensive material which has aroused psychoanalytic interest in this aspect of psychology. There is space for only a few other examples from the voluminous observations of all well-conducted analyses.

A man dreams, in part: "There were many little girls. No one special, yet I saw each vividly. I went from one to another, looked under their dresses. Very dimly there was an older woman in the background. . . ." In associating, the man recounts several occasions on which he satisfied his sexual curiosity with little girls in boyhood. No associations to the older woman occur at first, except that she appeared so vague as to be scarcely part of the dream, but he thinks there was something black on her head. He then recalls a black hat of his mother's when he was a child of four. The analyst comments that curiosity about the girls' genitals is apparent both in his dream and in his life experiences, but what little girl is a matter of indifference, for the important source of his curiosity was his mother, who is so vague and disguised in his dream as to be scarcely recognizable. After emotional ridicule of the analyst's "putting such ideas in his head," the patient suddenly has two vivid memories from about his fourth year: looking through the keyhole of the bathroom door when his mother was inside, and secret encounters with a little girl when they had urinated together.

A man who in adolescence had an outbreak of violent temper against an aunt, and in his adult phantasies zestfully visualizes himself spanking women, has a dream in which a living-room appears. He associates: "It was the living-room of an apartment from which we moved when I was very little. Now I remember a big vase in it. I used constantly to imagine myself breaking it to pieces. It had a narrow neck and bulged in the middle. It was exactly like a pregnant woman's abdomen. I had seen a pregnant woman once. Then too, women are round in front like they are behind." The patient goes on to accounts of his suffering from early knowledge that his mother loved a little sister more than him, and his fear of another similar rival if his mother should have another child.

Another patient refuses to pay his monthly bill and protests furiously that the analyst is ruthlessly mercenary. In his associations he immediately mentions his recent anger at a friend. This man had not given him a present he expected; many details show that the patient's feelings at that time were very similar to the present ones toward the analyst, and similarly disproportionate to the occasion. After these associations are mentioned, the analyst suggests to the patient that he unconsciously desired a present from the analyst, as he had from his friend, and displayed a childish resentment because he must give instead of being given. (The reviling of the analyst was a rationalization of these unconscious ideas.) The patient then exclaims: "Now I suddenly remember something vividly—how much I liked Mother to wipe me at the toilet. It felt nice, it was one of the nice things she did for me." This is a sample of an unconscious attitude of vital importance in his life. His memory of the infantile pleasure only occurred when he had suddenly become conscious of a strong desire to have something done for him. Further analysis showed how this early "anal pleasure" had been replaced, as a result of bowel training, by a normal feeling of disgust for all things related to anal function. But he had come to feel not only this disgust, but disgust at everything "down there," so that not only feces but the genital organs as well were "dirty, filthy, loathsome" things. As a result of this unconscious association of bowels and genitals, he had rejected most thoughts and activities associated with the other sex. No amount of logical arguing with himself, nor his intellectual agreement with the common-sense exhortations of his friends that "sex is normal and natural and beautiful," had affected its actual function in his life. Only after recovering from his unconscious the infantile wish for passive anal pleasure was he able gradually to develop a capacity for experiencing genital pleasure without disgust, and for giving pleasure without resentment.

Analysis of a woman's hysterical speech difficulties had disclosed that they were precipitated by violent conflicts of love and jealousy for an unfaithful lover. This tension she would relieve by masturbation, but always accompanied this by lifting her blanket to the side of her head in a special way. After many months' analysis she suddenly remembered that this detail, and several others as well, are identical, though unconscious, reproductions of details of the scene of masturbation in early childhood, when she would lift her blanket so as not to be seen from the parents' bed across the room.

The same patient is mystified by the fact that she must perform a certain ritual in preparing scrambled eggs, the most peculiar feature of which is the meticulous care she exercises in passing the eggs through a sieve. Though she recognizes this as silly, there is a compulsion to do it. One day she recalls that she is constantly forcing from her mind the thought that a rooster's sperm may be in an egg, and then shudders with horror on thinking that without the sieve she might inadvertently swallow the rooster's sperm. She then suddenly recalls night terrors at the age of four, when she had dreamed repeatedly that her father was chopping off the heads of chickens, and her curiosity as to the activities of farmyard animals, and especially her unanswered query: if eggs come out behind, how were they put in, in front? The emergence of these "memories" of infantile incidents and phantasies from the unconscious of this woman appear bizarre to the stranger exploring the unconscious for the first time, but are significant to the analyst. For, except for her recent mild disturbances of speech, routine psychiatric examination would have revealed only one "peculiar" characteristic of this agreeable, robust, and feminine girl. This was the fact that several times she had rejected very suitable offers of marriage because of an irresistible feeling that she must never conceive a child. Only after these unconscious infantile phantasies of the origin of little chickens, whose lasting dynamic effect was apparent in her cooking ritual, had been adequately "worked through" in analysis did she for the first time find consciously acceptable her natural yearning for complete mating and maternity.

Many disturbances of adult genital function are shown during analysis to be the results of unconscious wishes to use the genital organ for some other type of pleasure which had been consciously renounced in infancy. A man who suffered from frequent impotence ascribed it entirely to the rigid sexual taboos of his Puritan parents and his Sunday-school discipline. One day during analysis he suddenly felt that in some vague way there was some relation between a toe and his genital; he then had a vivid phantasy of his "penis, suckling a nipple, like my mouth," and recalled that as a baby over and over again he had tried to suck his big toe and had always regretted the period when he became too big to reach his mouth with it. In many other associations and acts he revealed that his love climax before analysis was still dominated by an unconscious desire to suck, rather than by wishes conducive to normal male orgasm.

A male patient who had consulted the analyst as to the advisability of marrying, as he suffered from ejaculatio præcox, recalled standing, when about five, beside his father at the toilet, intensely envying him both his stream and his capacity to spit forcibly into the bowl. This had survived in his unconscious as a wish for virile gratification by urination rather than ejaculation. The unconscious preference for urination as a sensual function disturbed the normal adult genital act.

A man mentions in free association that his watch dropped on the floor yesterday and was broken, and then goes on to mention the details of the most satisfying love-experience of his adult life the same evening. Later he recalls that when he was a small child a picture had been broken at the time when special circumstances had provided especially abundant evidence of his mother's affection. The "coincidence" of special happiness both in adult life and in infancy with the breaking of glass on both occasions appears very extraordinary until he recalls in free association that he had observed the wristband of his watch was loose, yet he had taken no precautions to prevent the "accident." Thus he unconsciously duplicates, not only by enjoyment of his love, but by facilitating the glass-breaking incident, the infantile experience.

We need not multiply illustrations of this type of material. Its significance does not become apparent in this way; for the citations appear bizarre or morbid to those who are accustomed only to logical formulations and adult conscious phantasy. The analyst, however, sees an abundance of these mental incidents every day, sees the emotion that accompanies them, can observe the manifold ways in which each isolated observation of the unconscious phantasy is repeated in the analysis of different conscious material, and the constant relationships of one detail to others. When the same emotional situation recurs in the analysis, the same specific mental or physiological features often recur consistently. For example, a patient complains of symptoms of stomach ulcer sporadically, but each time the pain coincides with a struggle against his distrust of his wife and coincidental distrust of his analyst's honesty. Another patient becomes constipated at each recurrence in the analysis of a compulsion to ridicule and insult the analyst. The analytic scientist observes such details day by day, and the recurrence of specific phantasies, symptoms, and behavior when an unconsciously related situation recurs. He also observes a multiplicity of interrelationships between one mental event and another, and often notes a change in material when the analyst has made a remark, or an event in the patient's everyday life has affected his deeper feelings. It is the study of such "confirmations" of the analyst's original observation, or his interpretative deductions, which convinces him that these manifold correlations are not merely the result of chance. Nor can he accept the more temperate criticism that they are due to morbid personalities and abnormal conditions. For many similar observations of universal human experience are made which cannot be explained as due to the pathology of an individual.

The apparent peculiarities and "shockingness" of some unconscious material, to those who are not familiar with it, is a conscious consequence of the striking difference from the ordinary conscious content to which adults are accustomed to give attention. These elements in free association represent the kind of mental imagery and memory which is normally excluded from adult consciousness, even from the consciousness of the honest critic of analysis. What is unconscious in both the normal and the neurotic adult is identical with what was originally on the surface of the mind in childhood, but kept secret to avoid reproofs by adults. It is, then, these survivals of the undisciplined mind of early childhood which are subsequently revealed only by the skillful application of psychoanalytic technique. This was the revolutionary conclusion of Freud. It was a discovery which compelled us to abrogate completely the myth of the "innocent" child, the child normally unaware of sexual thoughts until the physical flowering of puberty, just as Darwin forced us to renounce the pious dogma that human ancestors were never conceived before the sins of Adam and Eve. For psychoanalysis of adults reveals endless evidence that the child has in his first five years of life experienced many of the impulses to phantasy and action of which adults usually deny he is capable.

True, the child in the infantile period does not know all that is going on with realistic exactitude, and his sexual phantasies are not always just like those of grownups. For example, sexual intercourse is often pictured in the infantile mind as a very violent and dangerous struggle. The survival of this infantile conception in the adult unconscious was illustrated in the dream of two Negroes wrestling. Similarly, the child realizes that babies come from the mother's body, but in the earlier years he commonly phantasies birth as an act of excretion, and impregnation as occurring through the mouth, the umbilicus, or other body orifices. Rabelais was quite familiar with these ideas, and Gargantua was supposed to have been born through the ear. The ultimate effect of such infantile ideas was shown by the woman who compulsively had to pass eggs through a sieve before they were eaten, and by the man's unconscious association of a pregnant abdomen with buttocks. In fact, psychoanalysts have rediscovered in the unconscious of individual patients all those infantile distortions of biologic truth which were presented in the phantasies of a race: the Greeks' mythology of the birth of their gods.

The essential difference between the adult and the infant is not that sexual knowledge, erotic wishes, hatred of rivals, and jealousy are absent in the earliest years, but that they are at first more intense, more specific, and less subject to immediate repression. For the child is too weak to avenge himself physically, and his sexual organs too undeveloped to accomplish more complete erotic satisfaction than that of masturbation, phantasy, and sexual games in secret with other children. But the passions are all the more intense at first, because only gradually does he learn to bridle the emotional need of the moment in order to ensure more adequate satisfaction later on. When an adult manifests this kind of precipitate, unbridled emotion, unless there be exceptional provocation, we rightly refer to him as "infantile."

What most adults prior to Freud failed completely to appraise is the extraordinarily accurate intuitive powers of the child. He is sensitive to emotional meaning, responds with exquisite accuracy to each change of feelings in those about him, even when they themselves are unaware of these emotions. He often reacts to what adults are feeling when they act so oddly embarrassed in experiencing feelings he later learns to label "sexual," and his outwardly "innocent" behavior is quickly learned in response to even unspoken disapproval of his trainers, years before he fully represses his own ideas. Later in childhood, as the development of rational intelligence usurps mental consciousness, these powers are very much attenuated and can no longer be fully appreciated by the normal adult. Yet the artistically gifted have often recognized them. The hero of Dostoevski's *Idiot* says: "It was not that I taught them. Oh, no, there was a schoolmaster for that. . . . I've always been struck by seeing how little grown-up people understand children, how little even parents understand their own children. Nothing should be concealed from children *on the pretext* that they are little and that it is too early for them to understand. What a miserable and unfortunate idea! And how readily the children detect that their fathers consider them too little to understand anything, though they understand everything."

The very small child can hate a rival who receives any love from those who are nearest to him. While he loves mother and father, he hates father for possessing mother after baby's bedtime, and mother for talking to father instead of him. He may hate at first the newborn child, who withdraws so much attention from himself, and only later come to love the little one. At about one year old and for some time later he has an insatiable urge to destroy and torture. He is extremely curious, and one way or another discovers or imagines something of the nature of coitus and pregnancy. There are few patients whose analyses do not disclose that such memories of belief in the stork fable or similar adult lies were preceded by knowledge which approximated biological facts, but had been repressed.

THE MALE ŒDIPUS COMPLEX

Eventually, usually as the fifth birthday is approached, the infant's need for all possible affection from his parents culminates in an emotional situation which Freud, following the accounts in Greek mythology and drama, termed the "Œdipus Complex." [1] At about this time the boy's emotional need for his mother normally shows new features. The little fellow, if astutely observed, will give evidence of becoming at moments a "little man," and, indeed, a "little lover." Feelings for his mother at this time are intensified, and occasionally are apparently "passionate." Instead of seeking predominantly to be given only mother's gentle attentions, he is sometimes more the man in asserting what he wishes to do for her or with her, and desires her passive acceptance of his importunities. While need for his father's love is not lost, it is less imperative than in preceding years, and is overshadowed at times by his hostility for all rivals, but especially this male parent-rival. Furthermore, at this first culmination of the boy's real love for someone other than himself, sensual needs are intensified. Besides seeking bodily contact and caresses, even the little child touches his genital for pleasure, and phantasies doing what he imagines grownups do, and sharing in the conception of a child.

---

[1] There is considerable evidence, emphasized in the late 1920's by Dr. Melanie Klein of London, that an earlier, transient, less intense phase of the Œdipus complex occurs at about the age of two. (See Chapter XIII, pages 270–1.)

Behavioral or verbal expressions of these phantasies are some-times apparent. But the child is physically immature; his genitals give him pleasure but not the capacity for the adult act. And he still is subject to the will of physically dominant "giants." Still more potent in compelling him to restrain the display of such wishes are the most stringent moral taboos of all mankind, taboos on incest, on phantasying incest as well as committing it, which every young male Œdipus inevitably encounters in even the most tolerant of parents. This is why the full importance of the sexual component of the Œdipus complex was only fully discovered through Freud's psychoanalysis of the unconscious phantasies of the adult, and not by direct observation of the child.

LATENCY PERIOD

These overt manifestations of the Œdipus complex subside quite rapidly after their climax during the boy's development. In-fantile masturbation and sexual knowledge and phantasies of this period are in part forgotten; consequently the succeeding phase of development was termed by Freud the *latency period*. Adults often report with conscious honesty that they only learned the facts of sex from high-school comrades, never masturbated before puberty or had sexual ideas in early childhood. At the same time as this *re-pression of infantile sexuality* sets in, between the years of five and six—the age-coincidence is not accidental—the overt behavior of the child undergoes marked changes. He is far less absorbed in himself and his parents, less satisfied with the amusements of the nursery, and requires more friends and playmates outside. He be-comes more and more interested in the real world and its practical techniques, whether they be the use of a screwdriver, an algebraic equation, or how a man changes a tire. Sexual interests, though not absent, are *relatively* dormant until their full thrust appears for the second time with the maturation of sexual organs at puberty. But between six and fourteen (approximately) the latent heterosexual interests are far less conspicuous than the desire to be what the parent of the same sex appears to the child to be. This is particularly evident in the manifold ways in which the child strives to imitate him. The boy typically conceives his father as extraordinarily big and strong—a hero; and the boy very often day-dreams that, when he grows up, he will do what father does; he plays games created by such phantasies, or tries to excel in skills or games as he pictures his father doing in adult conquests.

During the latency period, the Œdipus complex, as a dominating drive productive of conscious sexual thoughts, is no longer so much in evidence. But analysis discloses that the Œdipus complex and the psychological means by which it is resolved have played a decisive role in the individual's development, and that it survives in the unconscious, especially of neurotic people, and continues to exert a causal influence on the behavior, success, and happiness of adults. The most invariable and universal feature of the morality of the human race, the denial in every boy of these intense and secret wishes of a period of childhood for incest and patricide, is established during the latency period. And conscious moral indifference in any degree to these phantasies of infancy is henceforth "unnatural" and abhorrent.

In adolescence there is in both sexes the familiar psychobiologic thrust of sexuality which, when it is normal, analysts refer to as "genitality." Together with the full development of the organs and the physiologic capacity for complete coitus and procreation, mature sexuality becomes henceforth a dominating drive, associated with the love for the potential mate, tenderness, a need for reciprocated pleasure, and, in its fullest development, the desire for one particular partner's children.

FEMALE ŒDIPUS COMPLEX

The girl's "Œdipus complex" was never so clearly described as the boy's by Freud, and late in his life he conceded he did not

understand it so well. Possibly this is the explanation of that se-
mantic paradox of psychoanalysis that, in spite of repeated efforts
of purists to speak of the "Electra Complex" of the girl, they have
never made it stick; it is still the "female Œdipus" to almost all psychiatrists. This is all the more striking when one recalls that most
of Freud's patients in the first fifteen years of his psychologic work,
from the hypnotic investigations with Breuer to the first long published psychoanalytic case, that of "Dora" (*Fragment of an Analysis of a Case of Hysteria,* 1905), were cases of hysteria, and a
very large percentage of patients with this neurosis are women, and
particularly feminine personalities at that!

But it was entirely clear from analyses of women that in many
respects their development, especially its psychosexual aspect, is
similar to boys' though not completely parallel. Certainly the oral,
anal, phallic (clitoral), and other pregenital needs are as vital in
the girl's early development as the boy's. And certainly the coquet-
tish witchery of so many little girls in the second and third years of
life attests their special interest in the men and amusingly confirms
the evidence of early sexuality obtained from analyses of the adult
woman's unconscious. Possibly the girl in her infantile period is
even more intense than the boy in her partiality at times for the
love of the other sex, but it is not at all clear whether this female
"Œdipal" (or "Electral") reaction to her father reaches the definite
crisis at five, followed rather abruptly by massive repression and
the latency period, as does the normal Œdipus complex of the boy.
From puberty on there is less uncertainty. The intensification of
heterosexuality at that time parallels the boy's, but tends at first in
girls to be dominated by phantasies of rape; the conflicts of earlier
years, especially those of bisexuality and those based on sexual
differences, are revived; and there is an awareness of her own incestuous thoughts and the sexual consciousness of the males of her
family which some girls at least repress less completely than adolescent boys repress their incestuous thoughts.[2]

[2] For further discussion of the development of femininity, see pages
49–51, 57–63.

PREGENITAL SEXUALITY [3]

"Pregenital sexuality" is another fact of infantile sexuality of primary importance. Before an interest in the genital function has assumed the dominance it has when the Œdipus complex is fully developed, the child has already experienced quite similar interests in other body organs. The source of these is those portions of the body where sensual pleasures are experienced most intensely, the *erotogenic zones*. They differ from genital desires in being relatively independent of need for the love of another person.

The first of the "erotogenic zones" to be utilized for sensual purposes is the mouth. Sucking is not only a biological but also a psychological function, for it affords pleasure which is very intense during the first months of life. The adult derivatives of this "oral" phase are manifest in many features of normal tenderness and in receptive and submissive forms of love—for example, in the kiss. Somewhat later in infancy, most typically during weaning, mouth-pleasure becomes aggressive, and biting is its major expression. The babe puts everything which interests him in his mouth, and analysis shows that at this time love is phantasied as incorporating, as taking into one's insides, what is desired—the nipple, or bottle. Similar phenomena during adult life are to be found in the totem feasts of savages, who eat that very animal which is regarded as the most loved ancestor of the tribe, and in such lovers' expressions as "I could eat you alive."

Still later in the infant's life his anus supplants the mouth as the chief source of sensual pleasure. Its full enjoyment, however, is soon much restricted by toilet training, and his resentment of this frustration of his pleasure is expressed in phantasies in which defecation represents defiant aggression and destruction of the hated one. We have already seen an example of the survival of this "anal" period of infancy in the adult's unconscious, and the rage aroused

---

[3] Because of their relative complexity, we postpone a detailed discussion of two important aspects of pregenital psychosexuality, "narcissism" and "sadism," until Chapters VI and VII.

when gratification of an anal phantasy was withheld, in the unconscious memory of the patient whose refusal to pay his bill was analyzed.[4] Not only is there a new source of erotogenic pleasure during this anal phase, but there is also an important set of phantasies not usually recognized by the adult as associated with anality. Smell is especially a pleasure, and the adult reaction to feces as the stimulus of maximal disgust is only gradually attained. In infancy they are regarded with pride and the "look what I can make" attitude, while the demand of the mother that they must be flushed away and treated as worthless may be deeply resented. Many magical ideas are also intimately associated by the infant with excretions, as though this physiologic function were indeed the act of a god relying solely upon himself to use his own body in an omnipotent way.

Pleasure and interest in urethral excretion is also a conspicuous feature of pregenital sexuality—for example, in the man with ejaculatio præcox—but a period of sensual dominance of this erotogenic interest is not so clearly defined as that of the mouth and anus. In addition to sensual and excretory pleasure, urination is an important means of immature sexual exhibition, especially in boys, and perhaps the commonest sexual indulgence with playmates of both sexes during childhood.

The successive dominance of these erotogenic zones, called by analysts the "oral," "anal," and "urethral," and the role each plays in psychological development, have particularly engaged the attention of analysts because their derivatives have been most apparent in the typical neuroses. Obviously, however, the sensual needs of the infant are not confined to these. The skin as well as the mouth is a vital portion of his sensory equipment, and this is perpetuated throughout life in caressing, in pleasure in baths and sunshine, and in the response of many individuals to changes of climate. All the body orifices are lined with skin and mucous membrane and to some extent serve an erotogenic function, as is apparent in nose-picking, ear-scratching, and playing with the skin between the toes.

[4] See page 41.

The hair and fingernails absorb the interest of all infants at some time in their quest for new pleasures, and occasionally are of irresistible importance to adults. The vocal organs may well be regarded as belonging to the same category, for speech and song are pleasures as well as utilities, in some people compelling ones. Breathing itself is probably an exquisite pleasure for the newborn, and begins with a conscious experience of aeration of all his body tissues; this is mildly relived in a sigh of contentment and pathologically denied in asthma. But the very early psychological importance of respiration is more completely effaced than that of the external organs, though occasionally there are indications that it has been unconsciously preserved. On the other hand, vision is an obvious factor in the sensual constellation, and plays a prominent part in the love-life of adults as well as infants, in the need both to behold a desired object and to display oneself as sexually attractive to the eye of another. All these are sources of sensual pleasure which the infant discovers, and each contributes its share to total development.

At this point the fair and pointed question may be raised: Yes, we concede that before the child is disciplined to civilized attitudes, he is entirely the creature of desire for pleasures, and that he finds many essential pleasures in the sensitive mucous membranes of mouth, anus, and other body orifices and functions; but why should Freud designate these pleasures as "sexual"? The answer is his observations of the phenomenon of *displacement* of the dominant zone where pleasure is unconsciously phantasied and sought. Thus we have seen [5] how a man's unconscious phantasy of the penis is "displaced" by conscious phantasies about a chemical apparatus; and how a woman's unconscious phantasy of genital pleasure is displaced by conscious oral symptoms. These observations during analysis show that when an unconscious conflict arises which precludes the use of one of these organs for erotic satisfaction, the individual can then attain it from some other organ in consequence of this unconscious mechanism.

[5] See pages 33, 36.

When the alternative pleasure is derived from an earlier stage of development, the displacement is called *regression*. We observe this, for example, in the following incident of an analysis. The patient stops abruptly while associating very freely about a platonic experience with a woman. He tickles his ear canal with his finger, and the analyst calls his attention to the act. He is suddenly disconcerted, says he was unaware of the act, and says no more. Then, with signs of considerable emotional struggle, he says that he was not going to report what he had just thought, but then he said he would try. When the analyst had called his attention to his finger, he continued, he had wanted to put it to his nose. His associations then led to the toilet, and he recalls that he often wanted to play with his anus and to smell the titillating finger, and then other details of similar pleasures early in his life. In this incident there had been a genital interest evoked by memories of the woman; this had threatened to become conscious, and the association had stopped. The patient had then performed an act of which he would have had no memory had the analyst not spoken, and which was motivated by an unconscious wish for anal sensations and smells. This displacement of a genital wish by an anal form of gratification illustrates what is called "regression," the substitution of a psychosexual aim from an earlier period of development.

A commonplace, and almost socially permissible, example of regression occurs when one expresses his dislike of another by imitating flatus with his mouth, or slang suggesting this. It is also common for women in analysis to refer to feeling as though coitus were "sucking with a little mouth down there." Other examples of unconscious displacement of infantile impulses have already been given: the man who unconsciously wished to use his penis as a mouth, he who unconsciously regarded his genital as dirty like an anus, etc. In frank sexual *perversions* we observe without analysis how one of these organs has been accepted as a *conscious* substitute for adult genital pleasure.

This tendency for representations of the mouth, anus, urethra, and genital to displace one another as dominant sources of phantasied or actual pleasure is one of the most characteristic phenomena of the unconscious. It has compelled Freud and other analysts to agree that pregenital pleasure and genital pleasure have many varied and complicated interrelationships which preclude consideration of them as unrelated components of mental experience. The facts demand they be grouped together in any scientific view of sexuality, as elements of the mind with so many attributes in common they can replace each other.

An observation of no less importance to our understanding of normal sexuality is Freud's shrewd demonstration that isolated and dominant pregenital pleasures become the basis of *forepleasure* used by lovers in arousing sexual excitement during courtship—kissing, caressing, pinching, biting, spanking, looking, and revealing, for instance, before such love-play has aroused imperative dominance of the need for genital gratification. Thus analysis has shown the role of pregenital sexuality in the experience of the infant and in his development, its perpetuation in the normal conscious desires and behavior of lovers during courtship, its pathological survival in perversions, and most important of all, its unconscious perpetuation in neurotic compromises after repression.

THE PHALLIC PHASE IN BOYS

The development of "pregenital sexuality" ends with a period of psychosexuality which analysis describes as the "phallic phase." During the dominance of the mouth, and then of the anus and other pregenital zones, the penis has been an organ of pleasure and interest for the boy as shown by occasional erections, titillation, and exhibitionistic efforts to call attention to it. But ultimately—rather late in the infantile period, according to Freud and Abraham, much earlier than is generally supposed by analysts, according to Jones and Klein, of the London school—it becomes the dominant zone for sensual gratification. But the psychic attributes of this phase are clearly distinguished by analysts from those of penis primacy in the mature or "genital" period. For during the phallic phase the child's partial aims are like those of the anal and oral stages, in that they are concerned essentially with an "autoerotic," self-sufficient gratification. The desire to give pleasure to the female is not, as it is in the sexually mature man, essential to gratification of the phallic impulses; and they are not closely related to feelings of tenderness, as those of mature genitality are.

The immediate goals of the phallic phase—autoerotism of the penis—are, however, very intimately associated with two other sexual aims, those of genital exhibitionism and urethral erotism. The little boy admires his organ and seeks the admiration of others; his enthusiasm for the power he imagines urination gives him, and his pleasure in displaying this act, or in comparing it with that of girls, are intimately interwoven with his other phallic phantasies. Gradually the phallic phase merges with a new need to imagine or seek a feminine partner, and the primitive aim of the phallic phase—to give oneself pleasure with the penis—is supplemented by tenderness and the need to give pleasure as well as enjoy it. The boy's sexual instincts then demand "genitality" in a *psychological* as well as an *anatomical* sense, and reach their full maturity during adolescence.

The differentiation of phallic and genital periods is of primary clinical importance. Otherwise it would be extremely difficult to explain systematically certain types of cases. Many men whose histories disclose an active erotic life with women have nevertheless not attained a fully developed genitality. Analysis of them discloses that their unconscious phantasies are those of the phallic period, and that their primary and dominant aim is autoerotic and not a fully developed capacity to love a woman. Similarly, in women, prostitute-like behavior, repetitive tendencies to quarrel violently with men they have attracted, and obviously masculine drives of a sort which leave them thwarted in their hopes of being loved by men are shown in analysis to be problems of the phallic period. Many cases of frigidity and of abnormal social inhibition are due to a strong unconscious sadism, which survives in the unconscious from this stage of libido development.

INFANTILE SEXUALITY AND
FEMALE DEVELOPMENT

The psychology of the female has proved to be no simple problem for Freud and other analysts. She has remained an enigma, and the occasion of one of the most protracted and exciting controversies of psychoanalytic history. Few doubted that femininity existed; no one seemed able to prove with certainty how it had developed. The problem has been: in what ways does the psychosexuality of the *female infant*—her erotogenic pleasures, love, rivalry, phantasy-life—differ from that of boys; and in what ways is it identical? And how do these early differences, if they exist, affect the ultimate differentiation of what is psychologically masculine and feminine?

In retrospect, it is surprising that, during the first decades of analysis, these points had not been thoroughly discussed. Yet it is also easy to understand. The conscious sexual differences of adult men and women were not the new problems which confronted the analyst. He was studying with an unprecedented productivity the unconscious sources of conflicts which prevented a normal sexual fulfillment in many people. His early discoveries were of unconscious phantasies which were not a product of the mind peculiar to either sex. Bisexuality was common to both; female patients had phantasies of being men, and men of being women. Ambivalence, displacement, and sublimation characterized the sexuality of both. Oral and anal phantasies, and problems of infantile jealousy, and the Œdipus complex were as important in the analyses of women as of men. Thus the early investigation of the unconscious tended to focus the psychosexual identities of the sexes rather than the differences.

The problem arose when psychoanalysis sought to reconstruct from the unconscious of the female adult the normal sexual experience of infancy and its role in the sexual differentiation of her personality. Several questions then demanded an answer. In the first place, how did the change of preferred sexual object of girls occur?

The development of incestuous phantasies of boys is easily explained as a consequence of the progression of the sexual instinct from oral to genital aims, the mother remaining the first, if secret, choice. But girls are like boys at the breast, yet eventually their sexual phantasies center upon the father. And there is a change not only in the sex of the most important object of their love, but in the type of gratification which is sought. Though the girl shares the boy's aggressive pleasures, his sexually curious inquiries, his destructiveness, and cruelties, a time comes when her strongest instincts are the quest of passive genital gratification by a man. This becomes essential to her complete sexual experience and resembles in important ways (passivity, submission, and need of protection) the suckling's relation to her mother, whereas the dominant sexual aim of the boy is completely different. A final problem, closely related to both of these, is that of the need to be given babies, a doll, or a child to care for.

The bomb of controversy was exploded by Karl Abraham's classic paper, "Manifestations of the Female Castration Complex," [6] in 1920. The *castration complex* in women consists of those phantasies and desires resulting from the infantile observation of the genitals of the opposite sex and the resulting phantasies and resentments. If this visual discovery occurs during certain periods of a girl's infantile development it has a traumatic effect. Much psychoanalytic data of many patients showed that the infant mind reacts unrealistically to this visual knowledge at first: a boy by thinking the girl lacks what everyone else possesses; the girl by imagining that she has been mutilated, that the penis has been taken away to punish her, that she at one time possessed a penis, or that she sometime in the future will. The discovery of an external difference intensifies her curiosity about what is inside her, she often phantasies that what she lacks outside she will find within her body. Emotionally, there is envy and resentment for an injury she phantasies was inflicted upon her, and the unconscious survival of these feelings is an important determinant of the more personal conscious

[6] Karl Abraham, *Selected Papers,* No. XXII. (London: Hogarth Press and the Institute of Psychoanalysis; 1950.)

feelings which many adult women have about minor wounds and bleeding, about the "miserable lot" of women, about the unfairness of a "man's world." The vast amount of unconscious phantasy related to this infantile problem of the girl was familiar to every analyst. But Abraham's masterly survey focused the question whether this experience of the little girl is not only the source of many dissatisfactions but the decisive factor which turns her thoughts and striving for sexual pleasure toward different aims from those of the boy. The central problem of the controversy was whether the girl is *forced* to adopt a passive aim and seek a new object, father or brother, and a compensation in motherhood, because the anatomical difference of the sexes makes the pursuit of male objectives realistically futile and disappointing.

Freud's answer to this question was "Yes," and so it remained. Yet few of his conclusions have been disagreed with at so many points by other analysts. His argument was based upon the opinion that the instinctual development of little girls is essentially identical with that of little boys for the first few years. That their early needs for oral, anal, and sadistic pleasure are very similar to those of boys is never disputed, and that the love of both sexes is primarily for the mother is beyond question. The controversy centers in Freud's contention that the first phase of a dominant pleasure in the genital organs, and the phantasies associated with it, is psychologically the same in girls as in the phallic phase of boys. It cannot be denied that there is much in infantile and unconscious psychology to support this view. It is a fact that women, in contrast to men, normally have two important external organs, the clitoris and the vagina. The vagina is the organ of copulation and reproduction. But the clitoris plays an important part in a woman's conscious sensual experience; it is stimulated by erotic feeling and is a major zone in the preliminary pleasure of love-making. It is very commonly the source of onanistic pleasure, and frequently, when there is vaginal frigidity, the organ by whose friction orgasm is achieved. Biologically, the clitoris grows from the same embryological structures and is formed of the same tissues as the penis; it is as though nature had provided the human female with a small but sensitive penis with which she might enjoy the sensual experience of the male as a preliminary to womanly fulfillment. Equally certain is the fact that the unconscious, and sometimes conscious, phantasies of adult women that they are fulfilling desires to be the man in the sexual act are intimately associated with clitoral sensuality. These facts show that there is unquestionably a phallic phase in girls as well as boys, and that during this phase the sexuality of girls is very similiar to that of boys, both in its erotogenicity and also in the kinds of phantasies accompanying their phallic pleasure.

Freud's contention was that the psychologic function of the clitoris in the adult woman is a survival of a period of infantile psychosexual development in which the clitoris was considered the only sexual organ by the little girls; its pleasures were associated with phantasies of being like the father or brother, and clitoral sensations are therefore associated with phantasies of male-like sexual aggression. From this major premise Freud proceeded with his argument that these phantasies are renounced only because the discovery in infancy that boys have prominent penises makes their realistic fulfillment impossible, and so the little girl seeks instead to be given a penis, to value this in father and boys because she has not her own, and to want a child as compensation. According to him, the desire for vaginal receptivity is developed only after puberty, and her earlier pattern of father-love is largely a repetition of her own previous attitude to her mother. There is little doubt that Freud's reconstruction of the infantile sexual development of the girl describes the most important features in the development of some women; whether it is the usual chain of events is often questioned.

Before these views of Freud had been fully argued, an important new contribution to female sexuality had been made in 1925 by Dr. Helene Deutsch, then working in Vienna.[7] While agreeing with Freud's major points, she emphasized three others. First, she discussed at length the fact that a mature woman's sexual-

---

[7] Helene Deutsch, *Zur Psychologie der weiblichen Sexualfunction* (Vienna: Internationaler Psychoanalytischer Verlag; 1925). Fully developed in a two-volume work: *Psychology of Women* (Grune and Stratton, 1944–5).

ity, in contrast to the man's, extends beyond coital orgasm and is completely fulfilled only by childbirth. Secondly, Dr. Deutsch emphasized that unconscious phantasies of being mutilated and bloody were motivated by the events of menstruation, defloration, childbirth, and the menopause, and were fundamental to the deep psychology of the female. And, thirdly, she claimed that the female child's acceptance of her feminine sexual role after puberty established a masochistic need to suffer, which was primary in determining her femininity and her differentiation from men in adult life.

That these are important components of female psychology, though by no means absent in the mental life of men, is certain; and they have important implications. For example, is the pain of normal childbirth a biological mischance or an essential phase of the total emotional experience of motherhood? That some women are vaguely uncomfortable and suffer a painful sense of incompleteness when the conscious experience of labor has been eliminated by modern anæsthesia is certain. To how many women this statement may apply, however, is an unanswerable question. And it is further complicated by the fact that only among those of European culture is childbirth regarded and experienced as an agonizing and incapacitating ordeal. Certainly many voluntary experiments during the last twenty years in giving birth without anæsthesia have richly rewarded many women; they feel that conscious childbirth is a climactic experience not to be missed, and report that the pain of childbirth, though real, is uniquely tolerable, even ecstatic, and contributes to the total value of complete fulfillment. Similarly, it is certain that some women are never able to satisfy their love-needs until they have submitted to a ruthless, selfish, sexual aggressor, and most women sometimes have phantasies of being raped. Yet again the question how normal and nearly universal is this need of the adult woman to suffer through childbirth and other sexual events cannot be surely answered.

Throughout the 1920's and early 1930's other analysts, particularly Ernest Jones, contended that the wish of girls to be girls is primary; they are born girls and not forced to be girls by the psychological accident of imagining themselves "castrated" in infancy.

They agreed that Freud's arguments were based upon accurate data and were empirically valid for many women except at one point, that of reconstruction of early development of femininity. They claimed that his data were to be interpreted as a secondary, neurotic development in later infancy or childhood, and that the assumption that these data describe the early sexual development of all female infants is wrong. They pointed out that other facts than those derived from psychoanalysis should be given more weight, such as the usual behavior of little girls, their coquetry, their affection for dolls, their usual grace of movement in contrast to boys, and that such general observations contradict the induction that girls are fundamentally like boys in the first few years. The conscious as well as unconscious mental life of women points in the same direction—for example, their greater dependence upon approval and tenderness from the lover, their seduction of male initiative and pursuit, their greater attention to their bodies and their houses. Very early in the controversy Dr. Karen Horney tried to settle the issue by proving that infant girls, as well as women, are actually more interested in the vagina than the clitoris; but this has never been proven and she had to agree that it was as much a matter of opinion as the contrary arguments of Freud. Nor did efforts to settle the problem by direct observation of children yield a final answer; for the secrecy of the child is sometimes as difficult to surmount as the amnesia of the adult. Finally, the subject had been rendered still more complicated by the investigations of Melanie Klein and her followers in the London Psychoanalytic Institute; for they had claimed that the genital development and coital phantasies of girls are important as early as the second year of life.

Though this controversy was heated and lasted for twenty years, it has never been settled. There is still much uncertainty as to the exact development of the sexual instincts of the little girl in her normal psychological preparation in infancy for womanhood. It may be that the essential facts are yet unknown. It may be that the pattern is more variable than has been presumed, and that different analysts have recognized the facts of individual cases, but were unjustified in generalizing them. It is even more likely that their efforts were premature; for the controversy was focused by the analytic perspective of thirty years ago, when efforts to describe all psychological phenomena in terms of instinct were still predominant. It may be that the answer is not to be found so much in the similarity or difference in the instinctual constitution of infant boys and girls as in the organization of primitive wishes in behavior patterns and character, and that the rapid advance today in the description of the personality structure will solve some of these difficulties.[8]

Yet the controversy is not the really important thing. The amazing fact is that a survey of the extensive literature on these problems shows so little disagreement in regard to the data of analysis which are interpreted. Every analyst confirms by his everyday experience the fact of the castration complex. No one disputes the frequent occurrence of penis-envy, phantasies of maleness, unconscious misinterpretation of the anatomical difference of the sexes, the importance of the clitoris, the special interest of women in blood, mutilations, and phantasies of being injured sexually, medically, and in innumerable other ways. The frequent identity of the unconscious associations of women to anal, oral, urethral, and phallic interest in infancy with those of men is beyond question. No analytic observer doubts that women unconsciously associate emotionalized ideas of this sort with infantile experience as frequently as do men. Though schematic generalization of the secret events of a little girl's infancy has proved to be so much more difficult, yet the unconscious phantasies derived from her infancy are facts which all psychoanalysts confirm and are as significant in the therapeutic process as those of boys, whose early development seems so much easier to generalize.

INFANTILE PSYCHOSEXUALITY AND PSYCHONEUROSIS

The data of psychoanalysis have thus not only proved the existence of infantile sexuality in men and women, but have estab-

[8] See Chapter VIII.

lished the vital role it plays in all phenomena in which unconscious wishes are decisive, and given us abundant material from which to infer a probable theory of some phases of its development. In the analysis of such a symptom as the inexplicable irritability with his wife of the man we mentioned,[9] associations first disclosed many details of dissatisfaction with his adult love-life. Later associations showed the relationship of this to his infantile wish to derive pleasure from displaying his stream to an admiring audience. Though this had not been conscious previously, its dynamic power in his adult adjustment was manifest in many ways. At first he had concealed from the analyst his recollection of the experience; its eventual disclosure was accompanied by the release of very marked emotion. Then ensued a definite change in his emotional attitude to people about him in everyday life. Similarly, the infantile memories of the woman with the cooking ritual [1] showed a great deal about her present conscious emotional turmoil and those determinants, such as jealousy of her lover, which she had not previously confessed to herself. Thus only with the recovery of infantile memories and phantasies of a sexual kind does the "emotional rationality" of the situation become clear to us, and only then does the patient deeply desire and attain a different solution of a very old problem.

In the investigation of the psychoneuroses, therefore, psychoanalysis discovered the phenomena of repression, first by demonstrating the precipitating traumata of adult life. Further investigation showed that these are sometimes obviously related closely to sexual problems of adult life, and this led to the discovery of such unconscious factors as ambivalence, bisexuality, and displacement. Finally, it was learned that wherever such problems are not successfully solved by conscious adult adjustments, there is an associated unsolved sexual problem of infancy. This involves a wish which cannot be reconciled with the conventions of society and the realities of community living. It often concerns early sexual phantasies about the mouth, anus, or urethra, and not primarily the genital organ; it often involves secret infantile phantasies, that coitus is a dangerous assault, that babies are born through the navel, that girls

---

[9] Page 33.   [1] See page 42.

are boys who have lost a penis; it is generally related to parents and others toward whom the child is not allowed to express a sexual feeling. These, the infantile components of psychosexuality, are shown in analysis to be the most decisive factors in the unconscious causation of a psychoneurotic symptom or character problem. For they are those associated with the most intense and forbidden emotion, that which above all must be denied conscious expression as a result of the universal discipline of the child, and they are those whose *adequate* expression during analysis is accompanied by the most significant and permanent changes in the health and life of the adult.

Similarly, the thorough analysis of most dreams will show that one or another infantile sexual wish is an important element of the latent content. The earlier associations with the dream of Negro boys wrestling revealed an adult erotic interest in women which had been excluded from consciousness; eventually it was shown in the associations that the act of wrestling—the "choice" of it to represent coitus in the disguised manifest content—was derived from an infantile phantasy of coitus as a violent and dangerous assault and struggle.

The studies of neurotic problems, and later of dreams, proved Freud's *via regia* to the full exposition of the significance of infantile sexuality. But this is not only a factor in the adult unconscious. It is, together with self-preservation and other egoistic needs, with aggression, hostility, and rivalry, the driving force in the experiences of the infant. The balance between its gratification and its discipline will, to a very considerable extent, determine the individual's whole development. Probably no stage of maturity is actually reached without experiencing in some way or other each of its antecedent stages. And wherever one or several sexual problems of infancy are inadequately solved, there is a succession of corresponding defects in the love-life and social interactions of later years.

The problems of weaning, of when and how the most adequate and natural gratification of oral "sexuality" by suckling should be terminated, are not only problems of nutrition, but problems of vital psychological import. The effect on the child's development is determined not only by his inherited inclination for oral pleasure, and by the duration of breast-feeding, but by the degree of the mother's own unconscious pleasure in nursing, or her reluctance for it. We have seen a fragment of the evidence that the man who unconsciously had no wish to use his penis normally, but still desired above all the pleasure of suckling, was handicapped in his whole development, even though we do not know exactly what special conditions of heredity, nursing, weaning, and his mother's unconscious reactions to her infant made it impossible for him to renounce these and to find in later stages of sexual development an adequate amount of pleasure. We have seen how one man reacted to trifling situations with rage because the pleasure in special attention to the anal region was still sought unconsciously. Nearly every day of an analyst's practice discloses new evidence of the failure to give up, except by repression, the wishes of the Œdipal and pre-Œdipal periods, and the phantasies associated with infantile masturbation. And repression is only a partial solution, as the drive for gratification remains in the unconscious an important determinant of adjustment.

Psychoanalysts have found the details of early sexuality too variable, the determinants of each individual case, especially those which involve the unconscious of parents and nurses as well as the patient, too subtle and complex, to permit of any codification of them for educational purposes. In no case can an analyst give assurance that if an infant is fed, weaned, and trained in a certain way prescribed for a particular month of his life, the child will develop no neurosis in adult years. In regard to the prevention of neurosis, he can, except for a few inadequate warnings, state only that the emotional problems of infancy are fundamental, and hope that years of further investigation may some day lead to more comprehensive knowledge of how adult difficulties may be avoided by rearing infants differently. At present the analyst's knowledge can add very little to the intuitive balance of affection and discipline accorded the infant by the non-neurotic mother. It is not so much knowledge and method that affect the emotional development of the infant, as whether or not those who care for the child are themselves struggling with unconscious infantile problems which involve the child.

CONFIRMATORY EVIDENCE

The facts of infantile sexuality were first established by the laborious psychoanalysis of the unconscious memories of adults. Yet they are manifest in several more obvious ways, which we generally disregard until our attention has been directed to them.

First, direct observation of children confirms them. Mothers who are not too slavish adherents of the "innocence" myths more often recognize the factuality of Freud's pronouncements than do scientists. They have seen the erections of babies, have noticed the infant's masturbation, have perhaps been amused that when a little girl's hand was removed from her genitals, she put it in her mouth. They have seen the intense curiosity of the child in its excrement, have perhaps felt normal adult disgust at the undeniable fact that a two-year-old would even touch feces with apparent pleasure or put it in his mouth. They have observed a boy's pride in his stream of urine. Pediatricians have noted that sucklings will often urinate when their most constant attendant picks them up, but not when someone else is holding them. If the mother has not shown too intense displeasure, questions as to sexual differences and reproduction by the infant will be persistent. To those who claim that direct observation of children discloses no curiosity in sexual topics and no pleasure in the body orifices, the analyst can only answer: "None so blind as they who will not see," or, because of their own modesty, deny what they do see. And he will realize that the child is extraordinarily intuitive, compared with the adult, that he recognizes immediately a momentary frown, the slightest sign of displeasure, and very rapidly learns to keep his sexuality secret from parents who abhor the notion that it may be manifest in a child.

Secondly, the normal non-genital love-life of adults is replete with survivals of the infantile sexual needs. The kiss evinces the role of the mouth in love-pleasure, as do many verbal endearments such as "sweetie" and "honey-bunch." Playful biting and spanking

are conspicuous in love-making. Obscenity, though superficially taboo, is understood by almost everybody and is unambiguous in its
reference to infantile sources of pleasure. The expression of derision and defiance by references to flatus and other anal functions is
universal in the vulgar speech of all languages. Many references
may be acceptable in jokes, which produce an emotional release by
laughter, though the same thought couched in dignified language
would bring exclusion from polite society. But let him who wishes
intellectual confirmation of the relationship of tabooed organs to
sexuality keep it in mind whenever a "smutty" story is told.

Thirdly, the sexual significance of infantile pleasures survives
in those abnormalities grouped as sexual *perversions*. There we observe the adult experiencing what psychoanalysis discloses as desired unconsciously by other adults, and consciously by infants.

Fourthly, those sexual phantasies which psychoanalysis has
shown are common to the mental life of all human infants recur,
spontaneously and consciously, in the psychotic delusions and behavior of many adult patients and occasionally in the *manifest* content of the dreams of normal people (for example, the man's dream
of the sister with a penis).

Fifthly, the discovery of infantile sexuality is the only causal
explanation ever given why normal human beings display complete
forgetfulness of practically all events preceding a very definite period of their lives, usually a certain month in the fifth or sixth years.
Yet we all recognize by watching children that the earliest years are
those which are most replete with vivid and intense emotional experience. To say merely that the incontestable fact of infantile amnesia is "just natural" is only as adequate an explanation as to say
a person is neurotic because he will not listen to reason.

Lastly, to the analyst himself the most convincing confirmation of infantile sexuality is the reaction of both scientists and laymen to Freud's discoveries when he first announced them. Great
numbers of individuals, accustomed to dignified scientific discussion, became emotional, illogical, and sophistical, or refused altogether to consider this aspect of psychoanalytic science, even after
the presence of unconscious motive, repression, and the relationship

of neuroses to adult sexuality had been fully accepted. It is one of the few topics on which the observations of technically skilled scientists are met with authoritative negation by those who have not learned to use the same technique. The arguments these learned people repeat over and over are the same ones the analyst hears daily from his patients, the same ones whose analysis confirms many details of the work of Freud. Though he should accept and ponder the objections of his sincere and scholarly critics, the analyst can finally find no better explanation of the extraordinary protests he daily meets than the obvious one: that scientists are human, as subject to the taboos of mankind as other people, and consequently eager to deny that which their race denies—the sexual aspects of the first five years of life.

UNCONSCIOUS GUILT AND PUNISHMENT PHANTASIES

CONFLICT AND PUNISHMENT PHANTASIES

T H E first twenty-four years of psychoanalytic study of the neuroses by Freud and an increasing number of his students were, in the main, devoted to the elaboration of the free-association technique for investigating repressed phantasies and memories. The investigations showed the intimate causal relation of conscious-alien wishes to neurotic symptoms, to dreams, and to other phenomena, such as wit and art, as well. They led inescapably to the conclusion that neurotic symptoms result from an intra-psychic struggle, one of whose components is an unconscious wish which is directly, or through associative linkage, related both to adult sexual needs and to those of the infantile period. This struggle, this opposition between emotionalized mental forces, was termed a *conflict;* the incomplete solution of a conflict by the successful exclusion of an active thought from conscious experience *repression;* and the means by which the critical wish circumvented this repression and attained indirect expression in conscious experience—for example, as a symptom, as neurotic behavior, as a dream—the *return of the repressed.*

To produce such mental "conflicts," however, two "combatants" are necessary, two opposed forces within the personality. During the earlier decades of their pioneering work, psychoanalysts concentrated—and with what fecundity!—on the study of only one of these, the emotionally charged memories and sexual wishes which are kept unconscious by repression. But the opposing group of mental forces in producing a two-sided conflict, in forcing and sustaining repression, were usually regarded merely as undesirable obstacles to conscious knowledge, and psychoanalytic technique was developed for the purpose of circumventing or relaxing these formidable obstacles to the conscious expression of the repressed.

In his earliest psychoanalytic papers, originally in 1894, Freud had indeed paid some passing attention to the problem, speculating that a pleasurable sexual wish is repressed to avoid such conscious displeasures as shame or disgust, and this over-simple concept was later developed in the demonstration that such traits as cleanliness, thrift, purity, are often protective reactions to maintain the repression of conflict-producing wishes ("reaction-formations," see pages 233–4). But these explanations were insufficient, and in his greatest work, *The Interpretation of Dreams*, published in 1900, Freud discussed a theoretical *censor,* which excludes unconscious wishes during the daytime, and still preserves certain of its functions during sleep, to the extent of compelling disguise of the wishes of the latent content in the actual conscious imagery of most manifest dreams. This "censor" was assumed to be in the service of the egoistic, or self-preservative, functions of the individual, over which reason and volition were supposed to preside. They are apparent not only in the censorship of dreams, but in all manifestations of repression and denial of conscious wish-fulfillment.

And so, between 1910 and 1920, there was a definite theory of neuroses and sexuality based on extensive empirical knowledge of analyzed repressions, but an almost entirely theoretical explanation of the opposing force in conflicts. By the end of this decade, psychoanalysts were turning their attention to the empirical study of these other components of psychic conflict, the factors which enforce repression. The results comprise the "ego psychology" whose investigation has largely occupied analysts since. The empirical foundations of these later developments included three groups of observations of outstanding importance: the relationship of anxiety to repressed phantasies, the representation in the patient's adult unconscious of authoritative people of his childhood ("super-ego"), and unconscious "punishment phantasies." Though all are intimately related, I shall postpone detailed discussion of the first two until we have considered the anxiety theory of neurosis and the concept of personality structure (Chapters VIII and IX).

The investigation of punishment phantasies—our immediate topic—was given its momentum by Freud's publication in 1909 of the case history of "Little Hans," [1] a five-year-old boy whose terror whenever he saw a horse we have already cited. Here Freud's study of the actual events and imagination affecting the boy not only had shown that a secret hostility and desire to bite the father had been repressed, but that the repressed phantasies of the father had undergone "object displacement" and returned to consciousness as phantasies of horses, especially the fearful phantasy that a horse (unconsciously, the father) would eat him. It was therefore clear that, although the original phantasy was a wish to attack father, the necessity for repression, and eventually for phobic symptom-formation, had been the reactive thought of what father would do to him. Many later analyses have shown that, like wishes, such effective phantasies of being punished are often repressed and unconscious. It was another demonstration of the dominance of the irrational in many life adjustments, and a major contribution to the problem of the source of conflicts partially solved by repression.

In the further elucidation of unconscious punishment phantasies Freud had the assistance of several dozen colleagues, an advantage he had not enjoyed in his earlier, almost isolated work.

---

[1] Sigmund Freud, *Analysis of a Phobia in a Five-Year-Old Boy* (1909). English translation, *Collected Papers*, Vol. III; Standard Edition, Vol. X. (See also pages 266–7, this volume.)

Ernest Jones extended the observations of Freud, especially by the analysis of nightmares, and Karl Abraham led in describing one of the most common and important infantile punishment phantasies of both boys and girls—the phantasy that the penis will be damaged or destroyed if sexual activity is detected by adults (the "castration complex").[2]

These investigations—indeed, every psychoanalysis—show that, not only are phantasies of a potential pleasure important elements of unconscious life, but phantasies of a painful or abhorrent event as well. Moreover, as in Freud's case of "Little Hans," there was often an intimate relationship in the associations between sexual wishes the child could not gratify and these imaginary punishments which he feared. Though this functional opposition of the desirable and the dreadful are clearly apparent, ontogenetically they are closely related. They first arise in the same period of life, and they both originate in part as entirely automatous phantasies of the infant and in part from his specially interpreted and emotionalized experiences of the actual world.

Examples of unconscious punishment phantasies of adults have already been cited. The cooking ritual, for example,[3] cannot be fully understood by demonstrating its relationship to the infantile phantasy of conception (a "wish"). The compulsive ritual was a defense against the possibility that this phantasy would be consciously revived if eggs were prepared and eaten in the usual way. There is nothing unusual in any little child's tentatively solving his curiosity as to conception by such a phantasy; that is a normal response to infantile sexuality. The only occasion for our special interest is that it still represents an active wish in the unconscious of an adult and so participates in symptom formation. Further free association by this patient showed that this sexual wish is intimately associated with another emotionalized image preserved in the unconscious from the same period of infancy. This is the idea that hens fertilized by roosters have their heads chopped off and are themselves later eaten, and that she would be treated likewise if she ate and swallowed a sperm in an egg. This represents, in contrast to

---

[2] See pages 58 ff.   [3] See page 42.

the sexual phantasy, a thought to be dreaded and guarded against. No reader will understand better than the patient how absurdly irrational these phantasies are. But he should try to understand that in spite of this common-sense conscious appraisal of the infantile ideas, the anxiety which accompanies their appearance in the patient's consciousness is as intense as it was in infancy, and produced the need for intra-psychic defense by repression and symptom-formation.

Similarly, the analysis of the dream of Negro boys wrestling [4] showed not only unconscious erotic wishes, but also phantasies derived from an experience at seven years of age, when playmates joked about cutting off each other's "carrots," and a still earlier fear of scissors, following a threat to cut off his nose if he slept with hands beneath the bed-clothes.

The man who was so irritated by every obligation to give [5] showed not only a very active wish to be treated as pleasantly as his mother had treated him in her toilet care of him, but a phantasy of her simultaneous reproofs. The man who unconsciously ascribed impotence to his religious training not only preserved unconsciously his wish to suck, but retained vivid and painful memories of excessive discipline in using his hands, first as objects he liked to put into his mouth, and a little later in manipulating a knife and fork. Moreover, at the period of his analysis when he was most occupied with remorse for masturbation he associatively recalled the terrifying phantasies that had been stimulated by jamming his finger in a closing door—phantasies that that might happen to his penis if he masturbated.

The man who broke his watch while very happy with his sweetheart [6] unconsciously associated this not only with a period of his childhood when he was enjoying much affection, but with a picture broken at that time. This was a trivial incident in itself, but further analysis demonstrated its close relationship to infantile phantasies of being punished by breaking or mutilating his body.

Thus psychoanalysis became intimately concerned, not only with unconscious sexual and hostility phantasies, but with uncon-

[4] See page 20.   [5] See pages 41, 51.   [6] See page 43.

scious punishment phantasies as well. It established the relationship of these to the pleasurable types of phantasy, and showed that symptoms, dreams, and similar phenomena are *compromise formations,* representing in disguise both elements of the conflict, the wish phantasy and the associated punishment.

PUNISHMENT PHANTASIES AND UNCONSCIOUS GUILT

Psychoanalysis calls the unpleasant mental experience which is threatened by unconscious punishment phantasies *unconscious guilt.* For when punishment phantasies become conscious, during psychoanalysis or elsewhere, the individual experiences intense feelings he describes as guilt, or the derived feelings of worthlessness, inferiority, shame, disgust, remorse. That is, he suffers psychologically, and the phantasies which accompany this suffering are often identical to experiences or fears of punishment in childhood. "If I tell you this, you will leave me alone, I'll be all alone, I'll be in the dark!" a patient moans. As a child she had been sent to bed early for punishment and been terrified in consequence.

Some neurotic symptoms are defenses, not against the unconscious wish, but against the unconscious guilt itself. For example, the most common symptom of compulsion neurosis is a constant compulsion to wash the hands. Analysis of this symptom reveals the unconscious infantile phantasy: "I shall be punished because my hands are dirty," or "My hands do dirty things." This was understood by Shakespeare: "Out, damned spot!" The man who took a roundabout way to avoid his brother's door [7] was avoiding only secondarily the unconscious wish for his brother's death, but primarily the painful sense of guilt which the wish would evoke if it became conscious.

A striking example of how the wish phantasy and punishment phantasy which oppose each other may both be fulfilled in a single act is disclosed by analysis of a man's throwing himself into the

[7] See page 10.

water, simulating suicide by drowning. The occasion was his sweet-heart's rejecting him in favor of another suitor. At the height of his emotional distress he experienced the vivid conscious thoughts: "I cannot endure the pain of her preferring another, I wish to die by drowning!" In psychoanalysis the association of the idea of drowning with unconscious infantile phantasies of two distinct categories, sex and punishment, was demonstrated. In his associations to "water" he thought of moments of perfect peace when he felt as if "bathed in goodness," of feeling like being rocked in his mother's lap, of poetry referring symbolically to mother-love as the ocean, of the idea when swimming that "plunging in" was like the smoothness and sudden shock of entering a woman's body. But there was also a second series of associations which included recollections of "being ducked" by comrades in boyhood, often in play and once for a violation of the boyhood ethics of his comrades, and then a sudden memory of his mother's teaching him to bathe himself and threatening to put his head under if he did not do it. We find, therefore, the acuteness of his distress, the conscious feeling that life could be only painful, had effectively awakened the dormant symbolic sexual phantasy: "to go into water is to go into a woman." It had also awakened those phantasies signifying that to have the head immersed is to be punished by mother. The objection that in this instance the conscious motive is adequate to explain the act is invalidated by the fact that further analysis revealed that his sweetheart actually had given him ample opportunity to win her from the rival, but his capacity for masculine courtship had been paralyzed by the unconscious infantilism that was awakened, and made him reject the adult wish to take the woman from his rival. There were many correlated details, whose analysis led to resolution of the conflict and core of his inhibition of masculine sexual activity, and adequately confirmed the analyst's interpretation that to drown himself was unconsciously to commit intercourse symbolically and at the same time to be punished by mother for it.

The full significance and irrationality of "unconscious guilt" in consequence of punishment phantasies are revealed by the fact that they represent not only *fear* of punishment, but *need* of punishment. Analysis of many activities discloses that a painful experience may be unconsciously self-induced; for many individuals find it is easier to endure a pain inflicted from without than to withstand the pressure of unconscious phantasies, which, if they do break into consciousness, are perceived as torments of conscience or feelings of worthlessness. For example, a man who suffers the abuse of an "impossible" spouse may be praised by his comrades for his goodness in enduring all and sacrificing everything for her, while analysis reveals that she is endured because the suffering she causes satisfies such an unconscious *need of punishment*. Sometimes it will be observed that the death or divorce of such a spouse results in a marked exacerbation of a psychoneurosis, which previously had been absent or mild because the unconscious guilt was satisfied by the marital suffering; that is, it can be less painful to be exposed to the travail of a shrewish wife than to torment by conscious punishment phantasies.

A similar phenomenon is to be observed in people with physical illness who complain excessively. The real pain is utilized to assuage the unconscious guilt; therefore, the more they can suffer from it, the better they feel because of the satisfaction of the unconscious punishment phantasies. For this reason the suffering of a bad marriage or a chronic illness saves many predisposed people from a more obvious neurosis. Not infrequently, cure of a physical illness is immediately followed by hitherto quiescent neurotic symptoms.

In like manner, it was observed that many men who had suffered from severe neuroses in civilian life were healthy and happy when subjected to the tribulation of active military service. Very severe psychoneurotics who are analysed in a sanatorium disclose the unconscious phantasy that they are being punished by incarceration. This is one of the reasons why a patient may appear markedly improved under sanatorium regime, and show utterly no change as soon as discharged to everyday life. Again, self-inflicted punishment may be observed every day among neurotic lovers; when their incessant quarrels are analysed, the unconscious motive for such "scenes" is often shown to be the phantasy: "I can only have the joy of love if first I suffer for it." To gratify the need both for suffering and for love, they nag each other and then can share the delights of "making up."

August Aichhorn and, subsequently, Franz Alexander and Hugo Staub confirmed by excellent clinical material what Freud had previously observed, that some crimes, and especially those which do not seem justified by the materialistic gain, are definitely motivated, not by the desire to steal for profit, but by this unconscious need to be punished.

Two other occasions where analysis disclosed unconscious guilt as the decisive etiological factor may now be cited. In one a truly accidental injury was exploited in order to satisfy the unconscious guilt; in the other the injury was self-motivated. The first patient had begun analysis because of an acute exacerbation of a neurosis after meeting the wife of one of his teachers. He was seriously injured in an automobile accident; he had a definite feeling that he had brought it on himself. He continually rejected this thought, for it was utterly irrational and inexplicable. The teacher had been driving the car and he himself was in no way responsible for the accident; this he realized completely, yet the thought recurred constantly, and he could not rid himself of it. In analysis his associations led him to recollection of the telegraph pole with which the auto had collided, then to a fishing-pole, going fishing with his father as a boy, his passionate interest on these trips in finding snakes and slaughtering them, and finally boyhood wishes to do violent harm to his father. The patient then discussed his father's virile attractiveness to women and his own inability to deal with them, and he recalled that on this very auto ride he had been hating the man who was driving because he (like father) was so self-assured and assertive in the presence of women. These associations clarify his obsession that he was responsible for the accident. Unconsciously he had, at the moment of the accident, harbored destructive phantasies against the teacher whose virile attributes were unconsciously equated with his father's. The overt expression of these wishes in childhood would have brought him dire actual punishment; and the impulse itself, while provoking no retaliation from without, produced a similar intra-psychic revenge, a tension which only punishment could allay. The actual accident occurred, and he reacted to it as though he himself were actually responsible and getting his just deserts. Contrary to all logic, he had not been able to escape the obsessional feeling that he had brought his injuries upon himself. Preoccupation with this obsession had remained the only trace in consciousness of the underlying mechanisms of his hostility to the father-surrogate ("object displacement"), who was actually driving, and also his need for self-punishment.

Unconscious guilt thus may be a reaction to a chance event. More frequently, as in the case of the man who broke his watch, it finds expression in some mishap which is actually determined directly by the unconscious forces within the personality ("need of punishment"), though it is often ascribed by our reason to chance or external factors. For example, a man under analytic treatment mentioned that on the preceding night, as he was passing through a darkened hallway from a bathroom to the bedroom of his wife, he had accidentally struck his temple against the corner of a projecting shelf; the blow was severe enough to cause a small wound, and he had suffered for a moment severe pain and dizziness. During analysis he upbraided himself for utter stupidity, claimed he *ought* to have a bump on his head if he could not steer himself any better than that. His associations stopped abruptly, and then he asked himself why it should have happened on this evening rather than on any other evening in which the circumstances were identical. His emotions somewhat heightened, his associations concerned themselves with the charms of his wife, and he then recalled that, while in the bathroom, he had been thinking absent-mindedly of many temperamental similarities of his wife and his mother. When he had stated this, the patient stopped and, holding his fist near his head, impulsively jerked his head sharply forward so as to strike his temple against his knuckles. Then he mentioned that on the preceding night he had made an identical movement of his head in the hallway, and the severe blow against the shelf had been caused by an actual jerk of his own musculature. These associations made clear that the blow had not been a pure mischance, but a direct muscular action of his own, though an action not consciously willed. And, secondly, the unconscious self-punishment occurred on this particular evening and at this moment because the stimulus to unconscious guilt had been the recognition of the identity of feelings for his wife with those he had for his mother; this had been immediately repressed, and was recovered the next day through work with the analyst.

In example after example we see how unconscious guilt, as well as unconscious sexuality, is derived from the psychology of infancy. They show how there is a constant relationship of an infantile wish and a corresponding punishment phantasy. What the little child, according to the taboos of his elders, must not do or observe, think or report, without punishment, is what in the adult unconscious gives rise to the phantasy of punishment. We have seen how an unconscious conflict occurs between drives represented by an unconscious sexual phantasy and an unconscious punishment phantasy, and how a neurotic symptom is that condition which satisfies unconsciously both these needs by providing both a substantive gratification and coincident suffering. Such unconscious punishment may, therefore, participate in symptom-formation, as occurred in the man who tried to drown himself, or in a precautionary device such as that observed in the man who would not pass his brother's door, and in the woman who practiced a compulsive ritual when preparing eggs. Need for punishment may exploit another event for its fulfillment, as happened to the man in the automobile accident; or it may actually precipitate an act which produces pain, as it did to the man who involuntarily knocked his own head. But in every case the full explanation and most fundamental motivation of the irrational event is only apparent when the corresponding punishment phantasy which induces guilt is recovered by psychoanalytic technique from the unconscious.

CASE HISTORY

In the full analysis of any single case the relationships of the unconscious to symptoms, total personality, adult sexuality, precipitating traumata, punishment phantasies, and infantile sexuality are even more convincing confirmation of Freud's conclusions than the analysis of any single detail. To give some intimations of this perspective of the psychoanalytic clinician, I now present a very condensed abstract of the treatment of the patient whose masturbation and egg-cooking rituals have been discussed in several places.[8] These were incidents in an analysis which took an hour a day for ten months—adequate for a fairly comprehensive recapitulation of this patient's development. Her case is chosen for two reasons: first, its publication *in toto* involves no ethical indiscretion; and, secondly, she was an unusually unworldly woman, with few interests except her love-life. The sexual thread is, therefore, far easier to follow, though no more vital, than in more complicated or cultivated personalities.

She was an unmarried woman of thirty, referred by a physician to the clinic of the Berlin Psychoanalytic Institute, in 1928, for difficulty in uttering certain words, and for the sudden compulsive termination of telephone conversations for no reason she could mention. These symptoms had appeared two years before. They had been much relieved by a "speech specialist," but had recurred as soon as his treatment was discontinued. Except for orgastic frigidity and the presenting symptoms, preliminary examinations revealed nothing which would distinguish her from a large number of normal women. She was even-tempered, moderately sociable, attractive, inoffensive, and feminine in manner and basic needs.

During the first weeks of treatment she gave further conscious information about her life, which could have been obtained without special analytic technique. The words whose utterance caused her such difficulty were all words which suggested to her in some way either her mother or a female rival for her present lover. The thought which suddenly impelled the termination of telephone conversations was that the voice might be that of a rival woman. Her chief neurotic symptoms had appeared when she suffered intense jealousy after observing another woman in the embrace of the lover. He was a "Don Juan," an extreme sensualist, with little tenderness

[8] On pages 41–2, 43, 45, 53, 64, 73–4.

in his feelings for the patient or other women. He possessed a constant succession of variegated mistresses and made no effort to conceal this fact from the patient. The relationship of her symptoms to adult sexuality and to an adult emotional trauma was, therefore, in this case immediately manifest. But further investigation is necessary to understand why a cause for normal jealousy activated a neurosis in this particular woman, and why in spite of it she continued to accept a lover who constantly caused her such intense distress and very little happiness.

Six weeks after treatment began, the patient found it impossible to speak aloud about anything to the analyst except very rare comments on the weather, for a period of five weeks. Then one day the patient mentioned she had been watching the rain and lapsed again into silence for many minutes. The analyst finally repeated her comment: "Looking at the rain," and the patient continued: "I was thinking about rain on the Rhine." After this thought was expressed, she became very distressed, struggled unwillingly to tell her associations, and finally in a tense, fragmentary way uttered these: "The Rhine bridges . . . a trip on the Rhine . . . boats on the Rhine . . . [*much more distressed*] the smokestacks of the boats . . . they bend over, they're *cut off* when they go under low bridges, I can't help but think of them as penises! . . . Cut off!" Several comments were exchanged by patient and analyst, and near the end of the hour, the patient, even more distressed, told several new memories of her infantile life. The most important was her terror when, as a little child, she had seen chickens' heads chopped off. At the end of this session the analyst commented: "The boats lose their penises, the chickens have their heads cut off, when you were little you were afraid the same would be done to you."

Having admitted this recollection of the chickens' heads to consciousness, she then talked fluently for weeks. She told many details of her early menstrual experiences, her horror of uterine bleeding, an adolescent friend's precipitate abortion, and a long-forgotten miscarriage of her own mother's, which she had witnessed when four years old. She also communicated many unrepressed details of her love-life from adolescence onward. Her several love-affairs had been quite normal except that she had always refused suitable offers of marriage because of a fear of becoming pregnant. She had therefore rejected every lover, until her affair with the unsuitable "Don Juan." From this released material we have learned that the neurotic symptom which brought her to the clinic was a rather trivial aspect of a fundamental problem involving her whole personality, and that her current love-life is no unfortunate environmental accident, but the result of an inner neurotic "fate" which had prevented a more happy and permanent mating.

We could now understand that her choice of the "Don Juan" lover had been a compromise sexual object. His character satisfied not only her conscious need for a man who made love, but also her unconscious need for protection against the anxieties a consciously more desirable suitor would have evoked. Possible marriage threatened her with pregnancy, and this fulfillment of her womanhood unconsciously meant for her the fate of chickens whose heads are cut off, bleeding, puberty phantasies of menstruation, her infantile image of her mother's miscarriage, loss of a body-part, and the anxiety produced by these ideas when conscious.

In subsequent weeks of analysis the patient bit by bit recalled a forgotten period of her life when she had previously suffered hysterical neurosis. This had occurred when she was fourteen or fifteen; the most conspicuous symptoms had been low back pains and sporadic visual difficulties. The unconscious association of these problems with vital emotional experiences was gradually revealed. The back pains had been identical with the complaints of a pregnant woman she knew, and she now recalled the intense desires and phantasies she had repressed of being herself this prospective mother. The hysterical visual symptoms were unconsciously repetitions of symptoms of conjunctivitis during an attack of scarlet fever in her childhood and this had coincided with the death of another older woman associated with her mother. Eventually she recalled her earlier phantasies that, if this woman should die, she would then care for the surviving babies as though they were her own.

These data are valuable etiological clues. Their ramifications show that her puberty neurosis had been coincident with the repression of ardent desires to have a child and that the reason for the repression was that the wish had been associated with the childhood (latency period) phantasy of getting a child by replacing (or killing, in unconscious phantasy) the older woman. Still more significant is the fact that this whole complex of phantasies, previously repressed, was admitted to consciousness only after the infantile memories of her mother's miscarriage and the patient's phantasy of being punished like the hens had been explored. The consequence in early adolescence had been the back pains and visual symptoms. We have seen before how in dreams an unconscious image may be represented by one detail—"red eyes," "sitting," a "black hat." Here we see how in hysteria the unconscious image of being both the other women is represented in her symptoms by one detail from the somatic suffering of each. The mechanisms differ from those of dreams only in the symptom's occurring when awake, and in the fact that conversion involves the representation of a mental image by physiological function.

Furthermore, we can now understand that the adult neurosis represents a similar situation to that which occurred at puberty. Though the symptomatology is somewhat different, intense rivalry for the natural rewards of womanhood is in both the puberty and the adult neuroses the precipitating cause. And we now see how intimately symptom-formation is related to her adult rejection of love, children, and marriage—in short, rejection of mature "genitality." Though consciously she denied a wish for pregnancy, we now know definitely that this wish had actually been very intense, though repressed, and that the real dynamics of her life are represented by the unconscious associations: to marry is to be pregnant, but to be pregnant is to wish another woman dead, and to be punished like the chickens.

The desire to have a child is usual in pubescent girls, but why this should act traumatically in this individual is still not clear until suddenly, and with intense emotion, she recalls another forgotten but momentous event in the eleventh year of her life, just before puberty. She had overheard a quarrel between her mother and her father in the next room. Suddenly her father had rushed out and shaken her while grasping her by the neck with his fingers. Her excitement had been intense because, with an intuitive perspicacity an adult might have lacked, she had recognized her parents' quarrel as a sexual scene which had become a fight instead of love. The patient then corrects her reported memory, sobbing violently. "No! No! It was not I whom father grabbed by the neck, it was mother. But, oh, I wanted him to!"

The analysis of the masturbation ritual mentioned previously then leads to recovery of significant events of a still earlier portion of her life. The vivid experience at eleven was then shown to be an emotional repetition of her phantasies at four. She remembered she had lain in bed, masturbated, raised her blanket so as not to see or be seen, heard her parents quarrel, and had excited phantasies which we may express schematically in the less vivid words of adults (instead of her mental pictures) something like this: "Father, like roosters, gives mother babies by being rough with her and grabbing her by the neck as he does chickens. I want him to do it to me. I hate mother because he does it to her!" As, bit by bit, these infantile experiences, phantasies, and emotions became conscious, the patient told of other things which previously she had concealed, especially various devices she had practiced for spying on the amours of her unfaithful lover, and other details of that affair which reproduced those of the infantile scene.

In this recapitulation of a long analysis, I have tried to illustrate a few of the unconscious components affecting the life of this patient. Though she, like most adults, was unaware of the sexual phantasies and traumatic experiences of the infantile period of her life, these had continued to exert unconsciously a decisive effect. When the quarrel of her parents had occurred at eleven, several features of it, especially the hidden sexual significance, the persons who participated in it, and the action of her father, had coincided with her infantile phantasies: "This is how mother had a baby by father, I want a baby too." Consequently, scenes awakening her maternal instincts after puberty had also activated her old unconscious hostility for her mother (though she *also* loved her mother dearly and consciously) and therefore had to be denied to an un-usual extent. Denial meant repression of impulses which then could only be satisfied by neurotic symptoms and yet must be satis-fied some way because their impetus was so strong.

As she grew older, this denial led to frustration of each op-portunity for marriage; for marriage meant to her not merely nor-mal adult love and maternity, but the realization of the forbidden unconscious wishes of infancy to take her mother's place. It was not, therefore, chance that led to the rejection of suitable lovers and the acceptance of the unsuitable one, but her unconscious drive to reproduce the old infantile situation. Thus the man whom com-mon sense would reject actually fitted her infantile phantasy. He was a man who, like her father, left her for another woman con-stantly; he was a man she contrived to spy upon; and this was ac-companied by masturbation and other details which actually repro-duced incidental features of the scene when she was four years old. On the other hand, she could not leave him, because of the uncon-scious need to repeat over and over this experience. But the situa-tion, like the experience at eleven, tremendously enhanced her emo-tional tension. This precipitated symptoms which, though the occasion of neurotic suffering, at the same time did gratify her un-conscious wish: "I deny mother's existence by not saying words which mean 'mother' or 'mother-love' to me; I deny the presence of a rival by not listening to any telephone voices which might be one of them."

And the conflict of unconscious infantile sexual phantasies and infantile punishment phantasies had also been clarified. Every normal impulse to normal sexual love reactivated not only her ri-valry with a sexualized mother, but also the fate of the chickens that father attacked. It is noteworthy, in retrospect, that only when the associations to watching the rain revealed these charged ideas, did the analysis of her desires and symptoms progress.

Finally, the case illustrates a general principle of psychoana-lytic therapy: that symptoms are not the primary neurotic prob-lem, but are an indication of the existence of a problem. Many symptoms can be cured without the laborious tracing down of the unconscious motives to their origin in infantile experience. It is not primarily the symptoms, but the total adjustment to unconscious conflict, the incapacity of the patient who has such symptoms to find a reasonable place in life with a minimum need for neurotic self-punishment to avoid conscious guilt, that should interest us most as therapists.

PSYCHOANALYTIC DATA: CONCLUDING REMARKS

The purpose of our first four chapters has been, primarily, a glimpse at the analyst's workshop—an introduction to the empirical data of psychoanalysis and a cursory sampling of typical findings among the raw material which is the foundation of Freud's theories and conclusions.

The presentation itself has shown the difficulties of such an effort. Not only is much of the material foreign to that of general everyday conscious experience, appearing alien and phantastic to many whose own daily work has not made its constant presence, deep in the engine-rooms of human nature, a commonplace observation; not only can one no more than hint at its abundance, its manifold recurrence in various relationships, and the emotional nuances which accompany our patients' associations; but a coherent exposition has required the "threading" of the data on propositions which, in the strictest sense, are not incontestable facts.

For example, the "unconscious" itself is not something we actually observe; what we do observe are the statements and actions of a patient. Some of these he has always been aware of, whereas others are startling because of their previous absence in his current ruminations. But the constant observation of these and their interrelationships permits no other construction than that of a dynamic unconscious. Similarly, "repression" and "conflict" are, in the strictest sense, interpretative concepts, but ones which so inevitably follow from the actual observations as to have *almost* the same factual validity as what a patient has said. We reason in a similar way about gravitation, in that it is strictly a *concept,* not observed but induced from its effects. But its effects are so recurrent and consistent that gravitation seems more a fact than a hypothesis. There remain only two alternatives to accepting the unconscious and repression and conflict and displacement as valid facts: to believe that analysts do not observe what they report; or to generalize their observations with some other verbiage whose real meaning is identical with that which analysts now use.

In Part I we have shown how the data of psychoanalysis comprise the utterances, actions, and feelings of patients, especially those which occur when the technique whose fundamental principle is "free," rather than logical, association is used. The most significant of these data have been shown to consist in emotion-laden phantasies and memories of whose existence or pertinence the patient was previously unaware.

Those associations which have the greatest emotional value, and against whose conscious recognition there is greatest opposition, are usually sexual wishes, hostile wishes, or punishment phantasies, and especially those of infantile sexual activity and phantasy.

The empirical conclusions which psychoanalysts have drawn from the consistent correlations between such data and those of the characteristic conscious thoughts and acts of the subjects are: first, that psychoneurotic symptoms, many personality traits, dreams, and errors of everyday life are due to an irrational, but purposeful and causal, effect of those unconscious wishes which are associated with unconscious punishment phantasies, especially those of the infantile period of life; and, secondly, that no other useful inference can be drawn from these observations but that of an effective and dynamic unconscious portion of the total mental life.

PART TWO

THE THEORIES OF
PSYCHOANALYSIS

THE PSYCHOANALYTIC
THEORY OF INSTINCTS

A S in other sciences, the boundaries between fact and theory in psychoanalysis cannot always be defined absolutely. Most of what we have so far surveyed deals with facts, with direct observations or immediate inferences from them. But the need to comprehend these facts as fully as possible has led to a systematic theory of the relationships of feeling, thought, and behavior. The most basic has been the *theory of instincts,* a hypothesis which is necessary for the coherent and dynamic integration of the psychological data with each other and with the data of biology.

THE PSYCHOANALYTIC DEFINITION
OF INSTINCTS

General psychoanalytic usage has given the word "instinct" a special technical meaning. Except that it signifies an innate function, it has little in common with traditional definitions of "instinct" as a reflex response to *external* stimulus, or as an unmodifiable pattern of behavior characteristic of a species. The meaning of "instinct" in analysis therefore has no implication of a specific response to an external stimulus. In fact, its use by analysts is the result of an inexact translation of the German word *"Trieb,"* whose connotation is actually closer to that of the English words "drive," "urge," "impulsion," than to "instinct" as previously understood. An "instinct" in psychoanalytic usage is an "impulsion," producing a mentally experienced need of a human for a certain kind of pleasure, and activating behavior appropriate to the need. An instinct may be mobilized by an external stimulus, but the conception does not include the external stimulus itself. One perceives instinctual function subjectively, therefore, as need, not as the sensation or thought which provokes the need. "Instinct" in psychoanalytic literature means the energy which produces those phenomena which characterize the human being's need for specific experience.

The psychoanalytic theory of the instincts is a hypothesis which reduces all observations of the unconscious, together with those of the conscious mind and the organic processes, to common laws.

BIOLOGIC IMPLICATIONS

The instinct theory is primarily psychological. For it assumes that mind and personality should, when convenient, be studied independently of morphology and physiology, and it is derived primarily from psychological observations. Yet the concept itself is, from a more fundamental, less pragmatic viewpoint, both biologic and kinetic.

The psychoanalyst, though he studies mental phenomena, does not conceive *a priori* of any boundary between mental and physical, or any basic distinction between the energy which is manifested in somatic reactions and that manifested in those psychological events which he studies. "Instinct" to him is that energy which is discharged in all phenomena which constitute life. He fails to find justification for presupposing the possibility of a thought, an emotion, a symptom, or an act, which is unaccompanied by some physiological function, even though physiology at present is unable to describe it with any thoroughness.

The interdependence between somatic and mentally experienced energies can, for example, be clearly observed in a person who is physically ill. Assuming (but only for a moment) an arbitrary division of the two, we may demonstrate an inverse correlation. When more energy is utilized by bodily processes, during physical illness, for example, there is more heat production and an increased expiration of carbon dioxide. At the same time there is diminution in the energy expended in psychological functions, such as recreation, work, thoughts about friends, impulses to socialized activity. On the other hand, when the psychic functions are extraordinarily active, such as occurs when a man is very much in love, or absorbed by emotions of hatred and fear—in active warfare for example—a diminution of the self-preservative organic functions is manifested by relative malnutrition and physical fatigue. In his theoretical papers Freud did not overlook these reciprocal relationships.

He referred to each observable psychological phenomenon, such as an idea, a phantasy, or a memory, as an *instinct-representation* (*"Trieb-representanz"*); that is, as one of the observable end-results of a discharge of the biologic energy which he calls "instinct." The most relevant of these instinct-representations for his purpose are the "ideas" which constitute the unconscious; for it is these which provide our most accessible and direct data on the most complex (that is, psychologic) functions of the organism. Associations which reveal unconscious motivation are, theoretically, representations of physiologic processes, even though the physiologic processes themselves cannot be studied directly. Thus the analyst can claim success exactly at the point where physiologic technique has failed—for example, in reducing the hysterical conversion symptom to laws of universal validity. For physiologic technique, though possessing as a rule the inestimable advantage of quantitative methods, requires the isolation of relatively simple phenomena and is still inadequate for the direct elucidation of very complex reactions. The relation of psychoanalysis to physiology may, therefore, be compared to colorimetric tests, where the chemist, though aware of the presence of ions, does not attempt to observe or count them directly, but attains more valuable knowledge of their effects by studying the delicate alterations they produce in the color of a dye. So the analyst, instead of direct study of organic processes of such great complexity as to baffle him, studies their psychic "representatives."

QUANTITATIVE IMPLICATIONS

The psychoanalytic theory of instincts is also a *kinetic* (or dynamic) concept. It deals with the hypothetical energy which *impels* the organism to activity, rather than with the *form* this activity takes. It closely parallels the conceptions of thermodynamics, in that it hypothesizes a constant and indestructible energy which expresses itself in *either* biological or psychological function. This aspect of Freud's theory is obscured only by the analyst's inability as yet to devise any kinetic unit which can be objectively measured. Like the carpenter who is not provided with a rule, or the chemist who lacks a balance, he can only *estimate* those relative proportions of instinctual energy which are distributed in various manifestations of the personality. This he does by observing the objective evidence of emotional tension and discharge, and also, to a great extent, by trained observation of his own emotional resonance to them.

Although these estimates are still too crude to have *absolute* scientific validity, the analyst's conceptions and his mode of thought are already very definitely quantitative. In fact it has to be so; for in human nature there appears to be no "not at all." That is, there is no person so normal that there is no trace of psychosis; no hysteria so typical that some evidence of obsessions does not appear; no human being so interested in one sex that amorous inclinations to the other can never be detected. In other words, total personalities when thoroughly studied cannot be differentiated, except for convenience, in terms of what features are *completely* present or *not at all*. Rather, their psychologic functions must be described in terms of the degree in which each normal and abnormal tendency of human nature asserts itself.

During psychoanalytic treatments this supposition of a fixed amount of energy at the psychological disposal of the individual becomes a far less chimerical speculation than it must be for students of conscious psychology. If there appear to be wide oscillations in an individual's energy output from day to day, analysis will as a rule disclose that this is only an apparent difference, whereas the energy which has been withdrawn from one focus is always active somewhere else. A certain patient who is generally interested and animated during his treatment hour becomes apparently listless and disinterested. Analysis discloses that he has suddenly begun to tell his secrets to a woman instead of the analyst; so there is a definite quantity of energy producing the need to tell a person, though it is now directed to the woman. A patient usually very aggressive becomes suddenly depressed; careful investigation indicates that his antagonism (his wish to attack or hurt) is as active as before, but is now turned against himself instead of others, producing the mood and the mental content of depression. A patient suddenly is relieved from obsessional thinking; he becomes for the first time in months busy planning a party for his friends. But what gives the analyst confidence in this hypothesis is not so much the more obvious shifts of psychic energy, but those very occasions which appear to be an exception until careful analytic investigation reveals that the new focus for energy dispersion was not immediately apparent, and work had to be done to discover it. Thus, the amount of instinctual drive of a certain kind may remain approximately constant though its immediate objectives are altered and present a different picture to the observer.

THE PLEASURE PRINCIPLE

In the early formulation of his instinct theories Freud had been much influenced by the German physicist and psychologist

Gustaf Fechner, who strove in his study of sensations to establish his hypothesis that these psychological phenomena are reducible to physical laws. The most fundamental of Freud's laws of instinctual activity is that the psychological (and social) activities are determined by a constant need to reduce emotional tension to a minimal level. These tensions are the propulsive factor in human life, and the production of the tensions is the function of the instincts. They are consciously perceived as painful or disagreeable feelings; activity is initiated by the need to perform some specific function which will reduce this instinctually produced tension; and the fulfillment of this tension-reducing function thereby evokes the mental experience of pleasure. Freud, therefore, termed this fundamental law of instinct the *Pleasure Principle;* the somatic origin of instinctual energy, the *source;* the tension which serves as an *inner* stimulus to appropriate actions, the *impetus;* the need for that special function which will reduce the tension, the *aim;* and the instrumentality by which the aim is fulfilled—that is, the other person, the thing, or the portion of oneself which is acted upon, the *object.*

This induction of a fundamental property of mental life, derived from psychoanalytic observation and called the *Pleasure Principle,* coincides with the ultimate conclusions of scientists in other fields. For example, the physiologist Walter Cannon, after a life of investigation of organic function, maintained that all bodily processes are devised to maintain a definite physico-chemical equilibrium which he termed "homeostasis." [1] The essence though not the wording of Cannon's conclusions about "homeostasis" coin-

---

[1] Walter B. Cannon, *The Wisdom of the Body* (New York: W. W. Norton & Co.; 1932; 306 pp.)

To my best knowledge the first mention of the essential identity of the physiologic principle of "homeostasis" and the psychoanalytic "Pleasure Principle" was in the first edition of this book, page 93 (1934). It developed from my being shown, by a student of Cannon's, Dr. Norman Freeman, in October 1930, a reprint of Cannon's first tentative conjectures about "homeostasis" published in 1926: "Some General Features of Endocrine Influence on Metabolism": *American Journal of Medical Sciences,* Vol. 171, pp. 1–20. The concept of homeostasis was given definitive exposition by Cannon in "Organization for Physiological Homeostasis": *Physiological Reviews,* Vol. IX, pp. 399–431 (1929). We had no idea then that with the development of psychosomatic interests by analysts this identity of the Pleasure Principle and homeostasis would be discussed so extensively in later years.

cided remarkably with the significant statements of Freud's own most speculative work, *Beyond the Pleasure Principle*. Their investigations had been in separate empirical realms, yet their final conclusions in regard to the fundamental processes of life were the same: the psychoanalyst, that psychological processes are initiated by the need to restore an emotional equilibrium which is experienced as pleasure; the physiologist, that organic processes are initiated by the need to restore a physico-chemical equilibrium which is experienced as health.

The identity of the ultimate conclusions of two such leaders of scientific thought (to mention only two) evokes conviction that we have here statements of an essential law of functions constituting life, so far as it is yet comprehensible. The further conclusion seems justified, that it is only the unavoidable technical limitations in both fields, physiology and psychology, that have kept us from demonstrating empirically those relationships whose assumption hypothetically is unavoidable. Physiology is limited by techniques applicable only to gross aspects of the total function which can be isolated for laboratory experiment. Psychoanalysis is superior for the investigation of processes of a complexity and subtlety which baffle the physiologist, but is itself handicapped by the crudeness of its quantitation.

The Pleasure Principle is of prime significance in the theory of the psychoneuroses. For Freud's answer to the question why the personality creates a symptom or adjustment to life which entails suffering was that this very situation entails the minimum suffering (the minimum degree of disagreeable tension) of which that particular personality is capable. A psychoneurotic represses a wish that is denied direct and normal release of tension, Freud concluded, either because recognition of that wish is too painful or because it produces such painful consequences as guilt or anxiety. But the frustration of instinctual needs, even though it is unconscious, produces an increment of the tension itself, which, in accordance with the Pleasure Principle, must in one way or another be reduced. As this cannot be accomplished directly, because of the frustration and repression, it is accomplished indirectly by the neurotic symptom. In terms of the empirical "instinct-representation" of the instinct in the mind, which we discover by free association, we describe this as a substitute gratification of the unconscious (repressed) wish. In terms of the instinct theory, we describe it as reduction of instinctual tension.

The later investigation of that group of instinct-representations which have been referred to as "unconscious punishment phantasies" permits us a theoretical amendment to this formula for symptom-formation. For we now see how the condition of conflict between a "wish" for pleasure and a phantasy of punishment is, theoretically, the opposition of *two* opposed instinct-systems. Besides the sexual "wish," and opposed to it, is that kinetic factor described as "need of punishment." Not only, therefore, is a neurotic symptom in part the unconscious gratification of a sexual or hostile impulse, and therefore productive of pleasure (more exactly, *less* pain) by a reduction of tension, but this gain in pleasure is always accompanied by suffering. The suffering itself, however, is the gratification of the second instinct-system, and is pleasurable in the sense that it is easier to bear than the corresponding degree of tension, especially if this reaches a level where the threatening guilt would erupt into consciousness. All cases of neurotic symptom-formation appear in analysis to be reducible to this formula: they are compromises affording gratification to both the instinct-systems, that represented by sexual phantasies, and that represented by punishment phantasies. Therefore it is always formed in accordance with the Pleasure Principle, in that the tension of both systems is reduced and the aims of both achieved. Neurosis is the most pleasurable, or the least painful, adjustment possible for a personality with such a conflict of instinct-systems. And even the suffering of neurosis is "pleasure in pain," in that the tension of the guilt-system is reduced. This is also the basis for the common observation of pleasure from masochistic gratifications.[2]

We may illustrate the Pleasure Principle by analogy with a simple water-system (Fig. I). Water enters at A; it is directed un-

[2] See "Sadism and Masochism," Chapter VII.

der pressure by the pump at B; and the normal tension of the system is maintained by release of the stream at the outlet C, whenever the pressure becomes sufficient to raise the water to that level. If, now, the normal outlet is blocked by a valve at D, the water-pressure increases to a point which compels some alteration of the dynamics of the system. Either the obstacle at the valve must be released, the pump must be demobilized, or a break in the system which secures the reduction of tension must occur, in the vent at X.

In the psychoanalytic theory of instincts, the water of this system represents the "source," or physico-chemical activities from

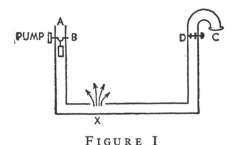

FIGURE I

which all life energy is derived; the pump represents the instincts which organize and direct this energy through channels normally leading to some specific and pleasure-giving activity which reduces the tension, represented by the outlet, C. Thus, for the fully mobilized adult sexual instincts, C represents orgasm; for hostile instincts, it represents the injury of an antagonist; for the ego-instincts, the ingestion of food or an act of self-preservation.

The valve, D, represents obstacles to the free discharge of this energy, and psychoanalysis has discovered that it is in the instinct-system "sexuality" that neurotic obstruction in the form of taboos has occurred. The valve is, therefore, itself controlled by the guilt-system, which, though more complex, itself is constructed on a similar dynamic plan to that of the sexual tensions. Occasionally the release of the tension produced by the conflict of the guilt-system with the sexual system is secured by release of the obstruction to the normal outlet. Thus a fortunate love-affair, an unusual friendship, or a vital new interest may cure a neurosis, though usually cures of this kind prove to be patchwork, and the neurosis returns at some later date. At other times the pump is ruined by the back-pressure, instinctual life becomes disorganized, and we have that demolition of usefully directed systems which constitutes psychosis. At other times the pressure produces a break at some weak internal point of the system, and there is a release of tension at X. As in the water-system, such a psychoneurotic symptom serves the desirable function of releasing the pressure without total disruption of the personality, but does so at a point where no normal function is served, and generally with more or less "flooding of the bathroom floor."

The Case History (Chapter IV) illustrates admirably the type of material from which these inductions are drawn. The study of this woman's conscious life showed a rejection of marriage, a fear of pregnancy, and a group of psychoneurotic symptoms. These features appeared inexplicable, irrational, and without purpose until psychoanalysis revealed the repressed *wish* to have a child as the dominant determinant of her life. Psychoanalytic theory would describe this unconscious wish as the psychological representative of an instinct corresponding to the water system. Repression of the wish corresponds to closure of the natural outlet of this instinct through rejection of love by a man, a normal home, orgasm, and pregnancy. The "valve" was closed by the energy represented psychologically by infantile fear of punishment by a rival woman whose love was also desired. The conflict of these two forces had originated in the association of love of babies with infantile jealousy of her mother. The closure of the valve was apparent in the patient's repeated rejection of men she loved, while the increment of the un-released instinctual tension was apparent in her self-frustrated efforts to find love and home, and her final acceptance of a painful love-affair. Finally the system burst, and the dammed-up instinctual pressure was relieved by "conversion" into symptoms. These showed definitely the neurotic stigmata of pleasure in the release of tension through abnormal channels and concomitant suffering which satisfied the guilt-system. With the analytic data available, no other interpretation is possible than that this abnormal "pleasure in pain" was indeed the maximal pleasure, the maximal release of both the sexual and the guilt tensions, of which this woman was capable, so long as the normal valve was closed by conflict and repression.

THE REALITY PRINCIPLE

Freud, moreover, recognized that, though the Pleasure Principle represents a cardinal feature of instinctual function, it does not fully account for a multitude of observations. The most important modification of the Pleasure Principle he called the "Reality Principle." The Reality Principle is the capacity of human beings to dispense with immediate pleasure in order to ensure pleasure, or avoid pain, at some future time. This function is the hallmark of mature behavior and is negligible in the infant. It is not innate, but develops as the child gradually learns by experience that immediate pleasure may incur a subsequent pain, most often the pain of punishment or loss of love by a parent. Thus a child may derive pleasure from sucking his thumb. In accordance with the Pleasure Principle, he will perform this agreeable act on every occasion when the instinct urges. If, however, he learns that mother slaps him, or that mother withholds a kiss, when he sucks, he will eventually adopt the Reality Principle, and deny himself immediate sucking pleasure in order to ensure the greater pleasure of mother's affection in the future. The Reality Principle, therefore, is not opposed to the Pleasure Principle, but is a modification, learned by experience and characterizing emotional maturity, of the inborn Pleasure Principle.

We may represent the Reality Principle in our hydraulic analogy by making an addition to our simple system (Fig. II). Valve D may be closed, and the resulting overflow of water may be stored in a reservoir, E. When the pressure of the reservoir now rises, it will be relieved at appropriate intervals by releasing the valve, D^1, which represents the good judgment of the normal adult in appraising the consequences of his act.

The simple system, therefore, represents the innate instinctual urges of the pleasure-seeking infant, the reservoir system that of the normal functions of the adult personality. Valve D will then be closed to all urges which are associated with unconscious guilt; valve D^1 to that overflow which threatens disastrous *external* con-

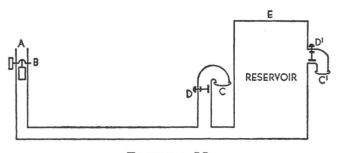

F I G U R E   II

sequences. The obviously infantile adult, such as the sexual pervert or the person with uncontrollable temperament, is he whose instinctual outlets through the reservoir system are closed at D^1 while valve D is open to impulses which normally are allowed gratification only in infancy. The psychoneurotic has a partial closure of both valves, D and D^1, so that release of tension is only possible by a rupture of the simple system.

In the mild neurotic the reservoir may be adequate most of the time. Such was true of the woman whose case we have cited. Had she been observed three years before her analysis, no neurosis would have been apparent, and only her frigidity and futile sexual history would have given the experienced observer a clue to the psychic situation which one day would result in the clogging of the system and the outbreak of definite symptoms. In other cases the capacity to apply the Reality Principle is so constantly limited as to produce chronic neurotic tension and infantile patterns throughout the greater part of life.

We may also cite the case of an intellectually talented man. Though he had attained honors in a technical school, and even been recommended for one of the best positions open to the graduating class, his life was tragically crippled by many very serious disturbances, of which the most serious were an inability to establish social relationships, friendships, or normal love affairs, constant preoccupation with day-dreams, and repeated episodes of impulsive, arrogant insolence to superiors. Wherever authority was represented, in amateur sports, in the company for which he worked, or with court officials, the patient first won affection and then alienated it by this uncontrolled need to express insulting defiance. In the analysis, the patient expressed this very attitude to the analyst, behaving as though the analyst had assumed (as he had not) the prerogatives of a disciplinarian. The patient would attempt to please, and then intentionally refuse to tell his thoughts, fail to keep appointments, and try various more subtle devices for enraging his therapist. After much laborious work the patient reported that when saying nothing he was imitating with his lips the sensations of bowel evacuation and flatus. This gave him the pleasant feeling of a specially vigorous insult to the analyst. Eventually he recalled several experiences of his mother's early care of him. At seven she had forbidden him to use the school toilet because boys said dirty things there; he had one day retained his excretions until after school was over, and while running home in pain had dirtied his trousers. After telling the analyst of these memories, he recalled her scrupulous personal attention to his bodily needs up to this age, the welcome affection she had lavished in this and many other ways, and the strenuous fear of violating her excessive demands for good behavior and bodily care. Later many vivid details of this training long before the age of seven were recalled, all of which reflected the same fundamental problem: on the one hand, an excessive need of being cared for by his mother, an absorption of his love-needs in this attitude; and, on the other hand, bitter resentment for her unusually excessive curtailment of his infantile pleasures, especially those of excreting, and fear of her punishments. In later childhood and adolescence this had resulted in complete paralysis of any demonstrable affection in his relationship to his mother, a constant source of anguished incomprehensibility to her. It had become the unconscious model for all his later attachments, to both men and women, to school-teachers, friends, and employers, and finally to the analyst. Even at twenty-four, he now narrated, he had reproduced the essential details of the seven-year-old scene. When consciously activated by feelings of warm affection for a host at a summer cottage, he had gone to walk in the woods at night and felt suddenly impelled to soil his trousers. Analysis disclosed the repression of memories of an occasion on which he had been slighted by this man. Of special interest had been the fact that it was generally occasions where some reference to cleanliness was made that precipitated his later insolence, thus always bearing the mark of the infantile restrictions his mother had excessively imposed upon him. On one occasion it was a friend commenting on the imperfection of his dress tie, on another an officer reprimanding him for the lack of neatness of his uniform, on a third a dentist advising cleanliness of the teeth.

Such a case represents an impairment of development more severe than is found in typical psychoneurosis. For the Reality Principle had never been well established, and the pressure for *immediate* gratification of instinctual tension was chronic. The pressure of the instincts is still confined chiefly within the primitive pleasure system. The functional capacity of the reservoir is very limited compared with that of mature adults. The Reality Principle is still subordinate to the Pleasure Principle, as in normal infancy. The individual has maturity of intellect and body. Yet he is not truly living in a grown-up world, but is constantly playing in imagination; emotionally he is a child to a very great extent. As a result, adult sources of instinct-gratification are impossible, and the maximal agreeable release of instinctual tension takes place in part at the psychic analogue of the valve D (by masturbation, ritualistic play, etc.), and in part through the explosive vent which his chronic insolence and defiance represent.

THE REPETITION COMPULSION

Finally, in addition to his early definition of the Pleasure and Reality Principles, Freud in his book *Beyond the Pleasure Principle* recognized another fundamental law of instinctual function—the "repetition compulsion." There is in human life, he finally concluded, a tendency to reproduce certain previously experienced emotional tensions, regardless of the capacity of the organism to derive pleasure from them, and regardless of their egoistic value. The repetition compulsion includes the traditional concept of "habit," but Freud's emphasis of its unconscious dynamics, its presence from the very earliest experiences of infancy, and its relationship to the instinct theory, involves much more than the renaming of this familiar observation. Freud had been impressed especially by such phenomena as the tendency of "shell-shocked" soldiers to repeat the traumatic event over and over, especially in dreams and in conscious waking hallucinations, as though reliving it, and by the endless repetition by children of even painful bits of play. And he was on still more intimate terms with the repetition compulsion as it was to some degree mobilized by every psychoanalysis as a repetitive obstacle to therapeutic success. This, he explained, became a decisive obstacle in a minority of cases which he called *destiny neuroses,* where the whole life of an individual was subordinated to the compulsive need to react to every critical situation offering potential pleasure in a way to ensure defeat. The case of the man just cited illustrates such a decisive compulsion to self-defeat, whereas the woman of the Case History showed a similar painful tendency, but limited in her case to the painful situation which endlessly prolonged the tension of her neurotic love-affair.

Freud finally concluded, in *Beyond the Pleasure Principle*, that this tendency to repetition compulsion of emotional ambivalence was not governed by the Pleasure Principle, but was better to be understood as a fundamental tendency of all instincts to reproduce reactions to past traumatic events by repetition. Whether or not this is a completely adequate answer to the problem, the repetition compulsion is unquestionably a vital problem of analysis, for to some extent every neurotic symptom or trait displays this compulsive need for repetitive self-defeat.[3]

CLASSIFICATION OF THE INSTINCTS

We now turn from the fundamental conception of instinct as biologic energy whose impulsion produces psychic tension and whose discharge produces pleasure, to the specific types of activity by which such discharge is attained. Freud's theory of instincts postulates an organization of such a kind that discharge of specific portions of the total energy is achieved by some specific activity. This specific activity is known as the *aim* of the instinct. Obviously not all instinctual energy is expended in the same type of activity, and therefore Freud classified different instincts in terms of their aims. Thus, in the discussion of those aspects of psychoanalytic theory which are most closely related to clinical problems, Freud came to use the word "instinct" in a derived sense. He sometimes spoke of instinct in terms of *how* it is manifested, while its original and biological meaning has reference to *what* is manifested. For example, he used the term "genital instinct" to designate that organization of biologic energy which requires genital activity for complete discharge of the tension. If we were indisposed to economize in our use of words we would have to say, instead of "genital instinct," "that component of the sexual group of instincts whose aim is genital function."

From the standpoint of a fundamental kinetic theory, in contrast to the descriptive classification of emotional nuances (which MacDougall, for instance, did so admirably in his theory of "sentiments"), all instinctual systems may be classified according to their

[3] This author has suggested ("Instinct and the Ego During Infancy," *Psychoanalytic Quarterly*, Vol. XI, Jan. 1942) that the repetition compulsion is originally a normal function compelling the practice of new motor and mental skills in the course of development, and normally disappearing when the skill is fully learned. Neurotic recurrence of repetition compulsion is therefore due to a defect in one of the mature ego-functions so that this stage of the unlearned function is reactivated.

aims in three major groups: the "ego instincts," whose aim is nutrition and self-preservation; the "destructive (aggressive) instincts," whose aim is hostile activity which injures, pains, or kills; and the "sexual (love) instincts," whose aims are to touch, to experience pleasurable sensations or their psychologic equivalents, creating, receiving, and giving. It is the "sexual instincts" or "libido" (as defined by Freud) which have been studied in most detail by analysts, and to these we now turn our attention.

CHAPTER

VI

THE LIBIDO THEORY

T H E "instinct theory" of psychoanalysis and the "libido theory" are too often considered practically synonymous terms. It is, however, worth recognizing that "instinct theory" is properly the more general term, as it defines Freud's concept of the biological source of all psychological drives, their essential attributes in terms of mental representation, the Pleasure Principle and instinctual tension, and also the quantitative implications we have previously discussed. This general hypothesis of instincts (or "drives"), discussed in the previous chapter, is therefore fundamental to the interpretation of all mental experience and behavior, regardless of how one may choose to classify and subclassify these instincts. Freud himself classified them in different ways at different stages in the development of his theories.

Freud originally gave the term *libido* to that group of instincts which specifically determine the psychosexual life of the individual. *Libido* is, therefore, a synonym for "sexual instincts." It is that fraction of the biological energy of the individual which produces sexual tensions and their mental representations; it denotes that group of instincts which produce sexual aims and the need for love-objects.

The sexual instincts, or libido, have as conspicuous a place in the theory of psychoanalysis as psychosexuality has among its data. This has resulted inevitably from Freud's concentration on those very neuroses in which sexual conflict proved to be primary, and from the more fundamental fact that the libido theory is derived from a mass of mental data which is not available for so adequate a definition of other instincts. For psychosexuality activates so much more of the imagination of mankind than do the relatively silent biologic needs, and it is also so much more subject to repression. The formulation of the libido theory is therefore inevitably the most detailed and adequate chapter of the instinct theory, for it includes those infererences which are most conclusively indicated by plentiful data.

The facts of sexuality—especially bisexuality, repression, displacement of object and aim, regression and sublimation—led Freud to consider all variations of psychosexuality as manifestations of one fundamental and closely related group of instincts with a variety of sexual aims. One of Freud's most enlightening and startling contributions was the recognition of the variety of interchangeable components of sexuality. The theorist's intellect had previously been presented with a problem not unlike a playroom littered with a variety of toys, and Freud with the libido theory was like the distraught but capable mother who picks up the toys, finds the right shelf for each, and gives us a picture of an organized and scientifically tidied room. The organizer is the theory of the libido, whose source is biological [1] and was indeed considered by Freud, decades before the data of modern endocrinology, a hypothetical substance which might some day be chemically identified.

PARTIAL AIMS AND DISPLACEMENT

That the libido is a reservoir of energy for sexual instincts with multiple aims is therefore a theory which takes fully into account the variety of sexual tensions and pleasures which have been recognized clinically. Freud conceived the libido to be unique among the instincts in that it is the source of energy for *partial aims* of the total sexuality, each of which is basically unconscious, but

[1] See pages 92 ff., above.

may be represented as a fully conscious wish, or by an aim-inhibited act, or as a symptom. We are clinically acquainted with many of these sexual aims, for example, the genital, oral, anal, phallic, exhibitionistic, and masochistic aims of the libido, and we have seen how each libidinal aim is specifically defined by the various forms of sensual phantasy, quality of pleasure, and guilt-reactions which are typical of it.

This concept of the libido being distributed among various "sexual instincts," each distinguished only by its partial aim, is important and necessary because of the phenomenon of *displacement*. We have seen (Chapters II and III) that the facts of unconscious sexuality show how readily a genital aim can be displaced by an oral aim, a phallic aim, or an anal aim. Thus the genital aim of the woman with the cooking ritual was displaced regressively by the infantile oral aim of conceiving with the mouth. The genital aim of the man who devised scientific apparatus [2] had been unconsciously displaced regressively by the aim of exhibiting his phallus in urinating. The masculine aims of the man who would not pay his bill [3] had been unconsciously displaced by the infantile aim to be stroked anally by mother. The man who tickled his ear in analysis [4] showed in free association the unconscious displacement of a genital by an anal phantasy.

Such phenomena illustrate not only a very important characteristic of the sexual instincts but a unique one. For displacement is not to be found in the mental representations of other instincts, and so displacement differentiates the phenomenology of the sexual instincts most decidedly from that of all the ego instincts. One cannot substitute the sky for food to satisfy hunger. But one can, under certain circumstances, substitute a good steak for the need for conversation with a friend, or even the sound of a violin for the cooing of a sweetheart. The libido theory takes full account of these possibilities through the theory of partial aims and their displaceability.

---

[2] See pages 33, 36, 53.   [3] See pages 41, 51–2.   [4] See page 54.

DEVELOPMENT OF THE LIBIDO

The definition of partial aims is essential in applying the libido theory to the problems of psychosexual development. For the libido theory is not only a theory of the psychosexuality of adults but a theory of its development. We have seen (Chapter III) that clinical psychoanalysis produces endless evidence that the conscious and unconscious pregenital aims of adults are residuals from periods of infancy when each of these is normally a dominant, and not a subsidiary, pleasure aim. And psychoanalysts have generally adopted the theory of Karl Abraham [5] that human biology dictates a definite sequence in the development of the aims of the libido.

This theory states that from birth throughout the first year or so of life the mouth is the dominant erotogenic zone, by whose adequate excitation, especially in suckling, libido tension is fully reduced, thereby affording the infant maximal pleasure. This is shown by the deep sleep, relaxation, placid contentment, and flushing which follow nursing—an observable psychologic complex strikingly similar, if not identical, with the sequelæ of normal adult orgasm. This period of psychosexual development is therefore called the *oral phase* of the libido, and itself includes an early phase in which the oral aims are passive, and a later oral phase in which activity by biting is more imperative.

The oral phase is replaced during infantile development by the *anal phase* in which anal aims of the libido are most conspicuous and manifested by intense interest in feces, and by a multitude of phantasies concerning the anus and excreta. This anal phase is considered to be dominant during the second and third years—and the more usual practices in the rearing of children, such as bowel training and elementary organization of clothing and washing habits, seem to correspond with this.

The pregenital development of the libido culminates in the in-

---

[5] Karl Abraham, *Selected Papers on Psycho-Analysis* (Hogarth Press, 1950) No. XXVI, Part II.

tensified desire to use the genital organs which characterizes the *phallic phase*. The penis then becomes the organ of maximal erotic pleasure in boys, and the need to experience this in phantasy and by masturbation becomes the dominant aim of the libido, supplemented by other phallic activities, especially the pleasure in exhibiting his power in urination and reinforced demands to be reacted to as a self-sufficient and important thing. In girls the clitoris subserves the same libidinal aim of this stage in libidinal development, providing erotogenic pleasure identical to the boy's and therefore serving as a source of phantasies similar to his, in contrast to the more feminine phantasies of the genital phase.[6]

Maturity of the libido is finally manifest in psychologic as well as anatomic *genitality,* which first becomes the dominant aim of the libido (at least in boys) when the Œdipus complex becomes dominant at the end of the infantile period. After the latency period (grade-school years), it is reactivated and intensified by the physiology of puberty, and reaches its full development during adolescence.

Normal male *genitality* requires gratification of the same sexual organs as do the libidinal aims of the phallic phase; but its aim is distinguished by the need to share gratification mutually with a mate. This determines a more complete differentiating of the dominant libidinal aims of the two sexes than occurs in earlier stages of development. The normally dominant aim of the adult male demands dominant activity for sexual fulfillment. In contrast, the female's primary aim is the seduction of this male activity in order to enjoy a more receptive role for mating to be complete; not only is orgasm sought, but conception has become the ultimate aim of the mature woman, while the active aims of her libido are fully satisfied in childbirth, the care of children and home, or in substitutes for maternity. Normal genitality, male and female, however, always involves essential secondary as well as primary libidinal aims, some of which are satisfied in the complete relationship of mating, especially the diversified forepleasures of erotic courtship, and some of

6 Chapter III, pages 53 ff.

which are satisfied in the "aim inhibited," or erotically denied, relationships which constitute friendship and are the basis of normal social relationships and sublimations.

But those libidinal aims of the genital adult determine not only his erotic fulfillment, but his capacity to love another person as well (*object love*). Complete genital fulfillment is inseparable from the capacity for tenderness, for over-evaluation of the partner, and inseparable from the need for the partner's pleasure. In other words, genitality creates the need of a man to love a woman sexually, and creates a woman's primary need for a man. This distinguishes the phenomenology of genitality most clearly from pregenital sexual aims. Especially important is this distinction between the adult whose actual aims are those of the phallic period and the genital adult; objectively the "phallic" man or woman is also impelled to enjoy the external sexual organs, but the partner is exploited and not loved. This is the underlying problem of many adult sexual relationships in which hatred and not gratitude is engendered by intercourse.

An empirical justification for this instinct theory of mature object-love is found not only in conscious erotic phantasies, and in the sensual fulfillment of coitus, but even more in its remarkable psychological and physiological sequelæ. Not only is the immediate erotic aim satisfied, but there is subsequently an awareness, objectively and subjectively, of bodily and mental well-being. A resolution of other conflicts which had been disturbing one's peace of mind has occurred. Irritability and inferiority feelings about other things have vanished for a while, though their external causes remain the same. Sleep is unperturbed. It is these facts that justify Freud's and Abraham's emphasis on a "genital object-relationship" whose libidinal aim is mutual orgasm as the dominant goal of the adult. Its disturbance by conflict is immediately apparent when coitus fails to solve other emotional problems than the need for erotic gratification because libido discharge has been incomplete. These facts of human experience, as well as others taken from the study of evolution, led Sandor Ferenczi to expand these theories in his "Genital Theory of the Libido." [7] In this speculation he claimed that the normal adult orgasm is not only a genital goal, but that it assimilates all the other libidinal aims (all the Christmas presents in one package, as it were). The genital and all pregenital aims, including the sadistic, are, according to him, simultaneously gratified in one climax, when it is complete.

The defects of the libido theory are those of every schematization of complex phenomena. The regular succession of sexual aims during pregenital development, and the separation of the aims of autoerotic and object love, are by no means so clear-cut in life as in the theory. Though there is little question that periods of special dominance of various pregenital aims of the libido occur in all human beings, there is in all periods the activity of a variety of aims, and not of just a single aim. Though sexual awareness of the mother and the desire of a little "Œdipus" for exclusive possession of her are especially apparent in a five-year-old, it is also certain he evinces such aims sporadically in earlier years, and it is probable there is a time during the second year when an earlier but less critical need for an Œdipal relationship develops. And finally, the libido theory of sexual development cannot take fully into account all the erotogenic zones, nor does it take into account many other aims of the libido which are not so specifically defined by an erotogenic zone—breathing, hearing, seeing, displaying, running, dancing, reasoning, and visceral experience, especially in the newborn, for example, are all important aims of the total libido.

But the libido theory has stood the test of time as an abstract concept which helps us to formulate and discuss systematically manifold clinical details and interrelationships of sexual psychology. As the source of the libido is conceived to be somatic, and the psychological facts are conceived to be its effects, the theory is basically biological. Yet discussion of the biological source is still confusing. Freud had expressed the hope in the preface to the *Three Contributions to the Theory of Sex* (1905) that new chemical discoveries would soon make the whole libido theory obsolete. The view at that

---

[7] Sandor Ferenczi: "Thalassa, A Theory of Genitality," in *Psychoanalytic Quarterly*, II, 361 (1933).

time that genital excitation arose in the seminal vesicles (clitoris and vagina in the female), and pregenital excitation in the other erogenous zones, seems entirely inadequate today. It is far more probable that the excitation is mentally referred to these localities, while the biological excitation itself, the libido, is a product of the total organism, whatever its paths of discharge may be. We love each other, not only with the genitals, but with our hearts and "guts." Chemistry, especially hormone physiology, has indeed vastly extended our knowledge of the physiologic basis of sexuality, personality, and behavior. But even these advances are still contributions to our knowledge of detail and not of the total processes, so that the libido theory of sexual drive is still very necessary. A comparison of the libido theory with the chapter on the facts of sexuality may well cause wonder whether it be not intellectually overscrupulous to call a formulation so much of which is demonstrated fact a theory at all.

THE EGO INSTINCTS

The *ego instincts* were originally defined as those which serve all the functions of self-preservation. For, in the early development of his theories, Freud had concluded that the instincts which impel to mastery of the outer world and to protection against its dangers are identical with those which are in opposition to certain of our drives toward sexual pleasure. He regarded the ego instincts as the forces which demand we heed the restrictions society imposes upon adult sexuality and heed its taboos of infantile sexuality, and as the forces which compel the intra-psychic repression of "dangerous" (conflict-threatening) impulses, whenever infantile wishes are still active forces in the adult unconscious.

The ego instincts were also considered servants of the Reality Principle, whose development ultimately enables the individual to do without the protection of his parents. But at the beginning of life sexual and ego instincts are both satisfied by the same aims of complete passivity toward the mother; the libidinal aim of sensual pleasure and the nutritional need of the ego both require the primacy of suckling. In the later infantile period the child's initiative is governed by autoerotic sexuality with other aims, generally in real opposition to the mother, who still supports the nutritional and protective requirements of ego-preservation. The two major functions of the ego instincts, mastery of reality and maintenance of repression, both become clearly manifest as independent functions of the individual at the same period of life when the child, renouncing the phantasies of his Œdipus complex, begins to face the world alone, and enters the latency period.

In the simplest terms, Freud originally theorized, psychic conflicts occur between variations of the impulses: "I must love," and "I must live"—of the need for pleasure and the need for preservation. Thus, in the early days of analytic theory, he would have interpreted the suffering of the patient who could not say "mother" as a blocking of her genital potentialities to enjoy life by the need to preserve herself from the phantasy of maternal retaliation. The man who dreamed of the Negro boys experienced a similar conflict of the wish to love women and the associated phantasy he would be injured.

The original hypothesis of the ego instincts constitutes by all odds the least satisfying and the least necessary part of the theory of instincts. In contrast to the libido theory, it is not based on an abundance of empirical data, as the "ego instincts" are not extensively represented in the mind. It is rather an early, hard-thought effort to provide an explanation of the counter-forces to sexual phantasies whose existence is manifested in conflict and repression. The theory of ego instincts is of interest to us in studying the first twenty years' development of Freud's enduring theories, especially the *Metapsychological Papers* (1910),[8] but the problems it attempts to solve have been dealt with more adequately in his later works on narcissism, the death-instinct theory, and especially the theory of personality structure.[9]

[8] Sigmund Freud, trans. in *Collected Papers,* Vol. IV.
[9] See Chapter VIII.

NARCISSISM

The advances in psychoanalytic theory since 1910 have to a great extent paralleled the extension of psychoanalytic investigation beyond the problems presented by the simpler psychoneuroses, dreams, and errors of everyday life. The first of these strides forward was the new and fundamental concept of narcissism (or narcissistic aspects of sexuality), dating from 1914. This was to some extent a product of the study of psychoses, for whose elucidation the formulations of repression, fixation, and regression were wholly inadequate. But the study of certain aspects of normal love-life also contributed to a theory which clarifies so many kinds of human experience.

Narcissism is any phenomenon in which oneself, one's person, one's body, or one's psychic attributes are the object of the libido. It is that supplement to the libido theory which deals with the *direction* of the sexual instincts (extroversion or introversion); it refers to those functions of the sexual instincts in which the ego is both active and passive, to those forms of love which are gratified independently of other people, or in which others are emotionally valued only for what they give to the subject. The narcissistic self is prepared to derive pleasure passively and receptively; it is indifferent to either the libidinal or the egoistic requirements of other people. Narcissism is the theoretical formulation of what we may term colloquially "self-love"; it is, therefore, the libidinal complement of "egotism" (in the more technical sense of service to one's own self-preservative needs). Thus, narcissism is the opposite of *object-love*, in which the fulfillment of another person's emotional requirement is indispensable to one's own pleasure. In many psychoses and markedly psychopathic types of personality, narcissism is even more complete. But some degree of narcissism is an important component of a great variety of psychological conditions, both normal and pathological.

Theoretically simple, narcissism is clinically a very complex problem. Not only is narcissistic libido at birth indistinguishable from the self-preservative (ego) instincts; not only (except in severe forms of mental or physical disease) is narcissism always mingled with variable degrees of object-love; but, besides these considerations, we find that the most common varieties of narcissism require the exploitation of another human being's love. This is obviously true, for example, of the adult types of love which more closely resemble the love of child to parent. Narcissism is a conspicuous component of what is one of the most typically feminine types of love, according to Freud, where the woman's chief requirement is to be adored and cared for. In the most typical (if there be such) loves of adult men for women, the role of narcissism is still more complex, in that the man's cherishing of the woman is so intimately related to the substitution, in greater or less degree, of the woman for himself as object of his own infantile (that is, narcissistic) needs. The love for children illustrates the same mechanism; for the adult finds in the child that intensity of narcissism which he cannot gratify adequately in himself, without frustration of the other instinctual needs of a mature personality, and so he loves the child's own infantilism. This component of child-love, when excessive, is largely responsible for the problems of parents who cannot allow their children to mature and become independent of them. Thus it is apparent that narcissism is a formulation not only of abnormal conditions, but of many aspects of normal adult love-life—as one indeed should expect from the fact that at the core of every human being is something of the infant, and every infant at first is completely narcissistic.

Narcissism, therefore, is one manifestation of the needs for love and pleasure grouped together as "sexual instincts." Its biologic source and general characteristics are identical with those of other currents of libido. It postulates only a difference in object and is, therefore, conspicuous in all sexual manifestations whose aim is not "genital" (and some that are, especially those of more passive individuals).

Following a much earlier hint of Karl Abraham, Freud showed how narcissism actually manifests many of the same characteristics which identify a libidinal process as love of another object. It is especially clear and important that both types of love give rise to the psychic over-evaluation of the beloved. The suitor acclaims his sweetheart's charms as unequaled and is pained at any injury she undergoes. The "narcissist," whose love is directed chiefly to his own person instead of another's, over-evaluates in exactly the same way his own importance and suffers the pangs of wounded hypersensitivity from all deprecatory opinions or any moderation in the affection bestowed upon him. The extreme example of pathological over-evaluation of self is seen in the megalomaniac, who has so completely "invested" his own person with his own love as to be indifferent to anything but his own greatness, beauty, or power. However absurd his claims may logically sound, they are emotionally true. He does not consciously lie about himself; he actually *feels* himself to be the greatest and most important of human specimens. The same instincts appear to be effective and produce similar types of "over-evaluation" in the lover who believes his sweetheart "the most beautiful girl in the world," and the megalomaniac who proclaims that he is Lincoln, Christ, or Napoleon. The difference is only in which object is invested by the libido, oneself or another, and in the tender components and solicitude which object-love always engenders.

Less conspicuous but convincing evidence of a "retreat" (or regression) from object-love to narcissism is evident in every variety of psychosis. Even that type of psychotic depression in which the individual proclaims he is the most miserable, the most useless, and the most loathsome of wretches, betrays his excessive evaluation of self in his use of superlatives and the excess of his demands for the reproaches of others. The schizophrenic patient betrays it in a different way when, sitting apart, doing, thinking, and feeling nothing in which others might share with emotional spontaneity, he shows how little outside of himself has subjective value.

Freud conceived the original relationship of the infant's libido to object to be, like the megalomaniac's, one in which only the self is loved. The babe knows nothing but himself, his only pleasures are his own body, lips, skin, internal organs, and eventually his special senses. Whatever external things he experiences, such as the breast, are at first conceived by him as part of himself and therefore psychologically *are*, to him, a part of himself. Only gradually does he learn that external objects are necessary for instinctual gratification, even of the narcissistic type. In the course of development this need of external objects becomes a major goal. It leads to everything about the human organism which is social, but is never (except perhaps in unusual moments of the most intense loving of another) so complete that there is not a residual narcissism in the most normal adults. An abnormal degree of adult narcissism is usually occasioned by some frustration of the object need. Thus the pathologically defiant man [1] was unable to love mother, teacher, sweethearts, or friends because of his resentment toward whatever person became the object of his love, and his narcissistic needs were thereby increased to an abnormal degree. But gratification of object-love may, conversely, be frustrated by excessive narcissistic trends. In this case, for example, it was frustrated because he must hate what he loved; but libido tension remains, and can then be satisfied only by a return to the infantile object, the self.

It is extraordinary that occasionally certain reasonably adult people may, for a few minutes during psychoanalysis, apparently reproduce the original narcissism which Freud presumed to be universal for the infant. For example, one patient feels he himself has the same thoughts and feelings as the analyst, and for a few moments reports some extraordinary associations: "I am so perplexed, so bewildered! I don't know, I can't tell whether you are I, or I am you. It is all the same—it is beautiful!" Another has a vivid phantasy of suckling and says that she must be feeling exactly like an infant; she "*knows* its sensations" and then complains of great confusion and uncertainty as to what is she and what is someone else. Both these moments, like all similar ones, occurred at times during psychoanalysis when conflict of love and hate for the same person made adult pleasure in a love-object temporarily impossible. They represent efforts to escape from a painful struggle to a pleasurable, if futile, childish peace.

There is another aspect of narcissism of special interest to

[1] See pages 103, 105.

medical scientists. This is the frequent identity of hypochondriacal and organic symptoms. A patient may complain of sensations in his heart because he has heart disease, or of heart disease because he has sensations in his heart. In hypochondria a patient loses interest in his previous activities and concentrates it on his organs; such a somatic concentration of narcissistic libido is mentally experienced as pain or as other abnormal bodily symptoms. In organic disease the pathology itself causes a concentration of psychic attention, and there follows a loss of interest in outside things. From the point of view of the theory of instincts, Freud argued, the distribution of libido appears the same in both these cases: in either hypochondria or organic disease we must account for the diminution of the concentration of the libido on the usual external sexual objects. Shall we not conclude that in both cases it is concentrated on the organs—more exactly the mental image of those organs—which have now become the "objects" of an unusual proportion of the total libido? This tight reasoning would seem confirmed by the striking fact that when either the person with physical disease or the person with hypochondria is relieved of symptoms, the libido is freed for the investment of other objects and the patient again has a need for other interests and other people than himself.

This is a conclusion congruous with the rest of our theory of instincts, which states that whenever damming-up of libido occurs, owing to the failure to gratify its aim, a tension results which is perceived psychically as some sort of pain. When the lover departs, there is no sexual object, gratification is denied, libido accumulates, and the person suffers, while his mental content becomes preeminently visual or verbal images of the object. When objects, and even thoughts of objects, are renounced, the self then becomes the object of love, and if this is not constantly gratified, pain is also experienced and becomes obvious to all in "spoiled-child" behavior. And when one's interest in both another object and one's own personality is lost, the libido appears, as in hypochondria and organic disease, to be concentrated in the mental representation of the organ involved; again the tension is perceived as pain, this time as physical pain, and the mental content is chiefly concerned with the object, now the organ. Such a postulated redistribution of the libido in conditions of physical pain, whether organically or psychologically caused, seems particularly clear when it occurs in a region from which the individual normally receives no sensations.

Thus the study of hypochondria and allied conditions leads to the conclusion that narcissism may be either a "sexualization" of one's own personality and sensations (self-love), or a "sexualization" of the organs and their functions; in the latter case the mechanics of life become the "object" of the libido, as do those of the newborn, who "needs" the breast both for nourishment and for pleasure. The concept of narcissism has developed since 1914 into one of the most valuable theoretical tools for the clinical understanding of personality and its ontogeny. It has enabled the analyst and psychiatrist to comprehend manifold observations on object-love, normal and abnormal egocentricity, adult and infant, and some physiological events, not merely as discrete phenomena, but as dynamically and quantitatively interrelated. In providing the theory of narcissism for this supreme intellectual achievement, Freud has demonstrated especially the value of using the libido theory for quantitative thinking when there are no exact quantitative data. For the essence of the theory of narcissism is the assumption that there is an approximately constant amount of libido available for any individual; that the more his libido is invested in the self, the less there is for object-love; that the more his libido is available for autistic ideas, the less there is remaining for realistic thought; and the more libido is invested in the mental representations of the body, the less there is available for interests outside the self.

SUMMARY

The libido theory, therefore, applies the general theory of instincts to the diverse facts of conscious and unconscious psychosexuality demonstrated by clinical psychoanalysis. It has proven itself the most adequate, valuable, and durable aspect of the theory of instincts for two reasons: first, it is induced from a quantity and variety of mental data whose abundance is not approached by the mental representations of other hypothesized instincts; and, secondly, it is immediately applicable to many phenomena with which clinical analysis is immediately concerned.

The libido theory provides us with an hypothetical explanation of the energy apparent in the impelling need to seek pleasure and love of many kinds. It enables us to understand how the repressed and unconscious psychosexual components of neurotic conflicts are not static but effect-producing, as is shown by their role in the production of symptoms, phantasies, dreams, and behavior. The theory of partial aims enables us to conceptualize a common factor, the libido, which determines many characteristics of typical experience at various age levels and the needs which activate many normal aspects of development. Finally, the theory of narcissism has become an indispensable instrument for the comprehension of several normal and abnormal personality types, the psychology of the infant, the psychopathology of psychoses, and the mental characteristics of physical illness.

For these reasons, the libido theory is today as indispensable to the clear thinking of analysts, dynamic psychiatrists, and those who apply analytic knowledge to other fields, as was the concept of ether to physicists until unforeseen knowledge of electronics finally made it superfluous.

CHAPTER

VII

THE THEORY OF
AGGRESSION

THEORY OF EROS AND THE DEATH INSTINCTS

T H E original theory of two distinct groups of instincts, the sexual and the ego instincts, opposed to each other in conditions of mental conflict, had sufficed to explain psychoanalytic observations of the simpler neuroses. But the recognition of narcissism, especially its role in hypochondria, psychoses, and organic neuroses, had pointed to certain inadequacies of this instinct theory. The Pleasure and Reality Principles had served to describe the purpose of instincts in the impulsion of most human reactions, but did not suffice to explain the repetition compulsions observed in some features of play, wartime shell-shock, and psychoanalytic treatment.[1] Another stimulus to a more comprehensive psychobiologic theory had been the increasing perplexity of psychoanalysts about the ramified phenomena of psychosexual sadism and masochism, and the relationship of these to other expressions of the sexual instincts. As a result of these further developments in the subject-matter of psychoanalysis, Freud, in 1920 (*Beyond the Pleasure Principle*), retracted his original theory that the sexual instincts (libido) and

[1] See pages 105–6.

ego instincts are primarily opposed and of different biological origin.

Freud now proposed the postulate, in partial agreement with Carl Jung (who in 1910 had strenuously disputed Freud's libido theory),[2] that the biologic energy which maintained all life processes, including those of self-preservation (previously called "ego instincts"), organic function ("organ narcissism"), self-love ("mental narcissism"), and object-love, was basically homogeneous. He proposed to name this energy *Eros,* whether it was manifested as "libido" in the service of the sexual instincts, or as "ego-libido" serving the functions of life-preservation. In "primary narcissism," he now thought, one sees clearly the primal identity of the two, typically in the gratification of both love and hunger in the newborn's suckling.

Freud now postulated another previously undescribed group of instincts, which were in opposition to both the sexual and the egoistic functions of Eros, as now conceived. These he termed the *death instincts.* The theory of the death instincts was justified by the tendency of all life to return to, or to repeat, the inorganic state. That is to say, the physiologic expression of Eros is anabolic, that of the death instincts is catabolic. Though no instance of direct representation in the mind of the inevitable biologic need to die exists, Freud postulated that derivatives of the catabolic instincts are included mentally in all destructive impulses and ideas. These, the new theory stated, are originally directed against the self and eventually produce death. As long as life lasts, however, and as a necessary condition for sustaining life, there is apparent a diversion of the primal death impulse toward outer objects, and it is this that provides the energy for all acts of aggression, hostility, or destruction and for sadistic or masochistic psychosexuality.

In many situations in social life this process is reversed, and there is a turning inward on oneself of the thwarted aggression toward others. This occurs, for example, in suicide and phantasies of suicide, and in incidents where a strong need to attack oneself is

---

[2] See pages 306 ff.

indicated by a mood of despair, melancholy, or self-depreciation. The occasions for such a reversal of destructive tendencies are most often those in which some need for love or pleasure is thwarted by another, and the primitive desire for retaliation inhibited. As retaliation is usually tabooed, consciously or unconsciously, in consequence of a fear of punishment, it is to be expected that most psychological representatives of self-destructive tendencies are closely related to those phantasies of punishment that have been discussed already (Chapter IV). The man who threw himself into the water in consequence of his stifled aggression toward his sweetheart is typical.

An overtly homosexual girl again illustrates this mechanism. She meets a former female lover who snubs her; she flies into a rage at the man whose attentions had deprived her of this girl, stifles it, and then behaves in so unusual a way that she is immediately discharged by her employer. She then complains for weeks that the unemployment, which her own actions precipitated, has shown her inability to cope with forces within her, that she is worthless, and failure is inevitable. Interpreted in terms of the theory of instincts, this behavior shows, throughout, the activity of that energy whose aim is destruction. She wants, first, the destruction of the man who has deprived her of her love-object, and when this is inhibited, she is compelled by her own unexpended need to provoke her own destruction. Freud would describe this as the activity of a *destructive instinct*, and this destructive instinct as a derivative of the death instinct, turned outward and then against the self, and the mental representatives of this introverted aggression are the acts that actually secured her own destruction in her vocation, and later the epithets which she applies to herself.

The theory of the death instincts is that theoretical concept which Freud himself advanced with the most caution and which was most disputed by analysts themselves. Its opponents presented two arguments. First, they claimed that postulating an instinct whose ultimate aim is death is antagonistic to the general concept of instinct, and that death is due to the exhaustion of the vital functions, a failure of life-processes rather than a fulfillment of innate biologic tendencies. The supporters of the death-instinct theory contended that this very argument is an expression of Eros, which opposes the "need" to die, and that if we can emotionally and tentatively accept that possibility, there is sufficient indication of an actual drive to accomplish death biologically as a positive aim. Perhaps this viewpoint is most simply expressed by the unmeditated response of a woman very busy at work, when she was interrupted by the philosophical remark: "Strange we work so hard, when death makes it mean nothing fifty years from now." "That's exactly why we work!" was her lightning-fast answer.

Secondly, the opponents of the death-instinct theory claimed it is unnecessary, as all evidence of a destructive impulse can be shown to be a reaction to a thwarted pleasure. This is a clinical fact and was undisputed, but the supporters of the death-instinct theory still contended that the observation leaves unanswered the theoretical problem of where these reactions to thwarted love derive the energy which impels the destructive effort. They agreed, however, that the practical work of the analyst is not affected by his acceptance or rejection of this death-instinct theory. Freud himself rested his argument on biologic rather than psychologic data, and saw in destructive impulses, whether externally or internally directed, the "compulsion" of living matter to repeat, or return to, the inorganic state (*Nirvana Principle*).

SADISM AND MASOCHISM

Whatever an individual analyst's attitude may be to Freud's theory that all aggressive and destructive needs come from a "death instinct," none can question the vital role of destructive tendencies, especially unconscious ones. Yet their theoretical formulation had for years been one of the more muddled aspects of psychoanalytic theory, a situation which the death-instinct hypothesis, whatever its shortcomings, formulated precisely and partially clarified.

The confusion had been due especially to the very intimate relationship, clinically and theoretically, of destructive impulses with those of the sadistic and masochistic phases of psychosexuality. For Freud in his original formulations of these problems had classified all sadistic and masochistic phantasies as pregenital wishes,[3] representative of "partial sexual instincts," first established, like other partial instincts, in the infantile period. The words "sadism" and "masochism" have subsequently been used by analysts in several quite different senses. As in general psychiatry, psychoanalysis refers to those specific sexual perversions in which the infliction of physical pain is a prerequisite of maximal erotic gratification as "sadism," and those in which the experiencing of pain is the prerequisite as "masochism." Freud discovered very early that phantasies corresponding to such perversions were conspicuous elements of the unconscious, and subsequently referred to all such wishes as "sadism" or "masochism," without implying thereby a manifest tendency to perverse behavior. From this it was only a step to the recognition of the similarity of many character reactions in which there was no immediate erotic goal. Chronic nagging, "biting sarcasm," temper tantrums, and similar phenomena were henceforth considered psychologic forms of sadism; and the various means by which the neurotic seeks and attains suffering, such as inferiority feelings, painful symptoms, the enjoyment of illness, martyrdom, the provocation of rebukes and unpleasant emotional reactions in others, were regarded as various forms of psychological masochism. *Sadism* (in its more general psychoanalytic sense) is, therefore, defined as the wish (conscious or unconscious) to inflict pain (physical or psychic); *masochism* as the wish to experience pain. They are manifest in conscious sexual perversion, in unconsciously perverse phantasies, in character traits and interpersonal reactions, and in "moral masochism."

In *moral masochism* there is a need to suffer, especially in ways dictated by unconscious punishment phantasies. It is a factor in all neuroses. From this standpoint it becomes apparent that unconscious (and conscious) guilt is not only a "penance," a punishment for tabooed wishes, but at the same time a special form of psychosexuality. Just as erotic sexuality occasionally finds conscious

[3] Sigmund Freud, *Three Contributions to the Theory of Sex* (1905).

pleasure in the conscious perversions, so psychosexuality, in the broader analytic sense, is constantly manifest in psychological sado-masochism. In the form of moral masochism this aspect of sexuality is closely related to narcissism. A person, for example, who retires from other people and is preoccupied with his own misery, is both subject and object of his own sado-masochistic drives; he is both inflicting pain and experiencing pain, and he is playing the dual role because he *needs* both. He has not succeeded in achieving the normal expressions of sexuality in full genital relationships to outer objects.

The man whose rejection by a sweetheart was followed by phantasies of drowning himself [4] illustrated as simply as possible these complex relationships. His capacity for normal sexuality had been apparent in his previous relationship with her. A traumatic frustration of this, however, was not coincident with diminution of sexual tension; as there was now no real object, the tension must have some other release. The result was a regression to more primitive sado-masochistic (self-destructive) sexuality. His impulse was to satisfy in one narcissistic act of drowning himself three compelling drives: (1) his mobilized aggression by turning it on himself; (2) his unambiguously sexual wish in a symbolic act (to plunge his body into the water); and (3) his unconscious guilt (moral masochism) by suffering from his own deed.

The dynamic relationships of the active and passive aims of sexuality, hostile destructiveness, and unconscious guilt are always very closely interwoven in such sado-masochistic phenomena.

Perhaps the most common intellectual stumbling-block of the newcomer to psychoanalysis is this problem of masochistic psychosexuality, the capacity of the human being to experience "pleasure in pain." What is painful cannot be pleasurable, is the reiterated and logical argument, and it is valid from the standpoint of the sensation of pain isolated from concomitant details. The "pleasure" of masochism is perhaps more exactly stated as those circumstances where pain is essential to pleasure, although—as classically in the chronic invalid who "loves" his symptoms—it is also true that one

4 See pages 75–6.

may also exploit pain for pleasure. These fine discriminations are, however, not the point. The point is that, when one considers the total situation, one must consider that ungratified libido tension always increases, and can be reduced by a masochistic experience. Though the act itself may not be a pleasant one, the tension-release is unquestionably *relatively* pleasurable. The pent-up individual, commonly observed, who relieves himself of suffering by furiously pounding his head, is an illustration of the tension-reduction achieved by more complicated masochistic phenomena—self-mutilation, an orgy of self-depreciation, provoking a lover to lose his temper, provoking an employer who is loved neurotically.

Unconscious sadistic and masochistic phantasies are derived from infantile sexuality, with whose development they are intimately bound. Hitherto we have discussed in detail chiefly passive (masochistic) aims of pregenital sexuality with specific sources of sensual pleasure. Now we must recognize that there is a sadistic aim corresponding to each of these. Karl Abraham pointed this out in a classic contribution to the libido theory (1924): that during the oral phase the child wishes to use his mouth not only to suck, but to bite. During the anal period he derives pleasure not only from passive stimuli of this zone, but from forcible expulsion. The reason why the peak of oral pleasure and the first peak of external aggression (for example, in tempers at weaning) should coincide, and why the peak of anal sensuality should be accompanied by the sadistic impulses which underlie such behavior as obstinacy, defiance, cruelty to other living things, and destructive rages, escapes further analysis. This, and the coincidence of oral sensuality and the oral type of sadism, apparently are constant and constitutionally determined events of infantile development.

This fact is the main reason for psychoanalysts' difficulties in the theoretical formulation of destructive trends. Clinically there are almost no observations of thoroughly studied sadistic or masochistic phenomena which do not show a sexual as well as an aggressive component. Wherever we observe conscious or unconscious representations of a destructive or cruel trend, we find a sexual component, a sensual pleasure-seeking aspect of the total situation; and wherever we find sadism and masochism, we find also evidence of a concurrent anal, oral, or other pregenital partial aim.

The man who had the illusion of crepe on his brother's door [5] had the concurrent phantasy of injuring him with his mouth. The man with the severe form of defiance of all authorities [6] manifested, coincidentally with his hatred, the powerful desire to express it by dirtying things, by being dirty, literally and in a derived sense. The first clues to these unconscious phantasies in the analysis were his imitations of flatus with his mouth, and his intentionally insolent display of dirty hands.

That such anal-sadistic wishes are none the less powerful forces in the unconscious determinants of behavior, even though conscious thought is a scrupulous denial of them, was clearly shown by a man who for a long period of analysis consciously made prodigious intellectual efforts to understand precisely each detail of the analyst's remarks and to report every association. But the analyst could observe that he himself, as well as the patient, was actually learning very little that was new and therapeutically valuable. Whenever his associations were especially "flat," he frequently placed his thumbs in a commonplace and unostentatious gesture in various angles of his clothing. The analyst finally suggested that he remove his thumbs. The patient, much annoyed, then gave mild vent to phantasies, previously unconscious, of playing with his anus and recognized that this trick was a mannerism that habitually occurred in situations where he desired, but feared, to assert his superiority over other people.

The derivatives of the normal oral sadism and anal sadism of infancy are apparent in many colloquial references to anger, such as "biting sarcasm," "henpecked husbands," "I will blow him to pieces," "he stinks," "the dirty rat"; most obscene expressions of derision and defiance include references to the excretory functions. The most severe case I have seen of psychoneurotic symptoms and character reactions determined by unconscious anal sadism was a woman of good family whose personality before analysis showed almost no capacity for tender feelings; every reaction to other peo-

[5] See page 10.   [6] See pages 103, 105.

ple was impelled by a conscious or unconscious phantasy either of causing them suffering or of provoking *their* sadism and thus causing pain and frustration to herself. Her general manner and boorish language were offensive and violated every ideal of good taste, and she had for a time chosen to be a prostitute in order "to see how filthy human beings could be." An interesting detail of her life had been the occupancy of two apartments during the same winter. One was in a good neighborhood; she cared for it immaculately and never received callers there. The other was in an undesirable neighborhood; she enjoyed its extreme disorderliness and general disreputability. Analysis showed that the two apartments represented, almost literally, unconscious phantasies of her own body. Her vagina was emotionally regarded, in her secret phantasies, as immaculately pure; and the capacity for voluptuous sensation there was unthinkable. But her anus was vile, and could be used sensually because of her wish to defile all men. Though physically she was promiscuous, actually she denied herself and her partners all normal genital gratification, and in those relationships used her vagina as an unconscious representative of her anal phantasies.

Oral sadism was hardly less conspicuous in this woman. On one day of her analysis she felt highly elated and wished to dance wildly; her association was that she felt as though she were strong and omnipotent, as though her very body was a penis, and she remembered dreaming the previous night of eating this organ. A violent temper tantrum in childhood had followed a glimpse of her little brother's penis.

A further illuminating aspect of her severe neurosis was the relationship of her sadism toward people to her "moral masochism"; though her promiscuous relationships with men were motivated by the passion to hurt physically and psychologically, she coincidentally punished herself by incurring the aversion and contempt of all her acquaintances. As unconscious need to suffer from every aggression was worked out in the analysis, her potentialities for experiencing normal feelings of tenderness and gratitude began to appear spontaneously in her everyday life. It was then demonstrated that her previous inability to reduce libido tension, except by regressive sadistic behavior, was due to a very powerful need represented mentally by a system of punishment phantasies, which may be condensed by the sentence: "I will be punished for any vaginal or tender feeling toward a man, even in phantasy."

Besides the oral and anal types of sadism, varieties which are characteristic of the phallic phase of infantile sexuality are important. These are especially to be observed in the problems of excessively narcissistic characters, whose dominant sensual interest is the use of penis or clitoris, but whose capacity for object-love of the partner is limited. The characteristic unconscious phantasy of this phase is not that the penis gives pleasure, but that it inflicts an injury. Men in whose character this phantasy is a dominant determinant often represent the penis as a dangerous weapon in their dreams, as others do occasionally. Such men are generally inconsiderate of the happiness of women with whom they are intimate, and may either exploit them only for their own sensual pleasures, or may be obviously women-haters, finding their chief human relationships in the company of other men.

Many women in whose character-formation the phantasies of the phallic period are dominant lead lives rationalized by the conscious philosophy, "It's a man's world," in the sense of men using women only for erotic exploitation, and ignore the evidence that for many of their own sex the erotic pleasures of love are mutual. Analysis will often reveal that this philosophy is developed from their unconscious wishes for the aggressive erotic role accompanying masturbation of the clitoris during the phallic phase, and that in childhood there had been many phantasies that they had organs like boys. The survival of these unconscious wishes in the adult unconscious is often apparent in the conspicuously competitive attitude of this type toward men. If they form warm attachments to men, their role is dominant, and if they desire a child as compensation for what they feel to be the rank injustice of being born a female, they have no yearning that it be the child of a particular man, hope excessively that it will be male and of unusual bodily and mental endowments, and often desire only one. They secretly but unconsciously wish it were practical to have a child without marriage.

Clinical experience also shows that sadism is a reaction to frustrated wishes of other kinds and thus satisfies in one act both the original sexual impulse and the desire for revenge. In adults without severe neuroses, the frustration may be an adult trauma. More frequently (though less obviously, for the subject's unconscious role in provoking the frustration will be strongly rationalized) it is wholly the result of frustrations imposed or invited by strong punishment phantasies. This is conspicuously so in adults whose sadistic trends are constant elements of their personality.

The critical frustration may be of a genital aim, as occurred in the suicidal man and in the woman with two apartments; more often the sadism is a reaction to the frustration of a passive pregenital wish. Other cases of sado-masochistic regression were illustrated by the man whose resentment was the sequel of denial of his unconscious wish to have his anus touched, and of the man whose marital irritability resulted from the excessive desire to have his genital gazed upon. In the pre-phallic years of infancy, sadism is always a reaction to the frustration of a passive wish—in fact, of almost any wish to be given some pleasure or to be treated with tenderness. Whether a sadistic reaction may occur without such traumata becomes an academic question when we consider that the requirements of rearing cannot dispense with a denial of many of the child's demands for pleasure. Unusual degrees of cruelty and temper, however, probably occur only in children some important aspect of whose need of love is either chronically unsatisfied or chronically so over-satisfied that the child learns to accept no frustration whatever. After the phallic period is reached, it may be the frustration of an active impulse which provokes the sadistic impulse.

Before a final discussion of the theoretical aspects of these problems, let us pause to summarize what are apparently the definitely established facts of sadism and masochism. We have found, then, that wishes to derive pleasure by the infliction or reception of pain are conspicuous dynamic factors in the unconscious, and decisive ones in many types of neurotic reaction. We have found that masochistic wishes are intimately associated with phantasies representing the need of punishment; and that sadistic wishes are generally, if not always, the result of external or internal frustrations of passive oral and anal wishes, or active phallic and genital wishes. Sadism and masochism serve, therefore, as libidinal aims by which pleasure may be obtained; and in this way they are like the other partial aims of pregenital sexuality, and are utilized repressively as substitutes for the genital function either when this has never been attained or when it is impaired by a psychic conflict. Coincidentally with the pleasure they afford, they satisfy the unconscious needs for punishment, and often the need for reprisal. Finally, certain varieties of unconscious sadistic and masochistic wishes of the adult, like other forms of repressed sexuality, are to be observed directly in the conscious phantasies and behavior of the infantile period, the specific types being determined by the dominance of one or another erotic zone.

SADO–MASOCHISM AND THE THEORIES OF INSTINCTS

Theoretically, then, in so far as sadism and masochism are forms of pregenital sexuality to which genital sexuality regresses in neurosis, these facts offer no unique problems. The libido theory is adequate for the purpose and explains the tension represented by a sadistic phantasy, and the pleasure derived from its gratification, as adequately as it explains other phenomena of pregenital sexuality.

The more difficult problems of theory are indicated in the most succinct way by a marked indefiniteness of terminology. Gradually most analysts, before and even after the publication of *Beyond the Pleasure Principle*, had come to speak of "masochism," not only in the senses we have defined but as practically synonymous with any and all passive, receptive, or submissive aims of the libido. It was even used generally to denote the aim of normal female love as "feminine masochistic." Analysts of this period were also habituated to thinking of any impulse with an active aim as "sadistic," whether it implied specifically lustful pleasure in hurting a love-object or, more vaguely, any form of activity or assertion, as well as the dominant sexual aim of normal male genitality, even when no primary need of a man to hurt the woman he loved was evident. It may be said that these confused usages of these important words had at least the excuse of a legitimate history; for it dated from Freud's inclusion (*Three Contributions to the Theory of Sex*, 1905) of psychological masochism and sadism in his original definition of pregenital sexuality.

Since the publication of *Beyond the Pleasure Principle*, analysts, including Freud, have gradually circumvented this terminological confusion by using more and more such words as "aggression," "aggressive instincts," and "destructive instincts." In the early pages of this book I have sometimes followed this example. The practice has led some analysts, and almost all dynamic psychiatrists who have adopted psychoanalytic theory, to create for themselves a new class of instincts, the *aggressive instincts*. In some ways, this has been a most fertile development, for a theory of "primary aggression," according with the premises of the basic theory of instincts, has stimulated a great deal of clinical investigation and discussion of those problems arising from a supposedly primary need for non-sexual self-assertion.

On the other hand, this trend of the last thirty years has created many vacua both in inductive theory and clinical acumen, vagaries that the adopters of the "instinct to aggression" theory have too generally been willing to ignore. With few exceptions, the difference between thinking in terms of an instinctual hypothesis or in terms of aggressive behavior is overlooked. The usual argument of analysts of the twenties and thirties who rejected the death-instinct theory was that all aggressions were responses to disappointing frustration, but they rarely faced the question of where the energy mobilized by frustrations comes from. Furthermore, the newer theories have led many contemporary investigators to overlook the unconscious sexual origins of many aggressions which were better understood by the older analysts. And, finally, though Freud himself in the last fifteen years of his work referred here and there to "aggression" and "destructive instincts," neither he nor other analysts worked out a definitive theory of "aggressive instincts" which compares in clarity and thoroughness with the earlier definitions of the basic instinct theory, the libido theory, or the death-instinct theory. The convenience of the newer terminology does not completely solve the old theoretical problems; and the existing difficulties created by extending the concept of sadism to all aggression, mental and behavioral, has not led to any adequate definition, clinical or theoretical, of when aggression is a derivative of sexuality and when it is not.

The very least that can be said for the Theory of Eros and the Death Instincts and its effect upon the further development of clinical psychoanalysis and its theory is that it is the most clear-cut effort to solve these complex problems of the theory of sado-masochism. For not only does it solve (if only philosophically and for the time being) the confusions resulting from the original theory of the relationship of the ego-instincts to the libido, and of both to psychic and body narcissism; it also postulates that, though in their most primitive state the biologic sources of death instincts and Eros are distinct, in the course of development a *fusion* of the two instincts occurs so that identical aims serve both impulses simultaneously. Partial fusion, therefore, has already occurred before even the earliest stages of libido function that we can observe in infancy. The degree of fusion at successive stages of libido development (together with the zone of erotogenic dominance and the extroversion or introversion of the impulses) would then determine the various partial aims, such as oral passivity and anal sadism.

The reason, according to Freud, why direct psychologic evidence of the death instincts is almost lacking is that they are "silent"; they do not manifest themselves in identifiable ways in the mind, in contrast to the sexual (life) instincts, which clamor for conscious recognition. Most of the psychologic evidence offered in support of this theory is, therefore, the destructive characteristics of sadistic and masochistic phenomena. These, according to Freud, when they first appear in the newborn child, are already products of a partial fusion, by which the same aims—that of biting, for example—serve both the need to destroy and the need to obtain pleasure. But this is a partial fusion only. Complete fusion of the life instincts (Eros) and death instincts is seen only in the fully mature impulses of the normal adult; its clearest manifestation is the erotic aggression of the male who loves the feminine object, an act which, theoretically, is determined by the neutralization of the destructive impulses by those of Eros as a result of complete fusion, producing an aggressive but undestructive act of love. Thus all genital aims of the libido interpreted in terms of the death-instinct theory represent complete fusion, while, conversely, the regressions, which determine many neurotic symptoms, involve "defusion," theoretically a partial split of the fused impulses into a mixture of destructive and sexual aims.

Freud's later theory of the death instinct permits of a simple formulation of the problems of the coincidence of suffering and pleasure, the differentiation of normal and sadistic aggression, and of sadistic and other forms of destructive drive. If one could prove that there exist certain forms of hatred and destructiveness which are not, coincidentally, regressive expressions of sexuality—and I am fairly convinced, though I cannot prove it, that certain manifestations of schizophrenia (the "world-destruction phantasy" described by Schilder, and catatonic rage, for example) are different phenomena from the unquestionably sadistic impulses of obsessional neuroses, and the aggressions of the typical manic psychoses—then these differences could be clearly explained as manifestations of an extroverted death instinct with which a very minimum of sexual fusion has occurred.

The reason why the theoretical problems of sado-masochism are so unsettled is probably the fact that almost all of the clinical problems with which analysts deal, and their observations of the associated conscious and unconscious aggressive phantasies, are manifestations of either a definitely sadistic or a definitely masochistic form of the sexual instinct. It is when interest centers upon the study of normalcy, on the one hand, or of psychosis and organic diseases on the other, that there is sound reason for doubting the universal adequacy of our present theories.

SUMMARY OF THE THEORIES OF INSTINCTS

The theories of instincts, therefore, have arisen from the universal need to clarify by inductively reasoned hypotheses the relationships of cause and effect operative in the data observed. The theories are based on the assumption that unconscious as well as conscious phantasies are the effects of dynamic forces whose sources are unknown chemical functions of the human organism. These hypothetical forces are called the "instincts" (or "drives"). For the explanation of the normal and abnormal phenomena observed in the study of the simpler neuroses, it was adequate in the earlier period of analysis to hypothesize two groups: the sexual instincts, whose source was called "libido" and whose primary aims are the sensual or equivalent pleasures experienced when libido tension is reduced; and the ego-instincts, whose aims serve the individual's need for survival, both by mastering the environment and by repressing the sexual impulses whenever the aims of self-preservation are in conflict with them. Later studies of more complex problems which involve unconscious guilt, the narcissistic gratification of libido, the psychoses, and the special relationships of sado-masochistic sexuality to other types of aggression and to biological considerations, led Freud to revise this original instinct theory. He then hypothesized a different dichotomy of antagonistic instincts: Eros, or life instincts, from which both ego-instincts and the psychosexual (libido) he had previously described are derived; death instincts, whose ultimate goal, "the return to the inorganic state," is successfully delayed during life by various degrees of fusion with Eros and whose lifetime effects are observable impulses to aggression and destructiveness, directed either at the world or at the self.

VIII

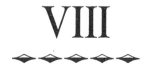

THE STRUCTURE OF THE
TOTAL PERSONALITY

T H E theories of instincts which we have discussed are *hypotheses* which explain quite adequately the dynamic forces whose effects are the actual phenomena observed in psychoanalysis and in life. The concept we are about to discuss is of a somewhat different order. It is not so much a hypothesis as an *abstraction* and a *synthesis* of the multitude of observations made. It bears much the same relation to the empirical data as algebraic symbols do to numbers. For the concept primarily gives generic names to several categories of psychological phenomena, to one or another of which general categories each isolated manifestation of the personality belongs. Secondarily, however, this new concept is hypothetical, in so far as these categories are considered as systems which control and organize the instinctual energies whose effects on mind and behavior we observe. This so-called "structure" of the personality corresponds roughly to the various systems of pipes and reservoirs of the hydraulic analogies we have previously used. (Figs. I and II, pages 99 and 102.)

A highly developed concept of personality structure, the result of years of creative thought by Freud, was first published under the title *The Unconscious* [1] in 1915, and in 1923 was replaced by an entirely new theory in his book *The Ego and the Id*.[2] These two

[1] Sigmund Freud, *The Unconscious* (*Collected Papers*, Vol. IV).
[2] Sigmund Freud, *The Ego and the Id*.

works were the foundation of modern *ego psychology,* the study and development of which has been the chief new interest of psychoanalysis for the last twenty-five years, and has led to a new and productive exploration of the unconscious determinants of the more highly integrated mental functions.

THE CONSCIOUS AND UNCONSCIOUS SYSTEMS

In the earlier contribution, *The Unconscious,* Freud had stated that it was not sufficient to formulate the personality in *dynamic* terms—by describing empirically the unconscious wishes and conflicts which analysis had disclosed; nor sufficient to formulate it in *economic* terms—that is, by appraising it in terms of the instinct theory, especially in terms of the libido tensions and quantities of pleasure-pain involved. An adequate formulation, which he now called *metapsychological,* should be from three points of view, the dynamic and economic, with which analysts were already familiar, and also the *topographical,* or structural. The third of these points of view, the structural, was new, involving a concept of "regions" of the mind, each region manifesting different laws of thought-association. These regions he called the "System Conscious" (capitalized in German to disignate its substantive meaning) and the "System Unconscious." [3]

The System Conscious includes those mental functions which have been ascribed to the "ego" in the later formulation of personality structure. It includes those agencies of the mind which deal with the outer world, control perception and reality-testing, and organize primitive wishes and behavior. The relationship of ideas in the System Conscious is controlled by the *secondary process,* which enforces such rational laws as the logical discrimination of identities and opposites (love and hate), and such elements of reality-testing as time, space, and sensory perceptions.

[3] Freud also, in this paper, discussed in detail a third system, the *"Preconscious,"* which he considered a part of the "System Conscious," consisting of those thoughts which were accessible to consciousness by an act of attention.

A barrier normally exists between the System Conscious and the System Unconscious. For no idea in the System Unconscious may become conscious (in the adjectival sense) by a mere effort of attention. All ideas belonging to the System Unconscious, in contrast to those of the System Conscious, are subject to the "primary process," [4] the laws of non-rational association of ideas first clearly defined in *The Interpretation of Dreams*.[5] Under the dominion of the primary process an idea's importance is entirely determined by the amount of instinct with which it is charged ("cathexis"), and the association of ideas in the System Unconscious is determined by the emotional linkages of these ideas.

We are already familiar with many examples of unconscious data showing these characteristics of the primary process. In Chapter I we saw how the associations of one patient showed that for him the idea "wife sewing" had the same value as the thought "Penelope weaving at her *womb*"; how for the man with the arm-tic, "Napoleon" was unconsciously the same as "I." The mental processes of the Unconscious are therefore unlike the secondary process of the System Conscious, in that they are uncritical and irrational; such processes as negation, logic, choice between opposites, and reality-testing are absent.

But during the next decade, valuable as this description of personality in terms of the Systems Conscious, Preconscious, and Unconscious had proved to be in advancing the perspective of analysis and the breadth of its investigation, it had become increasingly apparent that this early formulation of personality structure was both cumbersome and inexact. For example, the increasing recognition of unconscious punishment phantasies had shown that at times analysts were describing a conflict between two forces (represented by infantile sexual wishes and punishment phantasies), both of which were unconscious, as a conflict between the System Conscious and the System Unconscious. Furthermore, some things that were described as elements of the System Unconscious are not strictly un-

---

[4] Renamed "autism," or "autistic thinking," by Dr. Eugen Bleuler of Zurich in his classic studies of schizophrenic thought.
[5] Pages 18–21.

conscious. Examples of these are: the delusions of the schizophrenic psychosis, and some psychoneurotic phantasies of which the individual has been sporadically aware, though, when his attention is focused on them in the presence of another, he disclaims them. And, finally, many phenomena which functionally should be ascribed to the System Conscious are just not conscious at all. Many organized and rational decisions for actions, a great deal of the learning process, and many integrated habits are definitely processes which are unconscious in whole or in part, and these belong to the System Conscious. It is therefore just not so that the mind is sharply divided between a "conscious" portion, in which all thinking is rational and all action seemingly voluntary, and an "unconscious" portion, of whose content, ideas, memories, symbols, and wishes, there is never any awareness.

Nevertheless, the basic concepts of this first theory of personality structure constitute one of Freud's greatest contributions to clear systematic formulation and to the further understanding of the mind and personality as an integrated totality. For the first time he clearly defined certain postulates: that ideas of the Unconscious are related by entirely different laws of thought-association than are those which control adult rational processes, that these unconscious ideas have an instinctual charge producing impetus to enter the organized System Conscious unless dynamically opposed by a countercharge of the System Conscious, and that conscious thought, learning, behavior, and symptoms are processes belonging to a highly organized department of the mind. These are fundamental ideas which are perpetuated in the later concept of personality structure.

"THE EGO AND THE ID"

In *The Ego and the Id* (1923), Freud proposed a new method for generalizing all psychologic phenomena, whether conscious or unconscious. Psychologic data were described in terms of three systems, which together comprise the total personality. These systems he named the *Id*, the *Ego*, and the *Super-ego*. They may be succinctly defined as the "It wants," "I will (not)," and "You must (not)" departments of the personality. For each idea, symptom, or act could be described in terms of these three categories. Moreover, most dynamic phenomena, especially emotional tension associated with an idea, and all evidence of conflict between two opposed needs, could be concisely and adequately described as interactions between elements of these three portions of the personality. The use of this formulation for thirty years has induced the increasing conviction of analysts that it enables them to discuss the variegated observations of their science in a useful and systematic way. It is a device somewhat like the chemist's formula for molecular structure; by employing a high degree of abstraction, he depicts some relations of various atoms within a complex molecule.

THE ID

The *"id"* (literally the "it"; first named by Groddeck) is the "It wants me to," or, better, the "It impels me to" portion of the personality.[6] It is an expression which describes the ultimate sources of all impulses to feel, to think, or to act, that portion of the personality from which all observable effects derive the energy which makes them manifest. It is the source of instinctual drive, of emotion and tension. It therefore bears an intimate relationship to the system previously described less exactly as "the Unconscious." It comprises those elements of the personality which we refer to as most primitive and unrefined. It includes those features of human psychology which are most like the impulses observed in animals, a fact that is reflected by our need to refer to it ordinarily in the passive voice and not as something we will; we feel as though the primal impulses from within our minds were not truly part of our own personality, but rather something acting upon us. So, in ordi-

---

[6] Dr. Bertram Lewin comments on how the nuance of this idea is conveyed by such phrases of the German language as *"Es träumt mir," "Es brennt mir," "Es freut mich"* (literally, it dreams to me, it burns to me, it delights me; or, it makes me dream, it makes me burn, it delights me). This linguistic detail makes it all the clearer why Freud, writing in the German language, should have used the word *das Es,* translated the It or Id.

nary speech, references to what Freud called the "id" are most commonly used in the third person and imply no personal responsibility: "He is a beast," "That is bestial," for example. If I say: "He made me wild," *I* concede my wildness, but imply that the responsibility is *his*, although actually *he* would not have been an effective stimulus if it were not for latent primitive impulses within me. The sum of these primal impulses Freud called the "id."

The impulses of the id are originally independent of one another. They are not fused with other needs. For example, primitive aggression is the wish to destroy or kill; it has not been fused with libidinal components which make the desire to give or to create an element of many normal acts of aggression. At their source, they are not disciplined, attenuated, or controlled by morality, or by a fear of consequences. The impulses are not organized in a rationally temporal sequence, nor are they dependent upon real opportunities for expression. Thus, in a series of free associations, one frequently notes how an impulse of love originating in the id may at one instant be related to a present object, the next instant to the memory of an object of years ago, and a moment later to a phantasy of an object of the future. For example, in the following thought-sequence one sees throughout the impulse to love a woman, with a verbalization of logically and temporally unrelated objects: "I love (at present) my sister; she was very sweet coming home from school (years ago); sometime (in the future) I may marry an English girl." The instinct these associations represent is an impulse of the moment; the reference to a time is not a function of the impulse, but a rational subscript.

Besides lack of organization and primitiveness, the most striking characteristic of the id is its subordination to the Pleasure Principle. A need is at its source a need for immediate gratification; each of the component impulses of the id acts in accordance with the principle of the simple hydraulic system of Figure I; so long as it acts in full accordance with the Pleasure Principle, it represents the id directly, free from control by other parts of the personality structure. The concept of the id therefore includes the mental attributes previously ascribed to the System Unconscious by Freud.

It is that department of the mind where the primary process takes precedence over rational thought. Moreover, the Pleasure Principle was originally defined as a property of instincts and the tensions they create, but in the new theory of personality structure it is considered an important characteristic of the id. This junction-point of two theories, the instinct theory and the structural theory, is at times somewhat confusing, as the source of instincts is defined as *biological* whereas the id is considered a region *of the mind* where ideas are least organized but most immediately related to the biological processes which determine them.

In ordinary life, opportunities for the observation of id impulses which are not somewhat organized and refined by the other elements of the total personality are rare. But it is useful to consider them as independent agencies, if for no other reason than to systematize the discussion of their discipline and control. The id is the core of the personality, dominating all psychological reactions of the infant in full accordance with the Pleasure Principle, before he is influenced by socializing forces. The child who pulls off a beetle's legs with no remorse, no fear of punishment or other consequences, is giving direct expression to his id, as an adult rarely can. In certain forms of psychosis, which we call "manic states," we also see an almost "naked" id, with minimal evidence that other portions of the psychic structure are functioning. Such an individual is constantly active, constantly talking in a fragmented manner; there is no apparent rational relationship between different wishes, or between the wishes and their consequences. There is constant play of uninhibited feelings—laughter, rage, scorn; the patient one instant wishes to kiss, the next to defecate, the next to assault and injure. Such are the instinct-representations of the core of the emotional life of all of us, when stripped of those other portions of the personality which distinguish the emotional organization and the control exercised by normal and neurotic civilized men. In free association there is abundant evidence that at the core of even complex and highly civilized acts the impulse is primitive and possessed of those special characteristics by which the nature of the id is defined.

THE EGO

Early in life, however, the individual's experience leads to differentiation of perceptions of himself and his world. He also differentiates id impulses indulged without subsequent pain and those from whose indulgence he suffers. A "precipitate" of the experiences forms, and it is this that Freud designated the *"ego."* The ego is what each of us means when he speaks of "self," when he refers to "I." It comprises those elements of the personality responsible for perceiving, knowing, reasoning, feeling, choosing, and also doing.

This new concept of the ego included those primary attributes which were earlier considered characteristic of the System Conscious. The ego, as now defined, is governed by the "secondary process" which determines the reasonable association of ideas. It is, therefore, by definition, the totality of mental processes which are highly organized and whose function is primarily the integration of the personality and its environment. The raw mental material which is so organized by the ego, as chief administrative officer of the personality, as it were, comes from several sources.

First of all, from earliest infancy the ego records perceptual knowledge of the outer world and organizes these mental images of external reality. The ego is, therefore, the mental apparatus which develops the all-important process of *reality-testing,* a capacity preeminently characteristic of maturity and conspicuously defective only in infancy, in psychosis, and in sleep; it is the function of distinguishing fact from phantasy, wishful thinking from reason. The ego in this way serves the Reality Principle, and controls the dynamics represented by the "reservoir" in our hydraulic analogy (Fig. II, page 102).

The ego is also perceptive of the wishes of the super-ego (to be discussed later), and responds to the super-ego's moral mandates defensively in order to avoid conscious and unconscious guilt, punishment, and anxiety.

The ego is also the receptor of all representations in the id of instinctual needs, and is that mental organization which mediates between impulses and action by organizing wishes into pleasure-giving action-patterns, or else into symptomatic compromises, or by denying id impulses access to action through maintaining repression, inhibition, avoidance, or still more complexly integrated defenses.

Freud's later concept of an ego, therefore, is that department of the mind—or better, an aggregate of those functions of the mind—which integrates the perceptions of the external world that are reality-tested, the threats of real or phantasy-induced anxiety and self-punishment needs, and the demands from the id for aim-gratifying action. No function of the ego, therefore, is so simple it does not represent, as Hermann Nunberg and Robert Wälder separately pointed out in the early days of ego psychology, a "synthesis" of several dynamic components and a simultaneous, synchronized fulfillment of "multiple functions."

So far as this concept of the ego is theoretical it could have been philosophically created by non-analytic psychologists, and so far as it is a formulation of conscious rational processes it can be used and developed by any school of psychology. Its special value to psychoanalysis is that clinical analysis provides a mass of information about some ego-functions which are unconscious. A child's learning to speak a language without benefit of grammar, or a skilled auto-driver's immediate adjustment to emergencies, involve typically multiple, synthesizing integrations; yet first-rate skill in both adjustments involves integrative processes as unconscious as those of the woman whose severe neurotic conflict was resolved by living in two apartments, or the man whose triple conflict was synthesized in a quasi-suicidal drowning.[7] Comprehension of the end-results of some complex integrations that are unconsciously carried out makes the processes involved appear so rational that one pauses to wonder whether reasoning itself is so uniquely a fully conscious process as we are prone to assume, and whether the kinds of mental integration represented by the solution of a difficult mathematical problem, or the invention by John Dalton of the idea of

[7] See pages 75, 76, 129, 131–3.

atomic theory during sleep, are as truly exceptional feats of the unconscious portion of the mind as we like to think.

Let us illustrate these generalizations. An impulse of hate asserts itself. So far as this impulse at its source in the id is concerned, it is represented, consciously or unconsciously, by the wish: "I want to kill!" Under certain conditions the ego will direct this impulse into muscular action which achieves the death of the hated one. This is the only possible completely pleasurable outcome at the instant the impulse originates. Occasionally the ego will check this impulse temporarily and satisfy it completely on some future occasion when full gratification is assured and safe—by killing an enemy in battle, for instance. But usually this outcome will bring very painful consequences too: retaliation, or punishment from without, or remorse from within. It would then be the function of the ego, as agent of the Reality Principle, to curb the energy represented in the impulse, in order to avoid this future pain. This it might accomplish by a partial inhibition; the musculature would be utilized only to punch the nose of the hated one, or only to make a gesture. The impulse might be sublimated, by expression of this wish partially, harmlessly, and pleasantly in an aggressive game of tennis, by playing chess, or by hunting animals. The wish to kill might be partially gratified in a day-dream of assaulting and injuring, or the pleasure of partial emotional discharge might be achieved vicariously through responding to a murder mystery or watching a gangster movie. If, however, the wish is unconsciously associated with situations which have infantile values, even the conscious recognition of the wish and of an infantile punishment phantasy will be unacceptable to the ego, and the impulse will be repressed; it will then be excluded from direct motor action and from conscious thought. But if it is a powerful one, the impulse, in spite of the repression by the ego, will seek and achieve the partial outlet of a neurotic symptom. In the determination of any of these outcomes—direct gratification, delayed gratification, pleasure in phantasy, sublimation, or repression and symptomatic compromise—there is a perception of the inner impulse, and an integration of the component functions of the ego—rational appraisal, conflicts of wishes, defense against anxiety and guilt, and available mechanisms of behavior and sublimation—in the selection and organization of the most pleasurable, least painful, response.

THE SUPER-EGO

The necessity of restraining the immediacy and primitiveness of the id in one or another way does not arise, as we have already seen in the discussion of punishment phantasies (Chapter IV), entirely from the danger of external retaliation and disapprobation. The restraint of many impulses, especially those which could be executed with secrecy, is compelled by intra-psychic authorities which are entirely functions of the personality itself. In these cases it is not fear of society, but fear of remorse, fear of the threats imposed by the phantasies of punishment, that are effective. The aggregate of these prohibitory punishment-phantasies Freud schematized as the third component of the personality: he called it "the *super-ego.*"

These intra-psychic prohibitions of the super-ego are not innate; they are a result of development, a "precipitate" of experience. In this way, they are like the ego functions we have discussed. On the other hand, these functions are not those of acceptance, rejection, and execution of wishes from the id, but rather functions of authority, prohibition, and threat of consequences. The super-ego is a specialized portion of the ego, representing one aspect of the total personality function, much as, in the social organization, the courts decide what shall and shall not be approved, while the executive branches of the government make these mandates effective.

When super-ego function is conscious, we perceive it as bad conscience, or else as a compelling obedience to an "ideal." But psychoanalysis has shown, as we have seen in our discussion of unconscious punishment phantasies, that the mandates of the super-ego are not limited to those recognized as conscious morality, but include also many which are unconscious. Again we are indebted to Freud for showing that a portion of the mind reacts not only to the immorality of deeds which are consciously contemplated, but also to wishes of which we have no conscious cognizance. We may conceal a misdeed from society and escape its retaliation. But we cannot escape the reaction of the super-ego to any impulse, even one which is repressed. The impulse may be unconscious; the guilt may be unconscious; the occasion for the punishment may be unconscious and rationally trivial; but we cannot escape by will or logic the intra-psychic punishment, the irrational but effective penance of neurotic suffering which the super-ego compels the ego to impose. In some way or other, directly or indirectly, the unconscious apprehension of a guilt-arousing instinctual striving will have its due.

CLINICAL APPLICATIONS

The concept of personality structure, therefore, defines the total personality in terms of three systems: id, ego, and super-ego. Each psychologic detail and observation may be described as belonging to one or another of these systems or as a reaction between them. For example, the clinical samples of instinctive urges manifesting the "I wish" or "I need" functions of the personality are all considered examples of function originating in the id. In our Case History [8] the unconscious wish, "I want a baby"; the impulse, "I hate mother"; and the phantasy of impregnation by mouth, are all representatives of the woman's id. The repression of these wishes, the exclusion from consciousness of the infantile phantasies, the common-sense thought, "I should love a more suitable man," the act of seeking a therapist to cure her, all illustrate ego functions. They show an organizing mental apparatus mediating between the primitive impulses and the outer real world in a manner governed by the secondary process and generally recognized as characteristic of ego maturity. Id impulses have likewise been successfully organized for adult reactions in the normal aspects of her love-affairs, her platonic friendships, and her successful earning of

[8] See pages 81–7.

a livelihood. The super-ego is represented by such unconscious phantasies as: "You must not have a child"; "You must not share father's love"; "You must not touch your genitals"; "You must not hate your rivals"; "You will be cut." The analysis of the neurosis showed how the ego had consequently excluded (repressed) the wishes for home, love, and children from consciousness and from real experience. They were id impulses which the super-ego had countermanded because of the association of the normal adult sexual phantasies with infantile experience whose verbal or behavioral expression in childhood would have been disapproved by adults, and because of the unconscious association of love by a man and rivalry for a baby with her repressed Œdipal wishes. In this well-organized, socially adjusted woman the ego is therefore quite normal. The pathology of the case arises from the conflict of her unconscious id wishes and the punishment phantasies of her super-ego. The ego is functioning normally in maintaining repressions and dealing with the unrelieved tensions which result by symptom-formation instead of full genitality and love.

At times in analysis the validity of this "psychological geography" of personality structure is demonstrated very vividly by a patient who is representing different elements of his own personality by thoughts of different people. Periods occur in which a patient will consistently ascribe derogatory thoughts about himself to the analyst, then vehemently deny they are correct. Thus the lady who experienced an ecstasy in nature [9] for weeks ascribed the exhibitionistic phantasy-representatives of her own id to the analyst's obscenity, and by the conscious condemnations of others maintained the repression and served the unconscious taboos of her super-ego. At other times a patient will imagine the analyst's thoughts to be denunciatory; when this is not a correct intuition of the analyst's real attitude at that time, the patient is then disclosing his own unconscious super-ego functions in his conscious phantasies of what the analyst is reproaching him for. Occasionally the free associations of a patient—like many other phantasies of hu-

[9] See page 34.

man beings when alone and under tension—will take the form of a dialogue; a patient during analysis will sometimes use the words of a friend to express unconsciously impulses of his own id, and in his next associations denounce the friend to prove he himself is not like that. Such a division of the total personality in phantasy is a vivid representation of conflict within the personality structure, a way of disowning hatred or shame produced by an element of one's own personality.

All such mechanisms, in which a wish or a character trait or an ideal is consciously represented as something external to one's own personality, are called *projection*. This is one of the most common partial solutions of conflict. It occurs frequently in normal people and is the dominant psychological feature of the *paranoid* type of psychosis. It is clearly seen, for example, in acute paranoid states where a man is terrified by the delusion that some other man is eager to get him alone, assault him, and force him to engage in homosexual practices. Analysis discloses that by ascribing these wishes to others the patient is denying active homosexual impulses within himself. Projection which is not psychotic can also be observed in every group of adolescent boys, where one of a group is chosen for ridicule for "playing with himself" by those other boys who themselves are secretly engaging in the practice.

Projection is demonstrated by every dream. For dreams not only represent ideas, they represent them chiefly in the form of visual images. In these we probably witness nightly the most primitive form of projection, originating at a stage of mental development which antedates both the verbalization of wishes and the differentiation of hallucinations and the perception of reality. Thus, when a white man represents his own erotic phantasies by dreaming that Negro boys are wrestling, the patient projects his own wishes, and he does not consciously experience these wishes as his own.

Within the human mind, the pot not only is inclined to call the kettle black, but sometimes, by projection, even denies there is a kettle. One day, later in his analysis, this same man mentioned that he had heard a rumor about his friend Bob. But, he declared, he could not tell the analyst what it was, because it concerned, not himself, but a friend, and what his friend did; it was absolutely none of his or the analyst's business, he protested strenuously. As nothing else came to his mind, he was silent during the remainder of the treatment hour. At the end the analyst remarked: "In what way are you like Bob?" Then for several days the patient reported a profusion of associations which illustrated his own virtue, the analyst's "bad opinion" of him, and Bob's sins. They may be condensed as follows:

"You [the analyst] think I have sexual thoughts. You think I am vile, that I would hurt an innocent girl. You thought I had dirty thoughts when I spoke of what the boys did in school. It is the last thing I want. I've told you I chose my girl, three years ago, because she was then planning to move to California in three months. That would not give us time if I wanted to think bad thoughts about her. Besides we had gone to school together. We hardly ever kiss. I never see the crowd of boys and girls that had that club and did things. I never think any more those things about wrestling I told you of. My girl asked me to put my car in her garage, she never had before. I couldn't do it. I threw a cigarette butt in *her*—in—in—[very perturbed] I threw a butt in *the* fire-box."

[The patient pauses, has nothing to say. We observe the unconscious sexual symbolism of these ascetic lovers: she invites him to introduce a male symbol (car) into a female symbol (her garage); he refuses, but then verbally introduces a male symbol (cigarette) into a female symbol (box). It is as though these platonic sweethearts were reacting, though unconsciously, by specific acts to each other's sexuality, and the probability that some association threatens to emerge and reveal this to the patient's consciousness is indicated by his sudden perturbation in starting to say "*her* fire-box," and by the subsequent pause without reporting his associations. The super-ego's guilt-threatening function is aroused by this, and is manifest in the disturbed and irrational reaction the patient mentions next.]

He continues: "I worried all evening I might have caused a fire. [Patient is now experiencing conscious guilt but rationalizing it.] Couldn't get it out of my mind. You think there is something between us—no, she's a good girl, we're just friends. I am most fond of my niece [a child]. I watch her. Sometimes I wish I could play and put my arm around her. I never kiss her. I never kiss mother since I was grown up. We don't do those things. She's always doing things, like putting extra blankets out, saying I mustn't eat this or that, making me drink milk, and so on. Bob is so easy with his sisters, kisses them, and puts his arm around them. It's natural with sisters, isn't it? *You* wouldn't think anything of that. [With difficulty] They say Bob has had sexual intercourse with a girl. I don't know. . . ."

Finally the patient, more and more emotional, remembers that on the night before he had refused to speak of Bob's affairs he himself had had a nocturnal emission while dreaming that he held this niece in his lap.

Now the relationships of the other associations are clearer. Though in his waking life he denied it, in this dream his capacity for erotic phantasy about a little girl is not even disguised in the manifest content. His waking defense is: "Not I, but Bob, has such wishes, does such things"; and the primary, unconscious purpose of his refusal to mention a rumor about Bob's erotic life is not to keep this man's confidence, as he stated at first, but to conceal a fact which duplicates what he himself wants to do and has dreamed of doing. He also defends conscious revelation of his dream by arguing: "It cannot be I who criticize my own sexual wishes, for I have none; it is the analyst who blames me for what is not so." (Incidentally, we now see the relationship of his sexuality to the unconscious wish for his older brother's death. That component of his neurosis had been analyzed several months before when the sight of a coat hanging on the door led to his avoiding anxiety incurred by walking down this street. But it was only the analysis of the defense against revealing his projected sexuality that exposed the source of his repressed hatred in intense rivalry for his niece's affection.)

In these free associations we see that, by "projections," he had presented with graphic clarity Freud's concept of personality structure. What he consciously conceives of as himself is his ego, rejecting consciousness of certain erotic and hostile impulses and deny-ing participation in them. The super-ego, the element of the personality structure which compels the ego to do this by threaten-ing the punishment of painful feelings of guilt, is represented in the conscious mind by the patient's phantasy that the analyst is con-demning him. The id, the source of the sexual thoughts, is repre-sented by his phantasies of Bob's activities with girls, and by his in-terest in Bob's activities, and is undisguised in the erotic dream he finally reports. Thus his comments about Bob represent his own id, and those about the analyst his own super-ego. Without projection the same three structures would have been apparent in the free as-sociations, though their representation would then have been more "scrambled" and not so graphically simple to understand.

The woman who concealed the activity of sexual impulses from herself by repressing them and discussing instead her rhapsodical love of the woods disclosed projection in a different personality structure. A similar phenomenon is very common in everyday life, for example, in the moral aspersions of one woman about another whom she unconsciously fears is more attractive, or a man's depre-ciation of another whom he fears is more successful. The "Scarlet Letter" of Hester Prynne was the symbol of the cruel super-ego of the Puritan who projected his own repressed sexuality and pun-ished her instead of himself.

SUPER-EGO AND PARENT RELATIONS

These relations of ego to id and super-ego are the derivatives of the relationship of the child to his inner needs and to the outer world and his parents. For the adult's id continues the undisci-plined, uncivilized, unrealistic needs of the infantile personality, and especially its impetus for immediate pleasure. In the first years of life, the demarcation of id and ego is only gradually established, and the ego at first is largely occupied with the passive reception (and seduction!) of such gratifying stimuli as milk, warmth, and cuddling. As the ego matures, it acquires the function of reality-testing, and the control and organization of impulses from the id. And the super-ego becomes the agent of morality, the intra-psychic representative of those cultural ideals and interdictions which are imposed on the child by his parents.

To appraise further these characteristics of the super-ego, let us review in more detail some decisive experiences of childhood life and their effect upon development. The important influences (besides inborn potentialities) are the mother (and other nurses), later the father, and, to a less extent, teachers, relatives, and other grownups. These people minister to the infant's pleasures, and their affection and approval at first constitute his main experience of the gratifications mediated by other people. But they are also hated, because it is they who demand restraint on his autoerotic and sadistic pleasures (such as cruelty, soiling, masturbation, destructive play, infliction of pain on siblings, etc.). If he defies them, they either punish him or do not love him. At a still later stage, the Œdipus phase, he fears the revenge of one parent for his wish to take the other away. Moreover, these great people, like the giants of his fairy-tales, differ from him: they seem very big, all-powerful, all-knowing. The fear of their authority is intense because they appear to be so powerful; the aspiration to be like grownups is compelling because they are so "wonderful" and apparently can do whatever they will.

The various relationships of adult super-ego and ego duplicate these immature attitudes with amazing exactness. Those adult psychic functions of the super-ego which forbid and limit impulsive gratifications and, if unheeded, bring mental suffering and conscious guilt reproduce the roles of the parents toward the child. But the super-ego is also a love-object, and this is the basis of idealism— the wish to be like an idealized parent, the striving for an impossible perfection.[1]

This is more than a plausible theory. When other evidence of

---

[1] This attitude to the child's phantasies of important adults organized as the super-ego was recognized and clearly described by Freud as the *ego-ideal* many years before his final description of personality structure and his description of the super-ego as the source of guilt.

super-ego function is defective in the total personality of an adult, we actually observe that his emotional relationship to the environment is very much more like a child's than that of other adults—a naughty or abnormally good child's. Such a person is, then, not so fearful of feeling guilt as of getting caught. The analyst and scholar Hanns Sachs pointed out how apparent this was in the personality of the Roman Emperor Caligula, whom the Romans themselves called "The Little Fellow." His life was one of ruthless violation of all normal taboos, the perpetration of erratic, impulsive acts of rage and cruelty, the invention of childish games to play, actual incest, and utter disregard of consequences to himself or others. Similar characters are seen today among psychopathic personalities, who, though intellectually and physically mature, commit antisocial acts, pass bad checks, commit forgeries, run up bills, insult people unnecessarily, invite imprisonment and commitment to mental hospitals, though perfectly aware *intellectually* of the nature of their acts and their refusal to accept the responsibilities which other adults assume. When questioned, they show neither a guilty conscience, nor even any will to curb their impulses in order to avoid the consequences. They merely wish to do what they want to do when they want to do it; they are grown-up children of the Pleasure Principle, often with normal egos, but without fear of intrapsychic punishment because of defective super-ego functions.

One such man illustrated neatly his childish phantasies of being like powerful grownups by having on the letterhead of his fraudulent company: "I am not Napoleon, I am not Cæsar, I am not the President, but what I *will,* I *do*." (An insane man would have omitted the "nots" and believed himself to be Napoleon; the man with the neurotic tic already cited had repressed the phantasy of being like Napoleon and did not know he had ever experienced it, for it was represented consciously only by the symptom.) Another psychopathic individual was constantly occupied with inventing devices which gave bizarre gratification to his pregenital wishes—for example, a rubber balloon worn under his trousers to catch his urine, instead of bladder control. At unsuitable moments he would remove it from his trousers and display it with great pride—like the behavior many a mother has observed in a little boy's feeling of prowess in making water. The balloon also enabled him to enjoy the characteristically childish pleasure of urinating whenever it pleased him.

In contrast to such defects in the development of a super-ego, we often have in psychoneuroses and certain character types a super-ego which acts as an excessively harsh and cruel parent. An extreme case was illustrated by the woman who occupied two apartments; her parents had actually been very excessive in disciplining her as a child. A less extreme example is beautifully illustrated by the missionary in Somerset Maugham's story "Miss Thompson" (subsequently dramatized by John Colton and Clemence Randolph as *Rain*). The parentlike authority of his conscience, the cruelty of a love forbidden by this conscience, and at the same time the reverent wonder for the ideal he tried to represent—all these super-ego attributes were perfectly represented by the author. The inner authority said: "You must not love a woman sensually," and he banned such thoughts as well as actions from consciousness and used "projection" to express them by his violent tirade against the heroine's sexual sin. The cruelty of his acts of conscious moral duty led to his ruthless demand that she should suffer, and his complete submissiveness to a powerful ideal, represented in his religion, gave him an eloquence which converted the girl. When finally the force of his love for her (his id) compelled him to recognize his sensual phantasies, the ensuing torments of the soul (conflict of id and super-ego), whether to gratify his instincts or obey his duty, were solved only in suicide by drowning. The author has presented the same intra-psychic conflict and solution as that of the patient who threw himself into the water: the taboo of sexually winning his sweetheart from a rival had activated the "no" of intra-psychic authority, and partially inactivated the integrative functions of an ego.

IDENTIFICATION, PUNISHMENT PHANTASIES, AND THE SUPER-EGO

Freud also, in *The Ego and the Id*, described a most important unconscious process whereby the prohibitory attitudes of members of the environment toward many of the child's demands for pleasure becomes the adult's super-ego. He called this process *Identification*.

Identification is, therefore, the psychological assimilation by one individual of some emotional attitude or trait or idea of another personality. The most rudimentary kind of identification is imitation, as seen in a baby who crosses two fingers after watching a grownup do it, or who reproduces and repeats the vocal sounds made by another even before using them as meaningful words. We observe such behavior in the mimicry of children, or the conscious manners and fashions of the adult. But such conscious and ephemeral reproductions of the traits of another are very simple and transient precursors of identification; it is better to think of such imitation as a conscious means of immediate tension-release by play. "Identification," as used technically by analysts, usually implies a much more fundamental process in personality development; it is a reaction to important emotional experiences and is largely unconscious. Identification is not merely playing at being like someone else; it is *becoming* like him in some way. It is a complex *process,* a basic one in the growth of personality, not a transitory incident.

The emotional reaction to another which creates a determinative need to identify is usually that of a strong unconscious ambivalence; the object is both loved and hated, and his power is envied. This is a universal and important problem of every child; as when the child, for example, envies the loved parent's power to stay up after the child's bedtime. Such situations may evoke the need to identify, and result in the most complete and permanent solution possible of the conflict by the child's permanently acquiring the idea of being the parent in this way. Both the precipitating ambivalence and the identification are largely unconscious. They may, in the early stages of the process, be represented by conscious phantasies, for example: the child's "I want to drive the car like father"; the teen-age wallflower's "I wish I had as many dates as Anne." But that aspect of identification which transcends imitation or wishful phantasy is the actual unconscious creation of a permanent personality trait. It has then become a part of the basic reactions of the personality; and it is no longer a reaction to one individual in one situation but has become a component of his total reactions to all situations. Conscious psychology, pedagogy, and common observation have long recognized the importance of intellectual "learning" lessons which must be mastered in order for the adult to deal with the intellectual problems of his life. Identification is the emotional counterpart of conscious learning; it provides the personality with new individual mechanisms for dealing with personal situations of life; it contributes to the permanent resources of the personality, instead of limiting them.

Learning to talk, for example, is not only an intellectual process; it is developed by the desire to use the words first spoken by important people, until the words become part of the infant's own equipment and are available for social reactions as well as intellectual problems.[2] A little girl's first use of a sentence, "Mama go out," occurs when she is very distressed by her mother's leaving her; she had learned the words before, but she first used them to deal with a situation that had made her otherwise powerless. The little girl, struggling with her envy of the new baby, turns to her dolls with enhanced delight; though she is the baby's rival for the mother's attention, she may also identify with the baby and act more like one so little than she has in years, and at the same time identify with the mother by taking care of the baby herself, or showing increased interest in her dolls. A boy not allowed to drive a car may identify not only with the skills of the driver, but with the phallic power of the car; he thereby achieves one component of his ultimate capacity to exert power himself.

Analysts have unparalleled opportunities to observe how many

---

[2] See Ives Hendrick, "Instinct and the Ego During Infancy," *Psychoanalytic Quarterly,* Volume XI, pages 33–58 (1942).

of the subtleties of a person's mannerism and gesture are residuals of emotional relationships of early life solved by identification. Such data sometimes give a fairly complete picture, not only of the occurrence of identification itself, but of how it happened that an individual identified as a child with this or that trait of the personalities about him. Such analyses disclose convincingly how many "family resemblances" have been acquired by identifications—a "psychological inheritance," as it were. They prove that "blood" (germ plasm) is not the only factor which may account for them. An oldest son, for example, often resembles his maternal grandfather, either obviously in behavior or secretly in his personal ideals. That this is more likely to occur in oldest sons is a consequence of identifying with that man whom his mother, consciously or unconsciously, most loves: her father. Resemblances acquired by identification do not contradict the fact of biological heredity; one cannot execute identifications or any other psychological functions for which one has no inborn capacity. But they indicate that hereditary factors of personality are as much predetermined potentialities as inevitabilities. Heredity is the flour and water of human nature; emotion is the yeast; environment is the baker; and the mixing-bowl and oven are the earliest years of life.

Identification is a normal aspect of development. But it may also produce pathological symptoms and reactions. This was shown by the patient whose arm-tic was a fragmentary identification with Napoleon and represented the power the real grownups of his childhood seemed to have. When our illustrative case envied the mother her children, she showed her unconscious identification by developing back pains like those from which the mother suffered. Another woman became depressed and complained constantly that she knew herself to be evil, shallow intellectually, and without personality assets. One evening she enjoyed with voracious zest eating a plate of French-fried potatoes. These were associated by a chance external incident with a female rival, whom she then began to berate in terms almost identical with those she had been applying to herself. Analysis showed she had unconsciously gratified a desire to get the beloved enemy out of the way by devouring her. When the patient then became conscious that she had repressed the wish to be like her rival, she phantasied exultantly that she actually was. The depression was cured. It had been the result of verbally mistreating herself because unconsciously she had identified with an enemy whom she in phantasy originally mistreated.

Such instances of symptoms produced by identification are clues to the role of identification in the development of useful skills such as walking, talking, counting, for example, and so are clues to the role of identification in ego-development. But the most important product of identification—or at least that which was most adequately explored by Freud and is therefore first understood by analysts—is the super-ego. The super-ego is the composite of all an individual's identifications with the authoritative and prohibitive attitudes of other personalities, especially the prohibitors of what the child would like to do. Definite traces of real guilt and shame are observed during the infantile period; but by and large conduct is then controlled by the power of adults, actual and phantasied. The very little child is good because he fears the consequences of naughtiness which he is too helpless to mitigate, and because he fears that others will retaliate the primitive aggressions he imagines in kind— "eye for eye and tooth for tooth." In some adults this survives as the chief motive of instinct-control. But as children's activities outside the family circle become conspicuous, and adults can trust them with considerable supervision of their own lives (at about five and a half, the first school years), effective super-ego functions first become clearly determinative. Instinct-prohibitive authority has been internalized; the child is no longer controlled entirely by grownups, but by his own morality and his fear of bad conscience. It is therefore psychologically elementary and inadequate to state that a child "learns" to behave, that "good" behavior is entirely a result of habit-training. He does first "learn" to behave, or at least learns he will not be lovingly treated if he doesn't. But later he identifies with his preceptors' morality, with their unconscious taboos as well as their conscious ethics. This fundamental fact in normal adjustment to social standards was formerly overlooked by students of conscious child psychology. But it explains how a child who has been trained according to an excellent and intelligent plan may behave as badly, or abnormally, as an undisciplined brat. He has not failed to learn a habit, but new difficulties may result from his identifications with unconscious attitudes of his trainer which the child then perpetuates in a conflict between his super-ego and his id.

The formation of the super-ego by identification is a lifelong process. Those factors of social adjustment which distinguish the particular portion of society to which an individual belongs are those of the latency period (sixth to twelfth year). It is after the child has gone out from the family circle and is profoundly influenced by the daily human associations of schoolroom and playground that he builds, by identification with those he loves, hates, and emulates, the rudiments of his own particular "philosophy of life." The resulting blends of identifications of this period determine those standards of caste, of religion, of race, of culture, which are so decisive in the social configuration of the adult. Still later, identifications with personified ideals, those of art and philosophy, for example, add their components to the final character, and the unconscious restrictions he imposes on his instincts are elaborately rationalized.

But it is in the years preceding his extensive experience of the world beyond the home that the fundamental elements of character, the conformity of the individual to the *universal* restrictions of society—the taboos on murder, cruelty, theft, incest, and pregenital sexuality, for example—are established. And it is also in large part the identifications formed in those years that determine the specifically individual features of adult character, the specific ways in which he reacts to primitive stimuli, the degrees of moral stringency, self-sacrifice, idealism, and repression which determine, in large part, the relationships of adult life. In one individual the authority of the super-ego is excessive, and the adult then is a rigid, inflexible type, an impractical idealist or a psychoneurotic. In another, identifications may be inadequate, and the adult will defy social customs with guiltless impunity. Just how these individualistic traits of an adult's character are related to the love and discipline of the family circle of his infancy, only a very thorough analysis will disclose. For it is not only with those traits which are most apparent in other members of his family circle that the child "identifies"; this unconscious process is determined to a great extent by the portions of the parent's own super-ego which are themselves unconscious, and even by phantasies of the parents which are real to the child and emotionally experienced, but actually not characteristic of those he is phantasying about. Conspicuous traits of many personalities—for example, excessive unselfishness, over-solicitude, etc.—are often fulfillments in adult life, not of the child's wish to be like a parent, but of his wish to be like the person the child phantasied the parent should be.

It was by the analysis of punishment phantasies that the fundamental impetus to identification was discovered. Guilt, or fear of such intra-psychic punishments as remorse, shame, sense of inferiority, etc. are consequences of the anxiety that retaliation will be inflicted from without. Associations during analysis which represent the threat of intra-psychic punishment will sometimes reproduce with surprising exactness the words of disapproving parents. When the punishment phantasies have become very active and conscious in the current emotional life, patients then begin to speak, not of feeling disgusted or ashamed, as previously, but of being afraid. Sometimes there is a temporary phobia. Often there are nightmares, or groundless fears of insanity. Analysis of these fears shows that the patients are repeating, sometimes literally, fears which originated in the first five years of childhood. The illustrative case recalled the fear of being decapitated as her parents had decapitated chickens. Another patient dreamed of shears and eventually recalled that at the age of four he was terrified by being told that naughty boys who "played with themselves" would have their noses cut away. A man at a similar period of his analysis recalls terrifying dreams of revolving spirals when he was very little, and his father's taking him into the parents' bed to soothe him. Still another fails to solve the unconscious origin of his anxiety phantasies —for example, fears of dead animals—until one night his three-year-old boy awakes in terror and reports a dream of crocodiles rushing at him. The patient then feels as though the boy's experience was his own, and recalls his own night terrors, before the age of five, of robbers entering the room. Finally a detail of these dreams of his infancy, that the robbers always had red eyes, is associated with the fear of red eyes of angry real people and particularly his grandfather when in a temper.[3] An abundance of material further demonstrates an infantile terror that his grandfather would bite him; the thought, "Grandfather," had been displaced in his dreams and phobias by animals and robbers. It is the same type of phobia which was first studied intensively by Freud in the five-year-old "Little Hans's" fear of horses.

If, therefore, the conscious sources of guilt and feelings of inferiority are analysed to a point where the unconscious infantile sexual phantasies become conscious, the guilt will be replaced by anxiety and will reproduce the fears of infancy. For the basic elements of the super-ego are the permanent "precipitate" of identifications with parents, an enduring and rather rigid part of the individual's personality structure; and the unconscious guilt and "fear of conscience" are shown to be similarly derived from the actual original fear of the power and the punishments of these grownups.

Thus pyschoanalysis has shown that those aspects of the personality which represent the authority of society within the personality are developed from an unconscious process of identifications with parents and parent surrogates. We have at the core of all those *voluntary* moral acts which are the *sine qua non* of social maturity a super-ego which says: "Thou shalt not." The intra-psychic functions which compel the normal adult to behave with considerable conformity to the demands of his fellows are therefore modeled upon the parents and other authorities of the child's environment. If the child disobeys he is punished; if the adult disobeys he experiences conscious remorse or neurotic suffering, in consequence of the representation within his super-ego of those who first made their disapproval felt.

[3] See pages 19, 84.

PERSONALITY STRUCTURE: CONCLUSIONS

Thus Freud has given to psychoanalysis, to modern psychiatry, and to allied professions an intellectual instrument, a theory for describing the personality as a whole, whose potentialities have only begun to be realized in the last three decades. The foundations of psychoanalysis had been, and still are, the exploration of unconscious wishes, the conflicts and repressions they initiate, and the instinct theory for the dynamic clarification of these mental representations. The theory of personality structure provides a concept for understanding the impact of wishes and conflict on the most highly organized aspects of the personality, the ego and the super-ego.

The most far-reaching consequence of this definition of personality structure has been the study by Freud's successors of the *defense mechanisms*. The ego, by definition, includes most of these organized mechanisms for the control of threatening wishes—among them rationalization, repression, inhibition, symptom-formation, and especially discharge of neurotic conflict by rigid, compulsive patterns of behavior ("acting-out"). The formulation of ego-functions has, therefore, opened wide the gates for studying, not only neurotic symptoms, but *character neuroses,*[4] in so far as these are determined by repetitive patterns for avoiding guilt and anxiety and consciousness of conflict by highly organized behavior. It is in the clarification of these defense mechanisms that most of the new contributions to psychoanalysis have been made in the last thirty years—a most prolific achievement. For a while, this new development tended to ignore the importance of other functions than defenses in personality adjustment, but this was temporary. For the concept of personality structure includes all integrated thinking and behavior by which the individual deals with his environment, taking full account of the most effective and most valuable as well the neurotic. Today these executant aspects of the ego are being studied productively, especially by child psychiatrists in their recent exploration of the basic mechanisms in development,

[4] See pages 180–5.

by students of psychoses who recognize the serious defects in certain ego-functions of psychotic patients, and by psychological researchers in basic problems of learning and development. Both Freud's earlier and his later concepts of personality structure have resulted in a vista of new fields for psychoanalytical exploration.

CHAPTER

IX

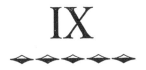

THE ANXIETY THEORY
OF PSYCHONEUROSIS

PSYCHONEUROTIC ANXIETY

F R O M the beginning of his psychological investigations the boundless curiosity of Freud's genius had been excited by the apparent inexplicability of neurotic symptoms—inexplicable in terms of common sense and the conscious wish of the otherwise normal patient, and inexplicable in terms of the medical and psychiatric knowledge of that era. This curiosity had led Freud to his hypnotic experiments with Breuer and to the traumatic theory of hysteria, followed by the exploration of repressed sexual and punishment phantasies, the understanding of conflict and repression, and the inductive creation of instinct theory to explain the dynamic effect of repressed ideas in the production of conscious symptoms.

In 1926, following within five years *Beyond the Pleasure Principle* and *The Ego and The Id*, Freud published the third of these three last major books, all fundamentally altering psychoanalytic thought, investigation foci, and technique. This last of the three books was called by Freud *Inhibition, Symptom, and Anxiety* (*Hemmung, Symptom, und Angst*), and by his translator *The Problem of Anxiety*.[1] In this book Freud undertook a completely

---

[1] *The Problem of Anxiety,* translated by Henry Alden Bunker, M.D.

new orientation to the etiology of the psychoneuroses. *His new thesis was that all psychoneuroses are responses to the need to avoid what is probably the most imperatively painful experience of the conscious mind—anxiety.* This new theory involved no new contribution to factual knowledge, and no abrogation of the understanding of psychoanalytic data which Freud had struggled thirty years to expound. It was based upon a new appraisal of this clinical material, most particularly of the facts regarding anxiety obtained from the *Analysis of Phobia in a Five-Year-Old Boy* ("Little Hans"), published in 1909,[2] and the relevance of these data to the material of other cases.

Conscious anxiety is a common human experience. It accompanies all types of neurosis, sometimes as the chief symptom, more often incidentally. Freud had consequently long been interested in the vicissitudes of this painful affect, and as early as 1896 had differentiated the symptomatology and etiology of psychoneurosis and *actual neuroses,* the latter including "neurasthenia" and "anxiety neurosis." [3]

It was, however, in the recognition a few years later of the factual reasons for defining *anxiety hysteria* that Freud really took the road which led eventually to the Anxiety Theory. There were a large number of such neuroses, he observed, whose most conspicuous symptoms were "phobias," or episodes of conscious anxiety ascribed to some specific thing or situation: the patient experiences anxiety, for example, when he encounters a certain person, or animal, or is alone in the street or in the darkness. Psychoanalysis of such cases had shown that their basic personalities were very like those of people with classic hysterical symptoms. He had there-

---

[2] See pages 266–8; also pages 37, 72, 166, 170.

[3] The symptoms of "actual neurosis" may be unrationalized anxiety, vague feelings of inexplicable apprehension, general uncertainty, chronic worry, impaired initiative, or only the physical symptoms of anxiety, such as heart palpitation, faintness, trembling, sweating, fatigue. Freud stated these syndromes were not psychoneurotic, but of toxic etiology resulting from physiologic abuse of sexual functions. This pronouncement was not further studied and modified by Freud in later years, and has largely been forgotten and replaced by modern ideas of anxiety neurosis, and is probably the most dubious of Freud's major clinical conclusions.

fore concluded that, though the chief symptoms of these two neuroses were different, the fundamental personalities and the kind of genital conflicts were of the same types in both conditions.

The analysis of phobias in anxiety hysteria and other neuroses had produced irrefutable evidence of the recurring coincidence of repressed sexual phantasies and conscious anxiety, and this had led Freud in the early years of analysis to conclude that such incidents of neurotic anxiety were direct mental manifestation of unsatisfied libido, that in certain conditions of repression, unconscious *sexual affect was transformed or "converted" into conscious anxiety*. A transformation of the emotion produced by libido tension had occurred. According to this theory, the back pains of the Case History [4] resulted from the physiological conversion of the wish to be the pregnant mother; and the patient who suffered anxiety about his sweetheart's fire-box [5] had converted his repressed sexual emotion (libido) into anxiety. The source of normal sexual feeling and anxiety was considered identical, but the anxiety was considered a transformation of the quality of the conscious emotional experience.

This theory of anxiety hysteria, however, had a much wider application than the explanation of one type of symptom. For it was also consistently observed during psychoanalysis that, whenever a previously repressed sexual wish became conscious, a feeling of anxiety appeared, and was often accompanied by transient symptoms such as phobias or nightmares. Analysis further showed that the latent content of these new symptoms was like the infantile wishes which had caused anxiety. We have seen a typical example of this common experience of analysts in our illustrative case: when the phantasy of going under the bridge was interpreted, anxiety and memories of pregnancy and phantasies of being cut erupted. The fire-box phobia resulted from interpreting the patient's denial of other sexual phantasies and his ascribing them to Bob.

The most important feature of Freud's book *The Problem of Anxiety* was the retraction of *this* theory that neurotic anxiety is a "conversion of sexual emotion." The anxiety of hysterias and of the

[4] See pages 83 ff.   [5] See pages 154 ff.

phobias of childhood and the transient anxiety symptoms which occur during the analysis of other psychoneuroses, Freud now stated, was *not* converted libido, but always actual, primary anxiety. Anxiety in psychoneurosis was like rationally conditional fear, the same subjective experience, except for the one fact that there was no adequate rational external stimulus. Neurotic anxiety was a response to an intra-psychic danger, a phantasy. It was a signal for defense, not against something tangible and external, but against a *wish* which might have invited actual punishment if it had led to forbidden acts in infancy.

For example, the anxiety of the illustrative case was a signal that she would be punished for infantile phantasies of having a baby. Again, when a patient sought help because he was in a panic lest people think him homosexual, analysis disclosed that the danger was a sexual impulse of the patient toward a homosexual object; the unconscious phantasy was that he would behave like a woman, and the anxiety was a signal for defense against an impulse which produced the phantasy. This theory, if it be a theory, is at present universally accepted by analysts and most psychiatrists who apply psychoanalytic knowledge and theory. It seems the best explanation of a great many interrelated observations.

ANXIETY, PHOBIA, AND PSYCHONEUROTIC INHIBITION

Though defense against the threat of irrational anxiety is the primary purpose of all neurotic reactions, the type of defense will differ with different conflicts and in different types of people. The simplest defense against incipient anxiety is one of *inhibition*. In order to avoid anxiety, a single act, a complex social function, or participation in situations where such acts or functions occur, is inhibited.

Freud had previously shown how the anxiety produced by a five-year-old boy's phantasies whenever he met his father was solved by a horse phobia. The fear of father had been repressed and displaced by fear of horses ("horse phobia"); thereafter, so long as real encounters with horses were avoided, the pain of anxiety was avoided. Similarly, a woman who is in danger of distressing anxiety or guilt from phantasies aroused by strange men looking at her can protect herself by avoiding public places, or by dressing herself so that no one will want to look. The man who blamed the rigid Puritan philosophy of his New England family [6] illustrated extensive inhibitions of this type. He suffered from defective capacity for self-assertion in his professional relations with his clients and in his social as well as erotic activities. He was only cured of the inhibition of normal social behavior, accompanied by a general masculinization of features, voice, and gesture when a series of primitive unconscious phantasies of *destroying* with his penis had led to the release of unconscious anxiety phantasies that his penis would be bitten off by a woman. The generalized inhibition of psychic functions prior to analysis had, according to Freud's final theory, been a protection against consciousness of this anxiety.

A second type of defense against anxiety, often combined with the former, may be called *retreat to narcissism*. To avoid the anxiety which threatens when impulses to love genital objects and friends are conscious, the individual may renounce love and camaraderie, and is then compelled to find pleasure predominantly in his own attributes, his phantasies, passive pleasures, and what he can induce other people to do for him. The man who was insolent to superiors as soon as he began to love them illustrates such a case. A very extreme example is that of a man who practically adopted, literally, the life of an infant cared for by his mother. For several years he stayed alone in bed, saw almost no one except her, would eat scarcely anything but milk which she brought to him, and forced her to carry off his excretions from the bed on diaper-like papers.

[6] See pages 42, 52.

ANXIETY AND HYSTERICAL CONVERSION

In the psychoneuroses, as we have seen, other mechanisms are utilized which are not so appropriately called "retreats" or "escapes" from anxiety. They may be said to "bind" anxiety by symptomatic, instead of direct, gratification of the wish.

The first of these mechanisms to be understood is the *hysterical conversion* symptom, where the requirements of the id and superego and their phantasy representations—that is, of instinct and unconscious guilt (anxiety)—are satisfied coincidentally by "conversion" of the wish into an abnormal and unpleasant physiologic function. We may cite the example of a functional headache in a man. In mentioning it the first time, he commented casually on the fact that he never made any attempt to reduce the vicious pain by sedatives or wet towels. Among his other associations were these: The forehead is conspicuous anteriorly like the buttocks posteriorly. Being spanked. When he was five, a little girl was crouching in a wagon so that he saw her bare behind; poking his head out from behind a barrel and being painfully struck in the forehead by a stone thrown by another little boy who was his rival in gaining from this little girl the privilege of seeing her naked parts. His mother's temper, her "socking" him over the head when he was naughty, her kind protection of him when a neighbor's wife tried to abuse him.

From these fragments we begin to discern an unconscious emotional relationship of the headaches to sexual experiences of early childhood and to experiences with his mother. Some of these represent satisfaction of his childhood love-needs by her, and others somewhat brutal punishment. A great deal of material in the analysis also shows a very strong masochistic tendency, the capacity for pleasure in pain; this child, for example, had found intense satisfaction, not only in his mother's protecting him, but in her mistreatment. The beatings were to the child evidence of her strong emotional bond to him.

These hints of a relationship of the headache to these childhood experiences were confirmed a few days later by a dream whose memory made a powerful impression: "I dreamt I was stunned by a blow on the head! I awoke in terrible fright!" Immediate associations are few, but significant. He recalls, as a boy, he took lunch to his father, a trolley-car motorman. One day the trolley was at the end of the line. The boy took the iron lever and stuck it in the switch. He suddenly recoiled in horror, feeling certain his father had struck him over the head; yet his father was some distance away. Could it be an electric shock from the cable connecting the two cars? He then said that he often spent hours taking out and putting in the electric plugs at home. The trolley switch, like these plugs, reminds him of a woman's organs, one part going to the vagina, the other to the anus. Sticking the lever in the switch was like inserting the penis. His father was a good motorman; the patient hated him for being always punctual, never losing a day's work.

The dream is, therefore, a repetition of a fragment of an actual forgotten experience which itself was tense with stored-up emotions of the guilty infantile period. In this the symbolism of playing motorman and inserting a lever in a trolley switch was a fulfillment of sexual wishes which are clearly differentiated from those of an adult type by their relationship to the infantile feelings toward the parents. Of this the patient was unaware, but nevertheless they activated the punishing function of the super-ego. Thus the patient endured as acute a punishment in an involuntary, vivid hallucination that he had received a stunning, cruel blow upon the head as if this punishment had actually been inflicted from without. As the hysterical headaches gratify both the unconscious wish to be treated sadistically by his mother and, at the same time, the need of punishment, they show the solution of both elements of the conflict by the same symptom. It is a typical neurotic compromise between the two tensions represented by sexual wish and punishment phantasy. This enables us to understand how the patient, suffering from his headache but not cognizant of its unconscious motivations, nevertheless accepted the pain and made no effort to relieve it. The pain was real and violent, but it was easier to endure than the anxiety reaction which the unconscious phantasies threatened to produce. The idea of a specific punishment—to be hit on the head—had been converted to the physiologic determinants of a headache.

ANXIETY, OBSESSIONS, AND COMPULSIONS

A second psychoneurotic mechanism of escaping guilt or infantile anxiety is the gratification of instinct and of guilt in alternating symptoms. This is the way of the obsessional and compulsion neuroses, closely related conditions in which a more or less large proportion of psychic energy is squandered in the constant repetition of absurd thoughts or useless acts. These symptoms are clearly distinguished from psychotic behavior and delusions by the fact that the patient is completely aware of the futility of the acts and the irrationality of the obsessions, strives to dispense with them in order to accomplish more satisfying tasks, yet cannot do so and is psychically compelled to repeat them over and over. Psychoanalysis has shown that compulsions are of two kinds: one kind of symptom is the expression, by either a compulsive act or an obsessional thought, of repressed wishes; and the other is a symptomatic "penance," or "atonement," which, like religious prayer, wards off the punishment of the psychic arbiter of "justice."

An example of the first type of obsession is illustrated by a woman patient who complains that the words "They turn up" keep coming constantly to her mind, and she cannot reject them and turn her attention to other things. She is greatly annoyed because the words have no sense at all; such foolish words without a meaning are too trivial, she declares, quite rationally; she shouldn't waste any more time talking about them, for there is much important work to be done in the analysis. The analyst recognizes that her emphasis on the triviality is a defense against some unconscious trend, and that her wish to leave consideration of the obsession and discuss instead something which seems to her excellent rational faculty really important is actually an escape to superficial considerations. So he urges her to think of the obsessional words:

"They turn up" and tell what comes spontaneously to her mind. She protests, but after many derogatory remarks concerning the analyst's inefficiency and stupidity, a memory-picture comes to her mind. She recalls a visit to an aunt when she was twelve. The aunt and she bathed together, the patient in the front of the tub. She recalled her wish to look at her naked aunt, the guilty resistance to the wish. Later she watched her aunt drying herself with a towel, and recalled the vivid impression when she momentarily glimpsed the older woman's breasts, and her tense curiosity in noting how the points stuck up. Then the patient went on to tell of her envy of the bodily development of a sister two years older. The two had talked much together in those years of puberty. Her sister constantly teased her with still having the figure of a boy; and, indeed, the immaturity of the patient's bodily development had persisted until adult years and had been the cause of grievously unsatisfied pride and shame to her. Further associations disclosed memories of earlier years, and especially feelings from early childhood that her sister had all that she herself desired, especially most of the attention and approbation of their father. She then recalled how at the age of four she had bathed with her sister and at the same time compared their bodies to their mother's. She felt as though she could re-experience the childish intensity of her interest in her mother's mature body, and some vague realization that there was a connection between this and the kind of attention bestowed by her father on her mother. At any rate the memory of her bitterness that she must sleep in the children's bedroom and so not have her mother's opportunity to remain with her father without interruption was very clearly remembered.

Here a significant train of events, memories with a common emotional basis which had been unconscious before the analysis, is revealed. We see how the senseless thought "They turn up" is an expression of a deep-seated desire. From a vast storehouse of emotional experience one single detail of the unconscious thought emerges to consciousness and takes over the instinctual energy of the whole unconscious trend. In the obsession to think over and over this senseless thought, the passion of puberty to have breasts like her aunt's, the unsatisfied longings to be possessed of the charms of her sister, and at the same time the survival since infancy of a longing to be made like her mother and not be excluded from the father during the night, all find a symptomatic expression.

We may illustrate the second type of compulsion symptom, that which protects directly against the guilt of infantile impulses, with a passing detail from the analysis of a man. At certain moments during treatment hours he would begin to speak with that heightened affect which characteristically accompanies the emergence of unconscious material in an analysis. Then he would abruptly cease talking altogether. If asked to continue, he would remark that there was absolutely nothing in his mind. Then he would begin to say: "I am looking at the wall. Imagining figures— 1, 2, 3; 1, 2, 3; 3 is a prime factor; 3, 5, 7; 3, 5, 7; 3, 5, 7." This was of special interest, because such a use of figures we know empirically to be one of the common manifestations of an obsessional neurosis. The man had had no conspicuous symptoms of this type of neurosis, and yet we were observing the actual origin of a typical though transient symptom during the treatment hour. The next day he recalled that he had recently performed a similar type of obsessional thinking in everyday life. He would sometimes stand before shop-windows and memorize the price numbers. Then, on his way home, he would repeat over and over the words: "17—95, 17—95." His next associations were that he took particular pleasure in walking about streets on a windy day; trolley-cars; his interest in a lady's stockings while riding in one the day before. It then occurred to him for the first time that the shop-windows where he began his obsessional counting were always those where lingerie was displayed. He now recalled a passionate interest during schooldays in secretly playing with the underwear of an aunt whom he visited, and then similar play in early childhood with his sisters', three and four years older than he. We now see how the repetition of price labels is essentially a defense against recognizing the emotions and phantasies aroused by the display of lingerie in shop-windows. The thought of the windows attracts him, the reason must be repressed. The guilt is strong enough to require such a neurotic defense rather than a normal reaction of pleasurable phantasy or turning to other activities; this is explained by the intimate relationship for him of lingerie and tabooed childhood sexual interest in his sisters. The supposition that association between the two indicates that a similar purpose is fulfilled in counting 1, 2, 3, and 3, 5, 7, during treatment is confirmed. Having overcome the obstacles to conscious recognition so far, he now tells us the associations which previously had been disavowed and restrained by the device of substituting a defensive obsessive counting during the treatment itself. The first time this occurred, he now states, was after the sudden recollection of sexual play with his younger sister at the age of four or five. This, he now reports, he had wished to forget immediately, before there was time to communicate it to the analyst.

THE ANXIETY THEORY OF PSYCHONEUROSIS

Freud's final conclusion in his gradually developed explanation of the etiology of psychoneuroses is that repression, and other mechanisms in the creation of psychoneurotic symptoms, are motivated by the need to escape an attack of conscious anxiety. Even as "real anxiety" (fear of a real danger) is a signal for defense against external danger, neurotic anxiety is the signal for defense of the personality against *internal* danger; this danger is a conscious repetition of anxieties experienced in infancy in phobias, nightmares, secret day-dreams, associated with phantasies of punishment for infantile desires. A drive which threatens to demand conscious gratification of an infantile wish in adult life, or its conscious recognition, therefore, is a danger or threat, because it is likely to produce the intolerable experience of anxiety, or at least its modification as guilt.

The basic data for this final conclusion are those analytic observations which show the relationship of every variety of neurotic symptom to the dominant symptom of anxiety hysteria: a phobia. Various personalities have various means of solving this problem of the danger of anxiety. The boy with the phobia, the man who could not assert himself, the man with the headache, the woman with the obsession "They turn up," and the man forced to repeat nonsensical figures, all show the danger of anxiety reaction to different unconscious phantasies. Each has a different mechanism for solving his conflict, but the final purpose, avoidance of anxiety and irrational guilt, is common to them all.

DEFENSE MECHANISMS AND CHARACTER NEUROSES

As with all major scientific discoveries, the long-sought answer to the problem of the relation of anxiety to symptoms opened many new important channels of investigation. The anxiety theory of neurotic symptoms has now been universally accepted, and subsequently analysts have been investigating its applicability to character-analysis. Our illustrative case had not only utilized such symptoms as stammering, frigidity, and the egg-cooking ritual to escape the anxiety engendered by her infantile phantasies; she had also rejected the adult fulfillment of her feminine nature by renouncing a suitable marriage and accepting employment by an unsuitable lover. From this adjustment she had suffered as well as from her symptoms; but inhibited activities of her life had unconsciously fulfilled the same purpose as her symptoms had: a protection from anxiety. Similarly, the man had not only solved by symptomatic impotence the anxiety problem aroused by phantasies of women biting; he had also avoided it by abstaining from platonic acquaintance with women and from executive duties in business.

Neurotic (irrational) anxiety not only leads to symptom-formation and inhibition of total personality function, it produces positive traits, which are distinguished from symptoms chiefly by their characterizing an individual's total reaction to life situations. A man always protrudes his lips and talks from the side of his mouth until he learns that infantile toilet training had led to his unconsciously imagining words are like feces, and that this mannerism is unconsciously repeating his infantile defiance of his mother by defecating in the wrong place. A woman chooses dresses with wing-like tulle in back, even when others are prettier, because unconsciously this perpetuates a favorite childhood fairy-tale of flying to a magic isle; this story had meant for her a phantasy of escaping with her little brother so that they might indulge their childish sexual games without being discovered by their mother. Many traits, such as modes of hair-brushing, perpetuate a boy's imitation of an athletic hero, long after an active interest in sports has lapsed, because unconsciously it also represents his infantile identification with a victorious father.

The most vital and complex social adjustments in life may be determined by such patterns, whose original and primary purpose was escape from anxiety. *"Character neuroses"* are people with rigid traits of this kind; their infantile desires to escape from associated anxieties are expressed chiefly in stereotyped patterns of behavior. Typically, they are "driven," compulsive people, who are repetitively defeated by environmental circumstance far more crucially than their capacity for achievement would warrant.

A woman of strong emotions and a brilliant and original mind was such a case. She had had unusual success in several vocations, but eventually was forced by circumstances she had unconsciously created to give up each. A clever idea had gained her promotion from salesgirl to manager, and her quick understanding of business principles won the respect and liking of male executives. She selected for assistant an inexperienced man of little independent ability; he adored her, and she diligently taught him to perform her duties, giving him "all she had." Eventually he revolted against her unconscious domination, vindictively challenged her right to conduct her own department, stole the business secrets, and she was forced by her own superiors to resign. During another period of her life she was equally successful as a schoolteacher and again was admired and supported by her superiors until one member of the school board refused to permit a valuable idea of hers to be put into practice. Her fight with this man created violent partisanship for and against her, and eventually a situation whose only possible solution was her dismissal. Each time her eventual catastrophe was ascribed by her, and by others who were well informed about the circumstances, to the malice of her antagonists, and the course of external events validated this belief. But analysis showed these events themselves were the inevitable consequence of unconscious patterns. Her successes were dependent upon her ability to create an environment of personally selected individuals who did not resent her peculiarities; and her failures always developed from the hostilities of people whom she could not exclude whenever the pursuit of a normal activity required her entering a community which was already established.

During her analysis, she re-experienced the panic and shame experienced at the age of ten when her father, a police captain with impetuous affections and violent rages, had whipped her. The most enduring unconscious effect of this experience was the terror resulting from helplessness because her father had held her so that she could not move her arms or legs. Though of strong character and consciously eager for children, her fear of pregnancy was intense because of the unconscious association that if she were pregnant she would be as helpless as when she was whipped. Her phantasies about the whipping involved not only an experience between herself and her father, but three people. The third person in her phantasy was a very powerful man who could save her from her father. A doctor had actually done this when she was twelve by forbidding her father to punish her; and earlier in her childhood this ideal of a protector had been realized by the behavior of her grandfather. But the phantasy of a strong man protecting her from her father was ultimately derived from very early childhood when her father himself had repeatedly protected her from abuse by an older brother. That was the father she loved as well as feared, the male protector.

She was a strongly bisexual woman, and in adult years not only did she re-experience terror in consequence of her desire to be pregnant and a need to be helpless in her relations with some men; but she also repeatedly acted the role of being the powerful man herself. Thus she was the affectionate and deserving little girl in her relations to the superiors in business who liked her and promoted her, and she was also the protector of the weak subordinate whose hatred eventually led to disaster. Repeatedly she acted the role of this powerful man when another girl seemed to be helpless and to need protection from an unpleasant man. Usually she attacked these men (unconsciously brutal fathers) with her wits, but sometimes she attacked them with her fists, and sometimes even by threatening to shoot. In these situations she was usually successful in dominating the man.

Her chief conscious problem in life was her frustrated desire for a feminine sexual role. This was associated with the whippings, and therefore with unconscious anxiety lest they be repeated; she must compulsively escape a man she felt to be powerful, and so the pattern of all her relations with men became an unyielding though disguised and unconscious demand that every man acknowledge her muscular strength, her businessman's mind, or the originality of an idea, before she could love him, overtly or indirectly, or accept what she wanted him to offer. A year after the whipping in childhood her father had threatened to punish her again and she had told him: "If you want to whip me, it's all right. But do it now, upstairs!" His acceptance of her suggestion unconsciously fulfilled her phantasy that she was stronger than her father, that her will had determined his actions, and this became the model of her technique in every human relationship. A terrible humiliation had occurred at a kissing game during adolescence; she had planned a trick to be kissed under certain conditions which she would control, but her trick was anticipated by the other children. Consciously she was shamed by the kiss, but unconsciously she was humiliated by the failure of her plan for controlling the game. In later years, expecting to be assaulted by one man, she struck his jaw with her fist and knocked him down; after that she could love him. Under similar conditions, as a last resort, she said to another insistent lover: "I shall jump down an elevator shaft!" He stopped short in his advances; she had known his sister had died this way and nothing could have thrilled her more than her success in paralyzing him by her clever remark. Her only pregnancy resulted from a ruse:

having agreed with her husband that conception was inadvisable, she then pretended for six months that she was pregnant; consciously her plan had been to avoid the use of contraceptives by pretended pregnancy, and so become really pregnant. The unconscious motivation of this rationalized behavior was that she could only permit conception if she could first deceive the man by a unique idea. At another time she involuntarily prevented introitus; she then told him exactly in what unusual manner she thought a woman must be stroked. He exulted in her "brilliant" idea, followed her directions, and there was no further inhibition. And afterward he, very happy, gave her a present; but she immediately responded by insisting that he first accept something from her. Thus she repeated the successful pattern of her sexual behavior in her reaction to the asexual gift: he must acknowledge her technique or her present before she would accept her husband in either way.

As she grew older, this pattern was more and more completely realized by clever devices to have the originality of really unusual ideas acknowledged, in order that then she could accept what she wanted various men to give her. In all these ways this talented woman was in every human situation demanding that a special idea of hers be acknowledged as a prerequisite to any relationship; for unconsciously these ideas represented the phantasy that she was the strong man saving her helpless other self from her father's whipping. Those whose personalities were capable of acknowledging this emotionally without hatred of her became warm and appreciative friends, and this was essential to her successes. But in every established community there were some whose personalities reacted negatively to her ruses; their hostility was evoked, no other pattern was possible for her, and in spite of her successes these enmities could not be avoided and made failure inevitable.

The pattern was quite unconscious. She was conscious of a thrill in her power of brain or brawn when the moments of victory were recalled; of a desire for men erotically like that of feminine women; of a capacity to think like men and act like men upon occasion; and of despair over her failures at certain times. And her whole physical appearance altered expressively in accordance with each conscious mood. But she was completely unconscious of the inevitable relationship between her successes of mind and will to her failures, and of the existence of a patterned unrealistic demand upon others to acknowledge her phantasy of being the man more powerful than her father.

Such a total personality pattern, because of its compulsiveness, its unconscious determinants, and its rigid repetition and inadaptability to various reality situations, is typically neurotic. That it not only is responsible for the adult's failures, but is his protection against repeating the threatening fear of infantile helplessness, is as true of such a character pattern as of simpler symptoms. Analyses have led to a recognition that repression, and its sequels—phobias, inhibitions, regression, displacement, and symptom-formation—are not the only mechanisms of psychological defense against anxiety. The study of symptoms had led Freud to recognize early in his work that some traits, such as obstinacy and defiance, were determined, like symptoms, by deeply repressed wishes. The metapsychological description of personality, and especially the basic concepts of personality structure, had inevitably further recognition that anxiety-producing conflict and repression are also decisive in the determination of many character traits, some normal and some neurotic. A component of character is deemed neurotic when it is sufficiently rigid to lack variability in adapting to variations in reality situations and interpersonal relations, and therefore engenders disaster and suffering. Such "character neuroses" are determined by chronic patterns for defense against infantile anxiety, and for the last thirty years analysis has been as much concerned scientifically and therapeutically with this kind of neurotic problem as it was in earlier years with typical psychogenic symptoms.

SUMMARY OF THE THEORY OF PSYCHONEUROSIS

In whatever way we approach the closely related problems of psychoneurotic symptoms and of character-formation—provided we neglect no opportunity for appraising the unconscious factors—we find they are means of solving conflicts involving the threat that either anxiety or guilt will become conscious. In every case the factors involved—repression, regression, symptom-formation, character pattern—serve to defend the ego from experiencing conscious anxiety, even though, at the same time, ego efficiency itself is impaired by the energy withdrawn from its mature functions by the conflict and its defense.

We have, therefore, three points of view from which to regard the etiology of the psychoneuroses and neurotic character problems:

I. The *empirical* observation (by study of free associations) of unconscious wishes, especially the sexual, hostile, and punishment phantasies and memories of the infantile period, and of their correlations with neurotic symptomatology and other conscious components of the personality.

II. The *abstraction* of these observations by the concept of *personality structure*.

III. The *induction* of dynamic factors, primarily biological, but represented psychologically by the empirical data, which comprise the *theory of instincts*.

In concluding this section on theories, I wish only to clarify the mutual relationship of these concepts. In discussing the theory of instincts (Chapter V), the analogy, though tremendously simplified, of the dynamics of hydraulic systems to the fundamental forces which determine emotion, behavior, and symptoms was discussed. If only it be recognized that personality systems are far more complex than our simple diagram, though the fundamental laws of instinct tension and release apply, we may accurately retain our analogy. The main groups of instinctual systems are then represented by the structural scheme of id, ego, and super-ego. An emotional conflict will then be one between super-ego and id, such as occurred in the illustrative case, or between two antagonistic impulses (such as love and hate, activity and passivity, love of a man and of a woman), both striving for acceptance by the ego. In psychosis, the primary conflict is between the total personality and a world whose reality is of diminished subjective value. The reservoir of Figure II represents the adult ego's capacity for delay of gratification; and a contraction of this reservoir, or prolonged blockage of its outlets, will produce an increment of the id tension, narcissism, and recourse to infantile and neurotic forms of pleasure.

The anxiety theory of psychoneurotic etiology is an important element in this synthesis. In the hydraulic analogy,[7] *anxiety is what controls the valves.* The sense of guilt, or fear of super-ego (parental) attack and punishment, closes the pleasure-principle valve, which permits of immediate infantile gratification. If the impulses are not fused, sublimated, displaced, or otherwise made acceptable to the ego, fear of retaliation by the outer world, of revenge, ostracism, etc., closes the valve of the reality reservoir. If super-ego or reality anxiety causes closure of all valves which give tension release through externalized activity, retreat to narcissism results, and if this be rigidly and consistently maintained, psychosis will break out. There are valves between all systems represented by the personality structure, and each is closed by the threat of intrapsychically motivated anxiety.

This synthesis of structural, instinctual, and anxiety theories appears best to fit the facts as they are known to us today. This is true of conscious as well as of unconscious thought and behavior, though the latter seems of far more significance for a deep understanding of human motivation. If *strong* irrational motives conflict with rational, the irrational are likely to win. Much that determines individuality, such as characterological trends, and whether a neurosis will be predominantly an obsessional or a hysterical defense against anxiety, is determined presumably by hereditary factors. For Freud—and he is often misquoted on this point—always considered heredity the explanation of inborn potentialities, and environment, especially the infant's, as playing a selective and sometimes decisive influence in the development or lack of development of potentialities. The confusion resulted from the usual tendency in pre-psychoanalytic psychiatry to use "heredity" or "constitution"

[7] See pages 99 and 102.

chiefly to disguise ignorance, in that everything which could not be explained was ascribed arbitrarily to it. When we find that an environmental situation plays a role in a specific maladjustment, the role of heredity is less emphasized; the disclosure of adult traumata which have become unconscious still further reduces its significance, and the demonstration of infantile repressions do so still more. At this point, however, analysts are compelled to join their colleagues in assigning what is still inexplicable to hereditary causes. There is no reason to doubt that an individual with sufficiently inferior germ plasm cannot escape mental illness under any life conditions; but it is also apparent that individuals whose heredity and infantile experiences are not unusually unfavorable may be made neurotic by exceptional emotional strain. Yet the discovery of psychoanalysis should be sufficient warning not to accept too complacently inborn "constitution" as the sole explanation of every human peculiarity. Fifty years ago hysterical people were believed to be just "made that way," to be "constitutionally weak," interesting patients but irretrievable. But Breuer showed the effect of adult emotional traumata upon symptom-formation, and Freud demonstrated the significance of infantile experience. In short, the more we learn of psychological facts, the less we need ascribe to unalterable heredity.

It remains only to emphasize that many of the features of the psychoanalytic explanation of the psychoneuroses are applicable to most other manifestations of human nature. Psychoneurotics are not peculiar in that their lives are governed by irrational forces of an unconscious nature—if anything, they are only a little more so, and the motivation of normal as well as of abnormal manifestations is subject to the same psychological laws.

PART THREE

THERAPY BY
PSYCHOANALYSIS

THE PSYCHOANALYTIC METHOD

TECHNICAL PRINCIPLES

T H E keystone of psychoanalytic technique has always been the free-association method of thought,[1] which the patient is taught and instructed to use to the very best of his ability throughout the treatment. Occasionally it is momentarily suspended for a rational review of the free associations themselves. But, though these intellectual interruptions of the usual procedure are indispensable, their function in the production of the cure by psychoanalytical technique is quite secondary.

Except for the consistent use of free association, the principles and practice of modern psychoanalytic therapy are fundamentally different from Freud's original procedure. At first he had anticipated that when the physician had discovered the patient's unconscious motivations, the communication of this knowledge to the patient, and its comprehension by him, would effect a cure. But repeated trials demonstrated to Freud that these expectations were wrong. He would succeed in learning the unconscious wish. He would inform the patient of it; the patient would agree and com-

---

[1] See Chapter I, pages 13–18.

prehend; this would affect the patient's intellectual appraisal of his problems, but not the emotional tensions themselves. Thus, early in his work, Freud learned a lesson which many who putter with his technique have not yet assimilated: that intellectual insight cannot control the forces of the unconscious, that repression is not simply the difference between knowing and not knowing, that cure depends on far more than making conscious.

Freud then observed that significant personality changes attended intellectual awareness only when this was accompanied by a discharge of the emotion which the unconscious idea was representing. Otherwise the situation was that of the passenger who boards the right train, but never arrives at his destination because no locomotive is attached. The locomotive, so to speak, of psychoanalytic therapy is the emotion which accompanies the ideas. It is not so important that the patient know as that he *feel* the forgotten unconscious experience or wish. And if this feeling is maintained, or the experience is repeated with different content or memories instead of complete repression again, a change in the patient's management of it occurs. What happens in a modern analysis may perhaps be most easily understood by consideration of experiences common to everyone's childhood. Thus, it is not the idea itself, the words, "My mother," that controls so much of the child's behavior —his toilet habits, for example—but the emotion: "I like her smile"; "she says I'm good"; "I make her happy." It is not the thought, "I am told not to play in the neighbor's garden," but the emotion, "I fear punishment," that is effective. It is not the picture of a college football-player, but the attendant affect, "I *want* to be a hero like him," that initiates the activity of a boy.

TRANSFERENCE

The emotion is of so much therapeutic value, not because it is actively induced by the analyst, but because it arises primarily and spontaneously from the patient's own being. Nothing in the clinical practice of analysis is more convincing than this fact, occurring in every case, with no effort by the physician to encourage it or determine its individual characteristics. For when a patient recounts free associations, he soon speaks of events or phantasies of vital interest to himself, and when these are told, the listener is gradually invested with some of the emotion which accompanies them. The patient gradually begins to feel that the sympathetic listener is loved or hated, a friend or an enemy, one who is nice to him or one who frustrates his needs and punishes him. The feelings toward the listener become more and more those felt toward the specific people the patient is talking about, or, more exactly, those his unconscious "is talking about." This special case of object-displacement during psychoanalysis is called *transference*.

Not only does the consistent narration of those associations which become conscious produce "transference" spontaneously, but the same phenomenon develops from emotionalized ideas that are still unconscious. This fact is extensively utilized in analysis; for by free associating to inexplicable and irrational feelings felt for the analyst the patient may arrive at the unconscious source of these in his actual experiences. Thus the strong emotional disinclination of a patient we have mentioned [2] to pay the analyst his fee developed before its unconscious source was known; free associations originating in this professional scene disclosed the previously unconscious memory of his infantile pleasure in his mother's care of him at the toilet. The patient simulating flatus with his mouth [3] in defiance of the analyst was reproducing an infantile scene before he had become conscious of it. The patient who distrusted the analyst's confidence [4] was combating a still unconscious desire to caress his little niece.

On one occasion strong affection for the analyst and phantasies of doing things *with* him developed in a patient who was an only child. Eventually it was discovered that this was a feeling of having a brother or sister, a playmate, another with whom to share love and secrets, when the parents left him alone. The patient's

[2] See pages 41, 51, 74, 110. [3] See pages 103, 105, 131, 173. [4] See pages 153–5.

childhood longing for a brother or sister had long been forgotten, but the revival of this unconscious need was expressed in the transference to the analyst before the childhood phantasies had consciously been recalled.

Phenomena with the typical features of transference during psychoanalysis occur constantly in everyday life: for example, in the frequent irrational resentment of subordinates toward an excellent executive. They occur in all other types of psychotherapy. The efficacy of suggestion and hypnosis depend on the childlike submission to adult will transferred to the therapist. The acceptance of admonition and advice depends on a similar unconscious wish to restore the childhood situation of being cared for and disciplined. It occurs in religious confession. Indeed, the early stages of some psychoanalyses, when the patient recounts with strong emotions thoughts he kept secret from all others, closely resemble confession, though eventually they differ greatly in that the real task of analysis begins where confession ends, in disclosing the *unconscious* sources of the conscious guilt and suffering.

It is, therefore, not the phenomenon of transference that distinguishes psychoanalytic therapy. The phenomenon is a fundamental property of human nature, and under the conditions of free association is as spontaneous and inevitable as water running down a hill to seek the lowest level. It is the *conscious, scientific utilization of transference as a dynamic force, and particularly the analysis of its unconscious sources, that distinguish its use in psychoanalysis from all other methods of psychotherapy.*

The non-analytic tendency to use "transference" as a synonym for "rapport," "friendly or erotic feeling," or a compliant attitude to the therapist is confusing. For transference, as understood by most analysts, is not a simple attitude of liking or disliking the analyst as a person, of loving or hating him for his personal virtues and vices. It is rather a reproduction of all the significant emotional constellations characteristic of the individual patient, with all the complexity and variation and fluctuation characteristic of human beings, which results from allowing him to express his emotional patterns spontaneously. It is as though those human relationships which are typical of his life, and especially the repressed, unconscious ones, were projected by the transference, magic-lantern fashion, upon a screen—the patient's subjectively distorted impression of the real personality of his analyst.

Many details of analytic technique are devised to maintain "as blank a screen" as possible. Before work begins, a definite hour and a definite fee are established. Any changes in routine which the patient subsequently demands will generally indicate a change, not in the objective situation but in the emotions of the patient. The analyst discloses as little of his actual self as practical; for every detail of the real person that is known to the patient will distort the transference picture of projected subjective situations. The analyst consequently refrains from analyzing intimate friends. Not only the actual facts of his life, but his temperament will be intruded as little as practical into the situation. He therefore usually makes what comments he has to make without display of subjective emotion, and refrains from expressing his own attitudes and biases. He will make no effort to direct the patient, morally or otherwise, to an adjustment which fits his own scheme of life and his own theory of what it should be like or how it should be lived. He will content himself with the premise that, if unconscious sources of tension are reduced, the adult patient will find the milieu and individual philosophy of life and relationship with others which best meet his particular needs more readily and more satisfactorily than by submission to the arbitrary, if well-meant, direction of the therapist.

Thus the technical devices of analysis which best serve for therapy also produce the best experimental situation yet devised for studying the more complex features of human nature.

Chemistry has discovered that there are a limited number of elements whose various transformations and combinations will result in the multifarious substances of our universe. The structure of a quart of gasoline, a lump of sugar, or a can of chloroform is not immediately apparent. The constituent elements of each are completely hidden by the properties of the compound, and we are accustomed descriptively to classify substances by those properties which are immediately apparent to the eye and senses. To understand the inner structure of a compound, the chemist subjects a small specimen to certain procedures. Under these conditions an analysis of its less obvious attributes and constituent parts can be made.

The principle of psychoanalytic procedure is not fundamentally unlike that of chemistry. The reactions of a human being are directly observable and classifiable, but the deeper motivations are not immediately apparent. Psychoanalysis is the test-tube of human experience. For one hour a day, for a limited period, a *sample* of human thoughts and feelings is examined under controlled conditions. A daily specimen of typical emotional reactions is taken. The endlessly involved complications of everyday life are reduced by the four walls of the treatment room; the multitude of people serving as emotional stimuli and instinctual objects are replaced by a single individual, the analyst.

With the use of a natural reagent, the transference, the therapeutic situation thus becomes a sample of life, and a sample under special conditions which permit of closer, more exact analysis than is possible in other relationships. The compounds of various dynamic instinctual attitudes which represent the patient's mental life and social behavior appear in typical form during the analytic hours. For everything which occurs in the analytic test-tube has three significances, each of which represents a typical organization of the component instincts. There is always an emotional relationship to the analyst; secondly, an emotional relationship to the people and activities of everyday life; and, thirdly, a past situation in infancy or childhood which forms the model for both life situation and analytic situation.

For example, during the first months of analysis that patient who would not go by his brother's door, who denied erotic feelings for women, and who would not tell his associations about Bob made little apparent progress.[5] Considered descriptively, he was "unco-operative," showed no ability or willingness to associate freely. In spite of his promise to tell everything which came to his mind,

[5] See pages 10, 37, 131, 153–5, 206, 212.

he constantly reserved conscious thoughts that seemed to him silly, irrelevant, illogical, or "none of the analyst's business." He seemed stupid, unable to understand the few very simple explanations the analyst offered. Eventually it was disclosed that he was hiding a profound suspicion of the analyst. He secretly thought that he was being exploited only for money, that the analyst cheated him by not talking more than five out of fifty minutes, that the analyst might communicate with his friends and do him injury; and when he heard the secretary's typewriter, he secretly phantasied that she was typing what he had told the previous hour. Simple statements of fact had utterly no effect on these suspicions. Occasionally he conceded that he was equally suspicious of everybody else, including parents, sweetheart, and friends.

After six months' treatment the patient had a dream accompanied by severe anxiety. Its manifest content was, in part: "An elevated railway station; a big junction with sheds; a gang of robbers chasing me. They chased me onto a roof. They took a rope and tied it around me, whirled me, and I dropped down an elevator shaft. I took out a gun and fired at them, but only at their legs, so as not to kill them. Then I was by the water. A motorboat with a man in it went by. My girl wanted something, led me to a house. I was in a funny thing of ropes, like a net. The gang was there. Two girls were together. Scissors were there."

Among many associations to this dream, all interesting in themselves but discursive here, the following were specially relevant. There were only a few elevated railway sheds like this, all of them important stations, like one in a prostitute-infested district of Chicago. The patient recalls vividly how trains come in and go out of the sheds; the roofs of train and shed fit tightly; it has often reminded him of coitus. He was whirled by the rope: as a boy, he used to tie a rope around stones and whirl them; once he broke a window, and his father didn't like it. Taking his watch out of his pocket, he said it only ran upside down; he was very angry at the watchmaker, but he decided after rumination not to act angry when he demanded better work (as he attacked the "robbers" in the manifest dream, but *only* their legs). In associating to the boat, he recalls various erotic incidents and a previous dream. The net suggests the special way packages were wrapped for Christmas, the girls cutting the strings, "window-shopping" with his sweetheart. The net terrified him, the gang was there. He thinks he knows why he dreamed this last night: a friend had told him his girl was unfaithful. He emphasizes that he is indifferent to what she does; he makes no claims on her, disregards everything he suspects unless he has proof. [The analyst here comments that in the latter part of the dream his sweetheart seduces him into a situation where men will injure him.]

The next day the patient tells many facts previously kept secret. His girl went out sometimes with a Russian. He wondered "how far" they went. People had told him they "went the limit." She had gone on week-end house parties. She had maintained she was the patient's girl; the Russian had said that he would like to meet the patient, they would have a good time. The patient felt that the Russian might want to fight it out. [The patient is then asked for his associations to scissors.] "Knives. It was a gang in the dream, because Russians go in gangs. This fellow might carry a knife. He might stick it in my girl. [Note the unconscious sexual symbolism of knife shown in this ambiguous remark.] Dirty stories referring to scissors cutting off the penis—I won't tell them to you. [The patient is reminded he should tell everything.] But I can't, because you don't know the words. I think of the language they use around street-corners. [Analyst is silent.] You wouldn't know what we mean by 'fairies' or 'broads'—going abroad, reading travel literature. Every time I've spoken of going abroad (a frequent phantasy), I've thought 'hopping a broad,' but didn't say it because you don't know what 'broad' means." [The analyst rhetorically asks if his parents hadn't understood the dirty words of small boys.]

The next day he recounts obscenities from his childhood, including a story of a carrot being stuck through a hole and cut off, and, finally, threats of his parents for infantile masturbation, and an anxiety phantasy that his father would cut off his penis with his mother's shears.

To recapitulate: the immediate situation is one in which he is consciously violating the rule of free association and keeping most sensitized thoughts secret from the analyst. He is preoccupied with sexual thoughts of his girl, suspicion that she is unfaithful, hatred of his rival, and fear that if she introduces them, the Russian will attack him. Conspicuous in his conscious attitudes are the denial of eroticism and of interest in his girl's other affairs, and his strong repudiation of aggressive wishes. These unconscious defenses are being weakened as the analysis progresses and the underlying wishes first appear consciously in the transference. He is suspicious that the analyst will injure him, and that the woman secretary (he has remarked before she has much the manner of his sweetheart) is participating in this injury. In all these matters he acts in the analysis essentially as he does outside, by scrupulous maintenance of good behavior, concealment of his suspicions, and denial of aggressive tendencies. Why these traits of character and behavior are so excessive is revealed only by the exactly analogous, though infantile, phantasy: "I am afraid my father will punish me with mother's scissors for sexual thoughts." But he protests in every way against this still active source of anxiety until it emerges in a dream representing all the associated emotions. An illustration of his defense is the rationalization that the analyst does not understand obscene words, and though the rationalization itself is derived from childhood discipline, it serves the patient's need for self-justification for the exclusion of crude sexual associations from the analysis for months. The transference, predominantly suspiciousness of the analyst, is therefore a duplication, detail for detail, of his emotions toward people in his outer life, and of a crucial emotional situation in his infancy, the phantasies they give rise to, and the activities they produce.

A second illustration is a portion of the transference of a man who came too late or not at all to his appointments. He was struggling to attain a degree essential to earning a good livelihood in his profession. But he had great difficulty concentrating on lectures and exercises; he missed many classes and seldom rose early in the morning. His social life was very limited; he rejected most opportunities for friendship. His mind was constantly occupied with the problem of proving his superiority, especially by intellectual declamation, with everyone he met.

In a short time the analytic situation became a miniature of this relationship to the world. When the time came for him each day to go to his analysis, he would procrastinate, do other trivial things, was always late; sometimes he would not go at all. It was a replica of his irresponsibility in his attendance at classes. He would devote a considerable portion of each hour of analysis to long discussions of political problems. These were highly intelligent, but obviously were unconsciously utilized to conceal recognition of the transference emotions, exactly as his phantasies of intellectual superiority had replaced emotional camaraderie and useful competition in classroom and social life.

The analyst's task was to demonstrate effectively how those brilliant, intellectual expositions served to conceal associations which lay close to his emotional life. Simply to explain the situation in general terms, to appeal to his keen intellectual faculties, was utterly futile; he would assent fully to the analyst's remarks and show the keenest intellectual interest, but no fundamental change in the analytic situation would occur. A better opportunity came one day when some emotion accompanied associations dealing with his envy of other men's success with girls. He then spoke of masturbation; he spoke of his mother's dressing him in childhood, his father's punishing him. He exchanged a few terse remarks, and he discovered his phantasies of intellectual brilliance were a substitute for the competition he had withdrawn from because of fear, now of all men, originally of his rigorous father. Behind his aloof intellectualism lay this hidden fear; he was afraid of any competition with men because his infantile fear of punishment for wishing to take his mother from his father had never been resolved and was unconsciously activated by each adult competitive situation with a man. The unconscious phantasy of being bigger than the analyst had produced excessive intellectual arguing and repression of facts and free association. The whole therapeutic situation became emotional instead of intellectual. Associations became free.

After this had occurred the analyst went away for several days. At the next appointment the patient was on time and his greeting was unusually warm and pleasant. His associations explained the change. He related a dream in which he was a child telling his mother all about his sexual worries. His associations dealt with the similarity between his dream and the relationship in childhood to his mother. The analyst remarked: "You came on time today; you are glad to see me. That was not so last week. Your dream and associations explain the change. Previously you were afraid of me because you felt toward me as toward another man— always competitors. Today you feel about me as you do about your mother. You have unconsciously fled from the attempt to master your fear of competition by going back, like a child, to the protection of your mother." The patient was silent. Then he said: "Maybe something that happened explains it. My teacher [a man whom the patient envied for the seductions of which he boasted] lost his job. I ought to have been sorry. I don't think I was. He was all broken up, and not bragging as usual." The teacher had lost his claim to prestige with the patient; he was, for the patient, no longer unconsciously a representative of the infantile rival whose claims must not be challenged. The analyst's absence had pleased the patient because he had unconsciously phantasied that it—like his teacher's— was a result of downfall. The patient's unconscious anxiety was much decreased; for, with the defeat of these rivals, teacher and analyst, he could accept his unconscious wish for mother without anxiety, and expressed this unconscious need in his unusual affection for the analyst. Coincidentally, there was notable improvement in his everyday relationships with other people.

This fragment of an analysis shows the correspondence between the emotions of an analytic hour and those of the patient's contemporaneous life. His reaction to the analyst was in its framework identical with the problem the world was presenting to him; his reaction changed entirely when the external situation changed, because the latter change had temporarily relieved his deep anxiety sufficiently for him to become conscious of these hostile wishes.

These few examples illustrate how individual the emotional

constellation determining each patient's transference must be. Indeed, there are as many varieties of transference as there are varieties of human temperaments, phantasies, and problems. Nevertheless, there are certain general features of the development of transferences common to all cases. These we shall now discuss.

First are the three phases of transference during the course of every typical analysis. Though these overlap and very rarely are so clear-cut as a textbook description, they can usually be recognized. We may call them the "initial phase," the "transference neurosis," and the "conclusion." The duration of each, relative and absolute, varies much in different patients.

INITIAL PHASE

We have already mentioned this initial phase of therapeutic analysis. It may last weeks or many months, and consists in learning to apply the method of free association, the gradual emergence of bits of unconscious material, and increasing indications of a transference of current emotions to the analyst. In general, the transference of this period is either predominantly "positive," when there is zest, interest, and pleasure in the work, or "negative," as in the patient who was suspicious at the beginning of his treatment. Then the work is difficult for both patient and analyst, and immediate evidence of progress is very slight.

When the early transference is positive, the patient becomes enthusiastic about the "wonder" of psychoanalysis, and there is often a rapid disappearance of his symptoms and an appearance of rapid cure. Such early symptomatic improvement has exactly the same significance as that which results from other methods of psychotherapy. It is the direct product of assuming a pleasantly dependent attitude to the therapist, divulging one's private thoughts, and gratifying unconsciously one's need of parental love and protection. Even though it is ascribed by the patient specifically to analysis, this is partly an illusion. It would happen under other therapeutic relationships where a strong rapport is quickly established. Thus, the patient with speech difficulties was "cured" of his symptoms for several months by the specialist in speech-training quite as effectively as by the analyst during the early period. The difference between this and the results of a complete analysis is that it is symptomatic, temporary, and dependent upon maintenance of the rapport with the therapist. If this is interrupted, the patient will generally develop new symptoms if he is neurotic, or get into new difficulties in real life if he has a character problem, and seek to re-establish a similar relationship with other people. Indeed, the use of free association without thorough analytic treatment of the total transference reactions often results in a habituation of the patient to the pleasurable aspects of the free-association method. In this case the treatment has given the patient more satisfaction in his illness than ever before, and the result of the treatment has been to make the patient more neurotic and more satisfied to accept this fact, and has not induced decisive improvement or cure.

In either case, whether the patient reacts positively with subjective improvement, or without immediate pleasure, the introductory phase will consist of experience with free association and the routine aspects of treatment, the development of ideas and feelings characteristic of the individual, and an increasing mutual understanding of the assets and life-difficulties whose analysis is our objective.

TRANSFERENCE NEUROSIS

During the second period of analysis the "transference neurosis" usually develops. The situation changes. A patient who at first was eager for better health, absorbed by the treatment for problems he objectively acknowledges, intelligent, mature, and adult in many ways, no longer shows those qualities consistently during the treatment hours. So far as his efforts reveal, he is no longer so co-operative, is more indifferent to what the necessities of the treatment are, forgets or disregards what he has learned in the introductory period, and makes little obvious progress. On the other hand, he feels distinctly that he is battling with the analyst, attempts to trick him into doing what he does not intend, disregards advice. Gradually it becomes apparent that his most compelling reason for coming to analysis is no longer to get well, but has become the need to win some type of emotional satisfaction from the analyst. He will not close a door himself, it must be closed for him. He will wear no coat and risk pneumonia unless the analyst orders it. In innumerable ways these efforts to secure one thing or another from the analyst, regardless of any relevance to the objective reasons for treatment, may for a time be manifested as the dominant emotional need.

Because this occurs with such consistency in analyses, we can understand that the transference has developed to a point where the transference emotions are more important to the patient than the permanent health he was seeking. This is the point where the major unresolved, unconscious problems of childhood begin to dominate behavior during treatment hours. They are now reproduced in the transference with all their pent-up emotion. The patient is unconsciously striving for what he failed either to gain or to do without in actual childhood. Only those who have observed it or experienced it themselves will appreciate how fully some of the reaction to the analyst at this period is like a child's. Petulance, irritability, defiance, a childishness in the tone of voice are frequent, even in people who are otherwise in their daily lives quite mature.

The three outstanding characteristics of the instinctual life of childhood—the Pleasure Principle prior to effective reality-testing, ambivalence, and the repetition compulsion—govern the situation. It is not the outcome of analysis, but the need of the moment that counts. It was the full recognition of the significance of this period of "transference neurosis" by Freud, as a result of failure with a case he analyzed in 1899 and reported in 1904, that marked the beginning of modern psychoanalytic technique. And it is its full comprehension and management that sharply differentiates the adequately trained from the untrained analyst, and tests the skill of the best. The transference neurosis is one striking manifestation of repetition compulsion, and gradually one situation after another from the life of the patient—each the same play, but with different actors in the cast—is analyzed until the original infantile conflict is revealed. Then the transference neurosis gradually subsides.

CONCLUSION

The *conclusion* of an analysis dates from this time. In one "text-book case" the transference neurosis very suddenly set in the day after a male patient recalled seeing a menstrual pad in childhood, and the same recollection, which had been again unconscious in the interval, after eight months' struggle with the transference neurosis, marked the beginning of the conclusion. The patient again becomes interested in the original purpose of the analysis; his emotions toward the analyst are less infantile and more friendly and objective. He begins to appraise the therapist, not as a transference picture produced by repressed phantasies, but as he really is. Material whose analysis was incomplete during the initial phase again appears in the associations. Memories occur which explain previously unsolved problems, and the transference subsides, while latent and new interests outside the analysis appear, are valued and dealt with more realistically, and absorb more and more of the energy previously sidetracked in the transference neurosis.

The conclusion is a gradual process, and never complete with the last visit to the analyst. If the unconscious source of major problems has been fairly well exposed, further associations will occur from time to time at emotional crises in the patient's everyday life, and he can then complete without assistance what was not entirely worked through with the analyst. After a variable period the temporarily accentuated awareness of the unconscious dwindles, useful repressions are partially re-established, and the former patient deals with life with less need of introspection and more satisfaction and maturity than in the years before analysis.

RESISTANCE

Besides transference and the eventual development of the transference neurosis, another important and equally spontaneous result of the use of free association is always to be observed. The most conscientious efforts to tell everything that comes to the mind are in nobody completely successful. After a few hours there are always thoughts which the patient will not communicate or immediately, almost before he has noticed them, represses again.

Similar signs of resistance are apparent throughout the whole course of every analysis. They betray themselves in innumerable ways to the analyst: the patient abruptly pauses, corrects himself, makes a slip of the tongue, stammers, stops talking, plays with some part of his clothes, asks a question and waits for an answer, becomes very intellectual, is late for appointments or finds reasons for not keeping them, scrutinizes the rationale of analytic therapy, can think of nothing to say, suddenly regards what comes to his mind as banal or irrelevant and not worth mentioning. All such phenomena are technically known as "resistance."

The laboratory experiments of Carl Jung, which led in 1902 to his interest in the methods of Freud, give the most simple demonstration of what we now call resistance. A series of words was given to a subject, who was asked to report the first single word association which came to mind. The association was noted, the time which elapsed before it was reported, and any special changes in manner or intonation in reporting it. Jung observed that a significantly longer interval would elapse in reporting associations to certain words, and demonstrated that this always indicated subjective emotional significance for those particular words in any individual. We now understand the delayed response is an indicator of "resistance" to communication of some ideas.

Typical examples of resistance have already been given: for example, the inability of the illustrative case to report her associations for five weeks; the suspicious patient's refusal to quote what was said about Bob, and his suppression of obscene words from his reported associations. Another illustration of resistance in clinical practice is provided by a woman who begins analysis while suffering acute and severe manifestations of neurosis, so that the emotions which will form the transference are already manifest before treatment begins and merely awaiting a therapist on whom to direct them. Consequently the first few days of analysis are very like the situation in many analyses after several weeks or months of work. She immediately reveals in all the personal relationships she mentions a constant struggle between the ambivalent wishes to dominate and be dominated. She dominates her husband, and then complains of not sleeping nights; then says insomnia is the way his mother, an invalid, gets so much attention. Similarly, she greatly wants to be helped by the analyst, but can scarcely endure being so "humble." On the third day of treatment she telephones that she can't continue analysis; she says she must attend exclusively to her practical affairs, must rigorously control her depression by applying her "philosophy of life," and not take time for therapy. A week later the analyst answers his phone and recognizes her voice; she had asked for a wrong number. A few weeks later, her emotional difficulties unbearable, she resumes the analysis. Here we see clearly the reproduction of the external conflict immediately in the neurotic opposition of the wishes to be helped by another and to help herself, the resistance to analytic work which causes her to leave the treatment, and the rationalized opposal of this to the transference, which compels her to telephone the analyst by mistake. When she had phoned the analyst, she later reported, she had consciously intended to phone her mother-in-law, whose attentions from her husband she had already mentioned.

The development of resistance in analysis is quite as automatic and independent of the will as the development of transference, and its sources are quite as unconscious. The emotional forces which give rise to it are opposed to those which produce transference, and the analysis therefore becomes a recurring conflict between transference and resistance, apparent as the alternation of free association by the patient and moments or days of involuntary interruptions of his effort to free-associate. The full significance of this for analytic therapy is apparent when we realize that this is a repetition of the very same sexuality-guilt conflict that originally produced the neurosis itself. We have already seen that those instinctual elements of the personality which demand conscious acceptance and gratification of a wish are opposed by those which prohibit and enforce repression. Neurotic manifestations have been shown to be compromises by which gratification of the instinct with coincidental gratification of the repressing forces in the form of suffering is attained. Transference and resistance in the therapeutic situation therefore represent those identical forces which reach their fullest development and antagonism in the transference neurosis. The transference itself can even serve the resistance, in that the wish for immediate pleasure in the analysis opposes the eventual purpose for which the analysis was undertaken, to increase one's potentialities for mature and happier adjustment.

The recognition and analysis of the unconscious sources of resistance are a major reason for the therapeutic superiority of the psychoanalytic method. For other methods, such as suggestion, hypnosis, encouragement, and persuasion of any kind, utilize unconscious transference, but completely ignore those opposing forces which appear in unconscious resistance.[6] They therefore do not affect one of the two groups of etiological factors at all; and this indeed was Freud's original reason for replacing treatment by hypnosis for the time-consuming method of free association. For in psychoanalysis both components of the conflict which causes the neurosis are made the basis of the whole treatment; instead of efforts of one kind or another to circumvent one of the responsible forces, psychoanalysis, in contrast to other methods, exposes them and deals directly with all etiological factors. Paradoxically, the analyst's close attention to resistance is also the best of arguments for the chief superiority that other methods do possess. For the analysis of resistance is the reason why the psychoanalytic treatment lasts so long. If one *must* treat a large number of patients and give only a short time to each, one *must* ignore unconscious resistance and do the best one can. Nevertheless, the "gaining of the patient's

---

[6] This paragraph is transcribed from the first edition of this book. The contrast between psychoanalysis and other therapies that. ignore resistance is not so true today as then. Modern dynamic psychotherapy has learned from psychoanalysis to deal with resistance (see Chapter XII, pages 261–5, "Dynamic Psychotherapy"). Nevertheless, it is still true that only in psychoanalysis can the unconscious sources of many resistances be thoroughly explored.

co-operation" by either emotional or intellectual suasion in other psychiatric methods should not be confused with an analysis of resistance; for this is only to win conscious liking and confidence for the therapist, and the co-operation of the conscious and intellectual faculties of the patient. This has little in common with the analyst's attention to the unconscious emotional sources of the conflict and repression, regardless of whether such attention yields immediate pleasure or pain, enthusiasm or condemnation of the treatment.

Recognition of the value of analysis of the unconscious sources of resistance constitutes a landmark in the history of the psychoanalytic method. The fact of disturbed communication when conflict is activated had been recognized during the earliest years of analysis, but its value had not; all varieties of resistance had been regarded as unfortunate obstacles to be overcome, as road blocks to be knocked over or avoided by detours. But finally, as we have already discussed in our account of "ego-defenses," [7] analysts came to understand that resistances were themselves important consequences of unconscious phantasies. Recognition of this principle not only radically advanced therapeutic technique, it also enriched psychoanalytic understanding of *both* components of many conflicts and the adaptations to both whose aggregate is the total personality.

The treatment of resistance constitutes the main function of the modern analyst. For many years he has not undertaken to "teach" the patient about his unconscious. For, in the first place, experience has shown that this by itself is ineffective. And, in the second place, both conscious insight and, more important, solution of the emotional conflict and permanent therapeutic effect come only from what the patient himself says and remembers. In other words, free association, if unobstructed, leads to significant wishes and memories. Once the process is at work, there is what Reik called a "compulsion to confess," which produces the unconscious material. At the end of an analysis, or months after its completion, it is common for hitherto unknown memories or phantasies, which neither analyst nor patient had ever suspected, to become conscious.

[7] See pages 180 ff.

INTERPRETATION

Resistance, however, is never absent, except perhaps in some very severe psychoses, when this absence itself constitutes a more serious abnormality than any neurosis. The analyst, therefore, has become essentially a technician in gradually reducing unconscious resistance. The chief implement in his technique is interpretation. This is no longer used entirely, as in the early efforts of psychoanalysis, for the purpose of instructing the patient about his unconscious wishes, but is also used to help him understand resistance to spontaneous and helpful self-instruction. In other words, the role of the analyst as interpreter is not to paraphrase what the patient reports, but to indicate at appropriate moments what he is *not* reporting.

The critics of psychoanalysis have frequently declared that analytic interpretation is *only* a form of suggestion. Analysts do not deny that every remark of the analyst is indeed a suggestion and may correctly be regarded as such, but they do deny that this is the whole story. What is correctly appraised by their critics is the similarity between interpretation in an analysis and the non-analytic suggestion with which they are familiar; the differences are ignored. In the first place, the analyst repudiates as far as possible the prerogative of authoritative infallibility and makes no effort to convince the patient that *because* the physician says so, the statement *must* be so. Furthermore, to the best of his ability, the analyst states what he believes *is* so, in contrast to the practitioner of suggestion, who states what is *not* so—"Nothing is the matter; you are all right; do what I say and it will clear up. . . ." At no time does the analyst promise cure, but he maintains that cure is to a considerable extent dependent on the patient's ability to perform his part of the analytic work.

The patient's reactions to interpretation during analysis are also very different. The immediate result of analytic interpretation is not generally symptomatic relief, and is often a heightening of the strain, and specific resistance. Experience shows that if mistaken interpretations are given, unless they are absurdly frequent or stupid, their effects are trivial and have no observable influence on the eventual course. On the other hand, it is constantly observed in analysis that when a correct interpretation is given at the right time, the patient reacts either immediately or after a period of emotional struggle with new associations, and these often confirm the correctness of the interpretation and add significant additional data, disclosing motivations and experiences of the patient, which could not have been guessed previously by the analyst.

Effective interpretation of resistance is a difficult technique. We can best explain it by a few illustrations from the clinical material already presented. When the man objected to paying his bill [8] and in his associations that day told of similar emotions toward a friend who would give him nothing, the analyst's interpretation was that his attitude to the friend showed his real objection to the bill to be the wish not to give but to receive. The patient first protested violently, and then vividly recalled the infantile pleasure from his mother's toilet care. This and other material at the same time confirmed the analyst's deduction that the patient was resisting the unconscious wish to be given something pleasurable and added an infantile memory of this type of pleasure, which had previously been inaccessible to consciousness, and unknown to the analyst.

The woman whose Case History we have given uttered scarcely an association for five weeks during one period of analysis.[9] This resistance was interpreted (or, better, resolved) by the following analytic experience. One day she was looking out of the window of the waiting-room when the analyst entered. When, as usual, she said nothing after the treatment began, he asked her what she was thinking when gazing out of the window. "I was looking at the rain." She then commented on the weather and deplored the absence of other thoughts. "But 'looking at the rain,' " the analyst commented. After ten minutes' silence she remarked: "I often look at the rain, I stand by my kitchen window and look out." A long pause, and the analyst asked her to say anything that came to her mind. "I see the canal from my window, and a bridge. The canal boats go by." At

[8] See page 193, 193 n.   [9] See page 82.

this point the analyst had some fortunate associations of his own to watching steamers on the Rhine, and, feeling they might be a clue to the resistance, he interjected: "They go under the bridge?" For the first time in five weeks the patient suddenly showed obvious emotional tension. "I won't say it! I won't say it! There was water trickling down the window—it always reminds me of urine. I always feel so pleasant when the canal boats have passed under the bridge. They put the smokestack down, and then it comes up again. I don't like the smokestacks to break off!" Then she reported very emotionally her association of the stacks cut off with penises, and recalled the similar scene of her father's chopping off hens' heads. She subsequently associated profusely for weeks.

In the case of the suspicious patient who apparently could not learn to associate,[1] the technique of interpretation was limited to asking quietly every few days for one of the names he withheld. Each time this was done, the patient for a few minutes showed a slight emotional reaction, until he eventually stated that he was going to seek medical treatment instead of psychological and then confessed his secret suspicions of the analyst's character.[2] In the interpretation of the dream which finally disclosed the unconscious sources of this suspicion, the analyst remarked only: "The dream shows you are suspicious and afraid that if your girl seduces you, she will get you into a situation where a man will injure you." The next day the patient confirmed this by confessing for the first time his suspicion of the Russian and his fear that his girl would introduce the two. At the conclusion of this day the analyst's interpretation was only a question implying that the patient's rationalized failure to report obscene words was like the small boy's reaction to his parents' discipline. The next day the patient not only confirmed this, but confessed the infantile masturbation-punishment phantasy (or event) which had been previously repressed.

The resistance of the pathologically defiant man [3] required more unusual methods. In order to analyze it successfully, the analyst was compelled to call upon his full reservoir of previous experience and to make several unusually radical, "deep" interpretations

[1] See pages 196–9.   [2] See pages 197–8.   [3] See page 193, 193 n.

of the patient's transference emotions before the patient's actual associations had pointed the way. Their correctness and technical value were confirmed by a diminution of resistance and consequent recollection of his mother's prohibiting his use of the school toilet, and the associations which followed. Until this time the possibility of cure had been very dubious.

It is not generally so much what the analyst discovers that produces progress in the analysis as his ability to help the patient to discover *for himself* by reducing unconscious resistance by such occasional, carefully selected interpretations at appropriate moments. Arbitrary pressure by exhortation from the analyst is ineffective; the only pressure of lasting therapeutic value is that of the patient's own instincts, and the analyst's chief usefulness is in modifying unconscious resistance to them by making their mental representatives conscious.

THEORY OF PSYCHOANALYTIC THERAPY

Modern psychoanalytic technique is, therefore, the product of trials for two professional generations and many errors. It is born of experience which has shown that when free association is consistently used, transference and resistance will develop spontaneously and produce an analytic situation which is representative of one individual's personality and needs and conflicts and, in its details, characteristic of no other. The unconscious wishes and punishment phantasies which have caused the presenting neurosis will be repeated during analysis, and will culminate in the transference neurosis, the skillful utilization of which by appropriate interpretation of unconscious resistances will lead to its resolution and free the natural forces which determine normal psychological development.

The course and results achieved by this technique can be fully described without the dynamic theory of instincts, and the instinctual value of repressed ideas, but hardly explained. For the analyst's theoretical concept of his role is a little like that of the diabetes therapist. By administering insulin, no necessary food is added and no deleterious element is removed. The insulin serves only as catalyst, which permits a spontaneous, biological metabolism of the nutritive substances already present in the body. It enables normal organic functions to pursue their natural course.

Similarly, the analyst's theory is that each individual is endowed with potentialities which cannot be altered by any therapist. Their most satisfactory realization is dependent upon the distribution of instinctual energy among those various systems of the personality structure which determine subjective experience, work, and relationships with other people. The total potential biological energy available for these functions of the organism which are mentally represented is constant for the individual and can be neither increased nor diminished by active interference. But the aims and modes of tension-release can be influenced. In neurosis and other personality difficulties an excessive amount of the total energy is absorbed by unconscious infantile problems, whose expression in greater or less degree produces "abnormal" symptoms or character problems, limiting the patient's total satisfaction. Successful psychoanalytic therapy consists in effecting, not an addition or a subtraction, but a *redistribution* of the energy, so that a significant reduction in the amount devoted to unconscious infantile objects, conflict, and the maintenance of repression results, and more is then available for mature, guiltless, less compulsive and stereotyped activities (friendship, home-making, work, art, erotic love, etc.).

To accomplish this, the original emotional infantile situation is reproduced by the transference during the course of analytic treatment. In the neurotic this reconstitutes an emotional relationship with another person which in his actual childhood was inadequately solved; there had been excessive repression, not a completely normal solution. In his adolescence, this childhood conflict had been reactivated and intensified, but only a compromise, a "neurotic" solution had been achieved, rather than a new, mature means of handling the problem. By reproducing the emotional features of this situation the transference neurosis provides the personality with an opportunity for a new solution of the old problem. In some cases the details of the mechanism by which this occurs in the concluding period of the analysis can be very definitely observed; in other cases the essential elements of the conflict must be sorted out from a less obvious mass of associations to be understood.

The basic mechanism of analytic therapy is therefore the basic mechanism or the neurosis itself. This is the repetition compulsion.[4] During analysis it becomes very clear that each neurotic repeats the pattern of his neurosis, and the situations where conflict becomes most apparent recur over and over. This feature of neurosis is less apparent to psychiatrists of other schools than to analysts; for they observe the patient's history with special reference to the effect of successive environments upon him. The analyst has vastly more opportunity to observe that the neurotic's *unconscious* emotional attitude to very different environmental situations and to different people is repeatedly the same. The same drama, sometimes a tragedy, is played day after day, with different casts and sets. What the patient needs is a better play, not the effort to make a success of the old play with new actors and scenery.

Our Case History [5] illustrated how the same emotions and neurosis were represented in the actual infantile problem, in the jealousies at puberty, and again in adult life. A more detailed account would illustrate how, in many other experiences of this woman's life, the same formula had been repeated, abortively or completely. Thus, two years before the onset of symptoms, she had renounced a suitable sweetheart because of preoccupation with sexual phantasies of her elderly employer which corresponded to those she later lived out with her lover. She had solved this by fleeing from her job. At eighteen there had been a similar situation, in which she terminated a normal heterosexual "crush" when a girl friend told her of her abortion and stimulated the emotions and phantasies with which the patient had reacted to her mother's pregnancy when she was four years old.

The outstanding feature of the theory of analytic therapy is that it enables those very tendencies of human nature which normally secure a solution of an infantile problem without producing symptoms to become automatically effective. The transference neu-

[4] See pages 105–6.   [5] See pages 81–7.

rosis, if maintained by persistent interpretation of resistances, gives these forces a chance to accomplish what they did not adequately accomplish in the childhood or adolescence of the neurotic. The analyst can in no way force this result, he can only give the forces of the personality a new chance to deal effectively with an old problem. It is much the same as an incision of an abscess; the surgeon cannot thereby produce the cure, but can merely produce a situation where the natural curative forces of the organism may be more effective.

Thus analytic therapy is not primarily the management of an external situation, nor is it indoctrination with mental artifacts and theories. It is based upon inherent laws of psychologic development which are active in normal development as well as in the therapeutic situation. Adolescence, for example, is essentially a process initiated by the biological intensification of personal conflicts of childhood before the total personality is fully prepared by maturity to cope with them. Adolescence therefore becomes a sequence of experiences, each requiring a solution; and adolescence leads to maturity in consequence of the development of new mechanisms for dealing with such conflicts in consequence of these experiences. In so far as these new adaptive mechanisms are adequate, maturity is real, but in every human being some conflicts remain which are solved over and over only by repression or a repetition of immature processes. The essential therapeutic process invoked by analysis when successful involves the same processes of personality development as those to which each individual is normally exposed. Analytic therapy may indeed be correctly defined as a technical procedure which awakens conflicts inadequately solved during natural adolescence, and by reducing the need for repression it provides a second chance for a better solution. In so far as treatment achieves no better solutions, analysis is a therapeutic failure, and at best it never achieves the perfect solution of all life's problems. But in so far as it does lead to a healthier capacity for living, there has been a successful reactivation of the normal processes of growth which are also conspicuously intense during adolescence.

Though *permanent* therapeutic effect is, therefore, only attained through the emotional dynamics liberated by the therapeutic situation, the practical procedure is dependent on the ideas which either accompany conscious affect or represent unconscious repressed emotion. Theoretically, one may argue [6] that it makes no difference whether the ideas which are the instrument of the day's work are revealed or not. In practice, however, it is found that so long as the key idea remains unconscious, a large amount of affect is never released, and the neurosis is usually uncured. A typical and successful conclusion of the analysis only eventuates when layer after layer of significant life experience is exposed in terms of ideas accompanied by emotion, until the ultimate emotional source of the conflict is reproduced.

The human being is more complex than the machine. Analysis is always intensely human, and human sympathy, as well as scientific understanding, contribute to a skillful technique. Rigid adherence at all times to the fundamental mechanistic principles of psychoanalytic technique is impossible. The immediate environmental situation may sometimes be so serious that the analyst must pay common-sense attention to its practical bearings. A few people whose lives have been extraordinarily deficient in affection must be given more praise and encouragement than strict analytic technique encourages. Very narcissistic persons, and the psychotic, must establish a strong personal feeling for the analyst before even an effective interest in cure can develop. But the experience of analysts is that every deviation from strict technique which such special conditions compel prolongs disproportionately the length of treatment and increases its difficulties. Perhaps this is one of the soundest reasons for their opinion that the theory approximates the actual reason for the effectiveness of analytic therapy in many cases.

[6] This was the argument of Otto Rank and others. (See page 336.)

XI

THE PSYCHOANALYTIC PATIENT

A S in medicine, therapeutic indications and prognosis are functions of both the nature of the disease and the capacities of the organism to resist it. Similarly, the results to be expected from a well-conducted psychoanalysis depend on both the nature of the condition treated and the capacity of the patient to perform his share of the psychoanalytic work and to tolerate the unpleasantness of its difficult periods. In other words, a recommendation to a patient to be psychoanalysed depends on both his *need* and his *ability* to utilize the method.

We may consider separately these two aspects of a preliminary consultation as to the advisability of psychoanalytic treatment.

INDICATIONS FOR PSYCHOANALYTIC THERAPY

The psychoanalyst is not *primarily* interested in the treatment of symptoms. For there is no technique for treatment affecting the etiological sources of symptoms independently of psychoanalysis of the total personality. Every case will demonstrate that the obvious symptoms are only superficial indicators of a basic problem, like the summits of mountains which appear as threatening reefs above the surface of the sea. Many aspects of the patient's social, professional, and sexual life are involved. If nothing else is changed, nature's remedy, the symptoms themselves, may even be the best for the patient. But if the basic personality problems are solved, the superficial symptoms are also cured, as a valuable by-product of the analysis. Many symptoms—those of hysteria, for example—may be more quickly eradicated by hypnosis or other forms of suggestion, or by persuasion, discipline, or some other psychological instrument dependent largely upon the authority of the therapist. Yet in a large number of cases symptomatic relief by these means is temporary, and the basic difficulty will recur as some new symptom or some other type of emotional maladjustment. Analysis can never replace these other methods, however, for maximal service to large numbers of patients in a short time, as in public psychiatric and mental-hygiene clinics, though it has contributed to a better understanding of the effectiveness of these other methods. And psychoanalysis can never be of value in unanalysable cases where no other psychiatric service than good custodial care can be utilized, or where there is no prospect of a partial social adjustment without the help of some form of supportive, reassuring, or mandatory therapy. When analysis is possible, it seems, to those psychiatrists who have learned to use it, always the best method. When it is successful, it ensures a new level of personality function, independent of further psychotherapy, that is not attained by other methods which have the advantages of simplicity and brevity.

However, a knowledge of the presenting symptoms and those divulged in a psychiatric interview is necessary in the formulation of an opinion as to the need and advisability of treatment. We shall consider such presenting symptoms in six groups: psychoneurotic symptoms, sexual perversions, neurotic character problems, narcissistic neuroses, psychoses, and organic symptoms.

THE PSYCHONEUROSES

Psychoneurosis is, for the analyst, a positive diagnosis, based on evidence of a fundamental need to suffer beyond what environmental accident or physical illness justifies, in a person with a well-developed interest in other people, a potential capacity for erotic, tender, friendly, and sublimated love, and actual or latent ability for useful work. Evidence of such need to suffer (unconscious guilt) may be overt, as in painful hysterical symptoms, strong repetitive tendencies to crucial errors of speech and act which bring social disaster, intense feelings of inferiority, constant dissatisfaction, recurrent incapacitating depression, etc. Or the evidence may be disguised, as it is in some marital situations where the need for suffering is satisfied entirely by torments inflicted by the partner, in obsessions and compulsions which protect the patient from immediate evidence of the suffering but at the cost of withdrawal of energy from activities essential for enjoying life, or in coincidental physical illness. It may be apparent only in extensive inhibitions which restrict pleasurable potentialities, such as limitations of social life, impaired vocational satisfaction, and erotic impotence or frigidity.

Psychoneuroses are of two kinds, those in which symptoms predominate and those in which neurotic character traits predominate. This distinction is descriptive and not fundamental, for there are always neurotic traits in people with neurotic symptoms, and generally (in the past if not in the present) neurotic symptoms in people with neurotic characters, and the unconscious problems of the two groups have important similarities.

The most common psychoneuroses, in which definite symptoms predominate and are the usual occasion for the patient's seeking medical or psychiatric help, are conversion hysteria, phobias without psychosis ("anxiety hysteria"), obsessional and compulsion neuroses, and neurotic depressions. Classic *hysteria,* more and more commonly classified as *conversion hysteria* since Freud described its mechanism, was the original object of psychoanalytic study and today is the best-understood neurosis. Its characteristic symptoms, occurring most often in women, are bodily symptoms resembling those of physical disease but not caused by physical disease—paralysis, anesthesia, blindness, some convulsions, pathological blushing, fainting, some headaches, etc. Unless very mild in a personality otherwise well adjusted these are positive indications for analysis. The typical course of their treatment is the early alleviation of symptoms and the recognition of basic conflicts produced by genital wishes; the analysis of these conflicts usually leads to fundamental personality development in addition to permanent symptomatic relief.[1] But a minority of cases of hysteria can be very difficult or even unanalysable, especially hysteria in women whose personalities are exceptionally baby-like, and some chronic cases in which the pleasure for many years from luxuriant "secondary gains" are too great to be renounced.

Anxiety hysterias present different symptoms, especially active phobias, in people whose personalities and conflicts are very like those of conversion hysterias. The indications for treatment and its course also closely resemble the problems of conversion hysteria.

The *obsessional neuroses* and *compulsion neuroses* are more common in men and are characterized respectively by the occurrence of odd and useless ideas which dominate and seriously disturb useful conscious thinking; or of repetitive rituals which replace normal, adaptable behavior patterns. These neuroses were the second major field of psychoanalytic investigation and yielded, during the first two decades of the century, a large fraction of psychoanalytic knowledge which had not been learned by analysis of the hysterias, especially fundamental knowledge of anal eroticism, regression, punishment phantasies, and unconscious guilt; of compulsive intellectualization as a neurotic defense; of reaction-formations, the role of infantile sexuality in the development of character, and other major determinants of ego psychology. But though psycho-

[1] Our illustrative case (pages 81–7) illustrates a typical course of treatment of the neurosis of a woman whose presenting symptom, inhibition of telephone talking, was a hysterical type of inhibition.

analysis has yielded so much knowledge of the etiology and unconscious processes of the obsessional neuroses, treatment of them is
usually much more difficult and protracted than treatment of other
neuroses, and they are not infrequently incurable. They do, however, produce serious disturbances in total adjustment, and long
analysis of a case usually repays the effort, even though the cure is
not theoretically complete.

Neurotic depressions are characterized by seriously unhappy
moods, preoccupation with self-blame for everything, extreme fati-
gability, and paralysis of initiative in speech, behavior, and all the
ego-functions. These cases too are common, and though never studied so systematically as the hysterias and obsessional neuroses, they
are well understood and often much helped by analytic treatment.

Overt sexual symptoms. Often sexual neurotic difficulties are
not entirely unconscious, but appear in part as presenting symptoms. They generally occur in individuals with other psychoneurotic
symptoms or character traits, but may occur without the other
symptoms being prominent. Symptoms may be excessive masturbation and much worry about masturbation in adults, impotence in
men and frigidity in women in any of their forms, such as disinclination for sexual intercourse, vaginismus, frequent difficulty or complete failure in attaining erection, prematurity of orgasm, partial or
complete failure to attain the acme of sensual pleasure, inadequate
feeling of satisfaction, tenderness, relaxation, and drowsiness afterward, or lack of tenderness and desire for love-play prior to intercourse. Frequently, psychoneurotic aspects of the love-life are not
conspicuous in the patient's original history; satisfactory sexual experience is reported, while important problems in this sphere are
apparent chiefly in the failure to encompass the various needs of
love consistently with one partner. Such a situation is often revealed
by an extreme and chronic tendency to infidelity or promiscuity, an
incapacity for adequate erotic relationship with a partner who is
loved tenderly, or a lack of tenderness for a voluptuous mate. The
most clear-cut cases are those in which a man, for example, is
impotent with his wife or women of his own social class, but potent
with prostitutes or social inferiors. It is almost the universal rule

that even those patients whose love-life has been a satisfying one attain both greater tender and greater sensual satisfaction after psychoanalysis than previously.

These symptoms of impaired capacity for mature sexual love usually represent the repression of fundamental conflicts in relation to people in childhood, and are usually permanently relieved.

Some other symptomatic psychoneuroses are much more resistive to treatment; for example, *adult enuresis, tics,* and *stammering.* Yet such symptoms are usually definite indications for psychoanalytic treatment; the result is generally a valuable relief of basic personality problems, even though the chronically established abnormal muscle habits are not entirely cured.

SEXUAL PERVERSIONS

Sexual perversions are closely allied to the symptomatic psychoneuroses, in that both result from neurotic compromises of adult sexual conflict, and both commonly occur in people who are mature and normal in many of their adaptations. Non-genital sexual passions have long been considered by analysts to be "perversions" only when some sensual pleasure usually playing a secondary role in fore-pleasure has replaced the need for genitally induced orgasm. The analyst, therefore, does not consider desire for other erotic pleasures, such as use of the mouth or other erotogenic zones, perversions so long as these are contributory to genital primacy and lacking in anti-social consequences. From this point of view, Freud pointed out in 1905, *"neurosis is the negative of perversion,"* for neurosis is often the consequence of the repression of non-genital sexual desires, in contrast to the primary conscious demand for non-genital orgasm which characterizes perversions.

Psychoanalysis has, therefore, contributed a great deal to the understanding of the perversions. But this scientific knowledge is not to be considered equivalent to certainty of cure. Some sexual perversions tend to be quite intractable, and excellent results are not so generally to be expected as in the treatment of psycho-neuroses.

The results of psychoanalysis of *overt homosexuality* [2] are comparable to those of the perversions. The indications for treatment of patients whose homosexuality is accompanied by psychoneurotic difficulties are much the same as for heterosexual neurotics, and the results, so far as the neurotic symptoms of the homosexual patient go, quite similar. But the cure of an erotic preference for one's own sex is by no means assured, in spite of the large amount of psychoanalytic knowledge as to its psychological causes. In general, the more indications there are, either conscious or repressed, of some heterosexual interest in the past history of the individual, and the less completely he has adopted the psychological traits and habits of the other sex, the better is the prognosis. Few of those homosexuals who suffer intensely from society's disapproval of their sexual practices are not worth a protracted effort to release their heterosexual potentialities by psychoanalysis.

PSYCHONEUROTIC CHARACTER PROBLEMS

Psychoneurotic character problems [3] are more closely allied to hysteria and compulsion neurosis in etiology and prognosis than are tics and stammering. Analysis reveals that in many of them the structure of the personality, the infantile conflicts, the therapeutic indications and prognosis, are identical with those of symptomatic neuroses. Only by the fact that a character trait instead of a symptom is the most distressing conscious representative of the unconscious conflict can these groups be differentiated.

---

[2] The psychoanalytic and psychiatric usage of this word is often confusing. "Homosexuality" is used, as here, in the customary sense, to define an abnormal conscious preference for actual erotic experience with a person of one's own sex. But it is also often used in psychoanalytic literature to designate that normal component of the sexual instincts which produces non-erotic emotional relationships with one's own sex, or an excessive desire to adopt the modes of gratification characteristic of the other sex. (See "Bisexuality," pages 27–31.

[3] Referred to elsewhere as "character neuroses"; see pages 180–5.

For example, women with *hysterical characters* are hyperfeminine, constantly display volatile and immature emotions with theatrical exaggeration, and sometimes fall in love with a succession of men, each affair terminating in a fiasco. Such individuals have unconscious problems identical with those which produce the functional paralyses, headaches, and other symptoms of conversion hysteria, and the phobias of anxiety hysteria.

The *compulsive character* is over-meticulous in dress and social manner, devotes excessive care to the collection of useless articles, is either brutal or coldly aloof, accepts and enforces a very rigid moral code, is often secretly superstitious and openly very obstinate, is with great difficulty diverted from a rigid course of sternly intellectual thought, and constantly experiences special difficulty in making decisions. Analysis shows the unconscious origins of such a character to be very similar to those of patients with definite compulsions or obsessions.

Besides these specific neurotic character types, there are a variety of traits of definitely neurotic origin which, when they are conspicuous and constant sources of tribulation for the patient and his companions, are positive indications for psychoanalysis. A few of the more common are: uncontrollable temper, chronic nagging, constant complaints about others or oneself, excessive diffidence or feelings of inferiority, lack of self-confidence, inclination to constant change of occupation, repeated unsolved difficulties arising in vocational life, a succession of unhappy love affairs, difficulty in concentrating on work and duties and finishing a job, inability to take much pleasure in recreation and avocations, deficient capacity to make friends, etc. An especially common complaint is excessive marital discord, which is the result of either a neurotic choice of partner or a neurotic reaction to a maturely selected spouse. The problems of divorce should not be settled before analysis by people contemplating it, as analysis will often show that the unconscious cause of the situation in the home is a curable neurotic conflict.

Neurotic character disorders today are far more common than clear-cut symptomatic neuroses, and comprise a large fraction of the problems for which analysis is recommended. The unconscious basis of many of these problems is well understood and can generally be significantly and permanently alleviated by analysis.

NARCISSISTIC CHARACTER.

Narcissistic character is the analyst's bushel-basket term for a variety of personalities distinguished by extreme egocentricity, defective interest in other people and incapacity for tender relations, marked hypersensitivity to withdrawal of affection and approval by others, excessive need of praise, and a paradoxical combination of over-evaluation of their own goals in life and feelings of inferiority evoked by the inevitable frustration of their over-ambitious phantasies. The milder types are closely allied to psychoneurotic characters, so that the diagnosis is often optional. Many overt homosexuals are extremely narcissistic; for often they can love only one who seems like themselves. Narcissistic characters may often be much helped or even "transformed" by analysis, but the therapeutic prognosis is extremely variable. The more evidence there is of definitely psychoneurotic problems in combination with their narcissistic traits, the better the prognosis. Those varieties who are very unassertive and readily accept entirely dependent and passive relationships ("anaclitic personality") are especially difficult. Mild *schizoid characters* may be much helped, but they and *paranoid characters* should never be treated by analysts without general psychiatric experience.

Still more serious psychological disturbances, such as *alcoholism, drug addiction, psychopathic personality*, and *criminality*, have occasionally been helped by analysis. But the benefit from therapy is too often limited because people with these afflictions are almost unbelievably excessive in their infantile demands; they are lacking in fully developed maturity of their sense of reality, capacity to endure disappointment and other tensions, deep desire for normalcy, and other functions of the adult ego.

PSYCHOSES[4]

The psychoanalysis of the psychoses must be discussed with still less certainty and with more reservations. Certainly the applications of psychoanalytic knowledge of the psychoneuroses, as well as special studies of psychoses by analytic methods, have vastly extended our understanding of psychoses.[5] Today a delusion or hallucination without brain damage appears no longer a bizarre and meaningless derangement of the brain, but, instead, a phenomenon of definite meaning with a purposeful causality. On the other hand, some aspects of the basic etiology and functional structure of psychoses are still very obscure or unknown.

Therapeutically, psychoanalysis first spoke with some authority of *manic-depressive psychoses*. The first thorough studies were made by Karl Abraham, who concluded that two types should be distinguished: those cases in which a careful history showed that each psychotic episode was preceded by a definite psychological trauma, most commonly the loss of a loved person through death, quarrel, or rejection; and, secondly, those in which no correlation of psychopathology and life events was possible. Abraham concluded that psychoanalysis is of no therapeutic value to the latter group, in which the biochemical constitution of the individual is the dominant etiological factor, but that psychoanalysis of patients in the former group, carried out in the intervals when they are apparently normal and neither extremely depressed nor excited, is often of fundamental value and succeeds in preventing future psychotic reactions.

The *schizophrenias* (dementia præcox) have evoked intense interest among analysts, as among other psychiatrists. Invaluable contributions to the understanding of their psychology were made

[4] For full discussion of the psychoanalytic study of psychoses, see: Ives Hendrick, "Psychoanalytic Contributions to the Study of Psychosis," *Journal of the American Medical Association,* Vol. 113, p. 918 (1939).

[5] See Chapter XII.

by Abraham, Jung, Freud, Tausk, Nunberg, and other Europeans during the first twenty years of analysis. But they were generally agreed that psychoanalysis was of no therapeutic value, a nihilistic viewpoint based on the assumption of organic and hereditary etiology and far more dogmatically upheld in Europe than in America. To this psychiatric prejudice the analysts of Germany and Vienna added a special pessimistic dogma of their own by erroneously assuming that a patient whose diagnosis was schizophrenia was *ipso facto* incapable of an emotional relationship (transference) to the therapist, and therefore incurable.

American leaders in psychiatry during the first generation of this century were not bound by the dogma that schizophrenic patients inevitably deteriorate, and had extensively studied the relationship of past situations and present environment to this disease. As a result, American psychoanalysts who had previously studied psychiatry under such psychiatrists as August Hoch, Adolf Meyer, C. Macfie Campbell, William A. White, and Earl Bond were far more progressive and optimistic in attempting the psychotherapy of schizophrenia and reported some results which fully justified their efforts. Younger psychiatrists—notably Lewis Hill and Harry Stack Sullivan—who studied psychoanalysis but used technique and applied theories which differed even more than those of other analysts who treat this psychosis, have demonstrated similar results. There can now be little doubt that skillful and prolonged psychotherapy definitely ameliorates or cures the more morbid features of some cases. The question is still open whether psychoanalytic technique is as specifically preferable for the treatment of schizophrenia as of the psychoneuroses. Theoretically, it would seem that the creation of a personal emotional relationship is a primary goal of schizophrenic therapy, at least in the first months of treatment, whereas this potentiality already exists in a non-psychotic patient and is not the goal, but the instrument ready to hand for psychoanalytic therapy.[6]

Paranoid psychoses have also been treated by psychoanalysis.

---

[6] This is transcribed from earlier editions. For expanded discussion, see Chapter XII.

My impression is that severe cases are less amenable to analytic therapy than many cases of schizophrenia, but that in those cases where the paranoid process absorbs only a limited portion of the patient's intellectual and emotional life, the probability of complete cure is considerably better.

ORGANIC ILLNESS[7]

The many intimate relationships between the theory and the practice of psychoanalysis and the organic medical sciences inevitably awaken interest in the therapy of bodily disease by psychoanalysis. "Reversible" somatic symptoms [8] are so common an accompaniment of psychoneurosis that cures incidental to the major problems of a neurosis are a common experience of practicing analysts, taken for granted by analysts long before "psychosomatic medicine" became a specialty and a slogan. All degrees of chronic and intermittent constipation, anorexia, and other minor ailments of the digestive tract are very regularly relieved as a secondary consequence of the analysis of personality problems. More frequent still are the cures of a variety of menstrual disorders, and sometimes sterility of long duration, coincidentally with the relief of the emotional conflicts of female sexuality. A therapeutic effect on a variety of other common complaints is also frequently observed, such as constant colds, headaches, insomnia, pseudo-pregnancy, functional frequency of urination, and skin eruptions.

Cases in which a serious organic condition produces the major symptom, whose relationship to disturbances of the sympathetic nervous system and to chronic and acute emotional tensions is recognized by patient and internist, may justify psychoanalytic therapy. Asthma, thyroid disease, disturbances of stomach and intestine, and some skin diseases come in this category, but each case must be judged individually. The reversibility of the somatic process will be a major consideration. If it is irreversible, psycho-

---

[7] See also Chapter XIV.　　　[8] See pages 299–300.

analysis may still be recommended on the principle of preventing the continuation of the destructive cycle. Or it may be inadvisable because the original cause is no longer a psychologic problem; the somatic process not only may be irreversible but can no longer be halted. In such cases the misery produced by the somatic disease and the social incapacitation have become the major problems, and the original neurosis is of secondary significance.

All the factors which may preclude successful analytic therapy of a psychoneurosis [9] affect the analytic treatment of psychosomatic disease. As with the psychoneurotic, need and theoretical advantage are not in themselves sufficient to ensure an adequate therapeutic return for a difficult analysis. Moreover, chronic diseases of the body are even more likely to produce a fundamental change in the patient's major goals in life than personality problems. He often has gone too far in his natural adjustment to an invalid's life and habituation to its advantages, even though he honestly believes he is still seeking health. In addition he has an easier avenue of escape from the different stresses of analysis than the neurotic—the logical denial that there is any personality problem, and the belief that psychology has nothing to offer for his ailment. For the human mind usually regards the internal organs as external to oneself, very much as a baby treats its toes as though they were little strangers. It seems inevitable that this should be so, because we normally have so little subjective experience of our internal workings; our minds only receive messages of their activities when there is pain, and then the mental attitude changes, and a person thinks of "*my* pain," "*my* stomach." This fact is much exploited by patients to avoid recognition of personality problems by arguing that their organs, not "themselves," have produced suffering.

To how many individual patients and how many organic diseases analytic therapy, in conjunction with medical therapy, may be extended we do not know. Certainly the list will grow as scientific knowledge of the different problems and practical experience in treating them accumulates. Already there is proof that selected individual cases of organic disease can be and have been cured or

[9] See pages 231–9.

arrested by psychoanalysis, after other therapeutic methods have failed. They include cases of asthma, stomach ulcers, migraine, epilepsy, essential hypertension, colitis, and arthritis.

ANALYSABILITY OF PATIENTS

Analysis, in contrast to other therapies, is not a procedure in which the patient is a passive recipient. The analyst's role is comparable to the "pro's" in golf; he may instruct and direct and indicate the reasons for failure, but the pupil makes the shots. The competent "pro" may help his pupil to improve his game, and sometimes very remarkably; but not infrequently a pupil will be so deficient in aptitude as not to warrant the effort and expense. Similarly, every human being has some infantile, psychoneurotic difficulty and some stamina and capacity to seek the normal gratifications of maturity. When either of these opposing elements is notably small, analysis need not be recommended; in the one case the need is insufficient, in the other the possibilities of eventual gain too small.

The patient in analysis undergoes a difficult experience. He must be able to accept at times a certain increment of misery in his immediate life because of the expectation of eventual benefits. Each discovery of things about himself so painful that he has previously completely denied their existence at first produces an exacerbation of tension and reinforced efforts to deny and disprove them. For temporary periods his friendships and family relationships may become sources of intense irritation and bitter disappointment. At other times he will despair of any favorable potentialities in himself, of any value in psychoanalysis, of any friendship or goodwill on the part of the therapist.

The capacity to undergo such stresses is an excellent indication of a person's capacity to face the *real*, externally conditioned difficulties of life after analysis. Its presence or absence is often not obvious, though the analyst, because of his experience in appraising unconscious reactions, can generally form some estimate in advance. In doubtful cases he may recommend a short period of "trial analysis" for a few weeks or months in order to appraise the problems and potentialities of his patient more completely.

A number of factors affect post-analytic potentialities. We shall discuss chiefly those of age, intelligence, "ego potentiality," "secondary gain," and "real situation."

AGE AND GENERAL INTELLIGENCE

Chronologic age is a rough measure of total life experience; the more mature a person's experience is, the more readily he will utilize the analysis. This is partly due to a general capacity to deal more effectively with childish impulses and to accept the inevitable difficulties of adult life, but even more to the fact that it is only the repetition, as years go on, of failures and suffering that brings to an intelligent neurotic the conviction that the trouble is with himself and cannot be ascribed entirely to ill luck or the faults of others. On the other hand, with advancing age the personality gradually loses its plasticity and capacity to adopt new attitudes and behavior patterns. So, in general, an analysis will proceed more quickly to an effective result in the twenties and thirties, but it is also often to be recommended in adolescence and middle age.

Though analysis is primarily concerned with instinctual and emotional reactions, and not with one's intellectual appraisal of them, intelligence is an essential instrument in securing this goal. The feeble-minded cannot be analyzed (unless, possibly, when the intellectual defect is due to emotional inhibition of a constitutionally sound intellect). And a high-grade intellect will facilitate progress very considerably, though it will also facilitate the rationalizing of one's inner difficulties.

EGO POTENTIALITY

Ego potentiality,[1] or, let us say, potential "strength of character," is an indefinite term to express certain factors which are hard to define, but are of the utmost importance in prognosis. By "ego potentiality" let us denote a certain capacity for fighting difficulties, "grit," the ability to come back and try again after neurosis has led to a series of débâcles. To speak somewhat more precisely, ego potentiality is the capacity to endure an excess of emotional tension, to strive for reasonable goals in spite of inner difficulties which tempt one to accept the decision, "I am just made that way, let the others make the most of it," as an excuse for withdrawing from the struggle. During analysis itself, these assets will be clearly apparent during the more difficult periods, when a neurotic patient must temporarily be able to accept a certain increment of painful tension in order to attain the ultimate goals of the analysis. Sometimes the old neurosis will seem temporarily a much more desirable state, a less painful solution of conflicts, than the immediate effort to discover its unconscious sources and eradicate them. People who are not very neurotic may best comprehend these matters by realizing that the most serious strains imposed by the outer difficulties of their own life struggle are duplicated and magnified by the inner strains of emotional pressure in the person with a neurotic problem. In other words, the patient's capacity to fight the neurosis is as great an asset in psychoanalytic therapy as in other life stresses, and it varies as greatly among individuals as does the degree of neurosis itself.

The amount of ego potentiality is not always immediately apparent. One reason is that it may be utilized pre-analytically in the structure of the presenting neurosis. This is notably the case in those manifestations technically known as *reaction formations*

---

[1] What was here defined as "ego potentiality" in the first edition of this book (1934), (and in the German translation of this section, "Die Stärke und Tragfähigkeit des Ichs," *Almanach der Psychoanalyse, 1936*), has later been called "ego strength," and by that name has been widely discussed during the last fifteen years.

against an infantile impulse. Thus, in some neurotic characters, the excessive pressure to dominate situations, to assert emphatically one's individuality in unsuitable ways and circumstances, is the most obvious evidence of conflict and the most persistent cause of failure. Analysis often discloses that this type of egocentric arrogance is the result of constant need to deny all passive wishes, especially excessive infantile needs to receive and to be supported. After a successful analysis, normally passive needs become acceptable and can then be enjoyed in relations with certain people and in certain sublimations such as "taking in" music. The former capacity for assertion is then no longer exhausted by the neurotic need to deny the passive impulses, but becomes available for useful and pleasurable forms of adult aggression. In other cases ego potentiality may be largely absorbed by the struggle to attain special privileges and attentions; assertiveness, though an asset in itself, is then utilized in a purely childish way. In still other cases the aggressive components of the personality are not utilized in "reaction-formations," but are more or less completely inhibited and unconscious. This is often so in cases of impotence and in cases of men who have relinquished more or less completely any authority in family affairs and then suffer from the unconscious revenge impulses of wives whose own feminine phantasies of a "real man" are unfulfilled.

Thus, very often those individuals who most resent undertaking psychoanalysis, such as the lady who gave up analysis and then telephoned the analyst by "mistake," [2] have the most ego potentiality and therefore the best prognosis. Such people will feel intensely that life is extraordinarily difficult because of personal problems, but will over and over reject consideration of an analysis because of their admirable but futile reluctance to accept help for problems they want to solve entirely without aid. Eventually the causes of rejection of treatment prove to be the potentialities of a strong character, and they are only to be regretted when the individual never comes to accept the fact that a perpetual fight against inner problems is foredoomed to failure more often than many of the most

[2] See pages 206–7.

difficult battles with outside obstacles. Honest skepticism about analysis is usually a good prognostic sign if it is not so extreme as to prevent making a determined effort to utilize whatever the method may have to offer. On the other hand, a naïve, exuberant conviction at the beginning of treatment that the analyst will surely point the way to an untroubled existence, that analysis is magic which dispels the cares of life, forebodes very special difficulties after treatment is well under way.

The potentialities of mature adjustment may be very limited in some individuals whose apparent neurosis is not especially severe. An understanding estimate of their personalities will show very meager indications that any portions of their personality are really adult, or that any strong drive to combat the infantile portions exists. For example, there are men who really have little wish for anything but to be taken care of, and no innate tendency to fight this inclination. And there are women who wish nothing but to be given presents, who have no strong desire, conscious or unconscious, that there be other children in the world besides themselves. Such women will always prefer clitoris stimulation to a real man's love, and they make an insignificant contribution to either family or social life. Extreme cases of this kind contra-indicate analysis; for there will be no portion of the personality striving to utilize the treatment for eventual maturity, and the patient will permit it to have no other significance than that of an enjoyable hour a day of the doctor's exclusive attention so long as he will put up with it.

SECONDARY GAIN

Secondary gain may probably be considered a special case of ego potentiality. At any rate, it is a very important factor in analytic prognosis. "Secondary gain" comprises the secondary benefits which people with neuroses strive to obtain from their symptoms. The etiological factors which we have hitherto discussed comprise a "primary gain," in that the symptom or other neurotic manifestation is itself the adjustment ensuring a personality struggling with this or that unconscious conflict the maximal pleasure or minimal pain of which he is capable. "Secondary gain" is the result of the effort to win from the neurosis itself a "bonus," consisting in additional pleasures which could not be obtained without it. Thus the primary gain of a hysterical symptom, as has been shown, is the solution of the tension between an unconscious sexual wish and the need for punishment. But, once established, the hysteric utilizes his paralyzed arm as an excuse to do no work, his nausea as reason for special attention in the preparation of his food, his tantrums as a threat to people who do not do what he wants them to do. Gradually, especially if the neurosis is severe and the ego potentiality small, he will discover one childish means after another by which he may get people to do what he likes and not to do what he does not like.

The most common of these "secondary gains" is the use of emotional masochism, so that in cases with marked secondary gain the fact that the patient can love his symptom and enjoy his misery and its effect upon others may be quite obvious to everyone.

Secondary gain is often, in chronic cases, more apparent than the primary symptoms themselves. It is often treated by the inexperienced as though it were the neurosis itself, and is largely responsible for the attitude of many physicians that neurotics are only annoying, undisciplined individuals who pick a fuss and act like spoiled children. The fundamental pathology of the personality is then ignored, and the will to understand and help the patient is paralyzed.

On the other hand, a large group of therapists treat the secondary gain by logical or emotional suasion. But the sum of the temporary improvements that result is often more than balanced by the habits of increased secondary gain which ensue. For undergoing treatment itself is generally a secondary gain. Some neurotics come to require someone's constant sympathy and interest in their symptoms, and after a few years they are going from one physican to another for a diversity of complaints, until the pleasure in medical treatment, or sometimes in quackery, constitutes the major evidence of the neurosis. On the other hand, the assumption of a harsh, intolerant attitude will merely send such patients to other physicians or to illegitimate purveyors of pseudo-medical help.

The analyst, in contrast to many other psychotherapists, does not regard the secondary gain as the primary occasion for treatment, but as an important obstacle to be circumvented in his work. Not infrequently, secondary gain is so great as to impede seriously or entirely preclude successful analysis. For the patient has learned to derive so much that is satisfying from such secondary gains that the advantages of illness outweigh the suffering. Completion of analysis requires more than a theoretical idea that it might be nice to be mature; it requires a reasonable expectation that life will be pleasanter with a minimum of neurosis.

Secondary gains of such proportions that analysis is rendered ineffective are especially easy for the wealthy to maintain. With sufficient funds, a neurotic may hire exactly the type of personalities he likes to wait upon him, demand whatever sort of pampering he may require from those he pays, and autocratically nourish the fear of dismissal in those who attend him, much to his own satisfaction. It cannot be denied that under such favorable circumstances a neurotic may work out a far more pleasurable existence than is granted to many a non-neurotic. Some of the largest incomes among graduates of our great medical schools are earned by specializing in ministering to the secondary gains of these wealthy invalids in luxurious cradles, and disguising it by the flimsy veil of some sort of medical terminology. Yet we should not overlook the fact that the privileges of invalidism are by no means confined to the wealthy, but are exploited with equal avidity by many who prefer permanent disability insurance, veterans' benefits, unemployment aid, or lifelong social-service help to health and responsibility.

Secondary gain increases as a neurosis becomes more chronic, and this is the chief reason for advocating analysis while the neurosis is still mild. Too often, every ameliorative form of treatment is tried first, and by the time the analyst is consulted, the patient's original ardent desire and will to be cured is smothered in the excitements of habitual illness and preoccupations with a variety of treatments.

REAL SITUATION

The therapeutic prognosis can also be impaired by life problems over which the patient has no control. It is true that the analyst discovers how many of the apparently accidental misfortunes of a neurotic's life are the direct result of his own specific unconscious tendencies. And it is also true that during and after analysis there is often a spontaneous shifting of personal relationships, and increased capacity to handle well necessary complications in everyday life. On the other hand, a natural tendency to work out more satisfying environmental relationships after analysis is occasionally thwarted by real external situations. Those very relationships with certain people, which originally were conspicuous consequences of the neurosis, can sometimes not be renounced, even though the patient no longer himself requires the infantile gratifications and the suffering they afford. Such, for example, may occur in large and concentrated family relationships, where a dozen or so other members are as neurotic as the patient himself; in exceptional cases they may practically compel a cured neurotic to resume his neurosis, as the only method of survival. Economic stresses may play an important role. In order to earn his own or another's livelihood no new arrangement of his life is possible. No individual is a self-sufficient unit, and not only are his mature emotions constantly mingling, stimulating, and responding to those of others, but this is equally, or more, true of repressed impulses. The infantile sadism of one personality—a husband, a wife, a mother, for example—responds to the infantile masochism of another, and demands it, even though the other, after analysis, unconsciously as well as consciously desires a more mature relationship. Thus a neurotic employer may unconsciously be incensed because his cured subordinate no longer utters tirades of abuse, and discharge the employee, really because he is no longer neurotic. A nearly cured alcoholic may have no other solution with a wife who can't endure his being a man. These are common problems of analytic therapy. Of greater importance in many cases is the empirical fact that analytic results usually affect favorably the neurosis of the patient's spouse as well as himself and their mutual marital adjustment is frequently improved by the analysis of either.

SUMMARY

Age, intelligence, ego potentiality (in modern usage, "ego strength"), real situation, and secondary gain are, therefore, a few of the factors, in addition to the symptomatic picture, the total personality structure, and the ability of the analyst, which determine therapeutic prognosis. In deciding whether or not to recommend analysis, the psychoanalyst himself is generally in a far more favorable position than other advisers. Not only has he greater experience with the various factors involved, but he can especially appraise more readily and to some extent predict the complicated *unconscious* dynamics. It is not always those most obviously in desperate need who have the least to gain; in such cases a person's basic resources may be hidden by the acute distress. On the other hand, those who most successfully hide the evidence of serious difficulties from other people, who would rather suffer in private than endure inferiority feeling from acknowledgment of excessive difficulty, often struggle against a positive recommendation but ultimately attain most gratifying results. Injustice may be done to other patients when referring physicians postpone a recommendation for analysis many years, trying every other kind of treatment first. For analysis should not be considered a treatment of last resort, to be considered only if everything else fails. A patient riddled with cancer metastases is not the test of surgical efficacy, and the unfortunate whose life is a *complete* disaster is not the only test of analytic therapy. Rather, it is in general those who can survive neurotic suffering as functioning, partially successful adults, and those who can be helped somewhat for a long time, or a great deal for a short time, by other methods of therapy who can be helped most decisively by analysis.

THERAPEUTIC RESULTS OF PSYCHOANALYSIS

A logic-tight demonstration of the therapeutic results of analysis is utterly impossible. Even in medical therapies the smaller number of variables and the questionable reliability of some of the data present an onerous and often impossible task to the scientific statistician. In psychoanalysis the variables in the people passing judgment, in the personalities, symptoms, and other factors affected by treatment, and in the criteria of "authentic" psychoanalysis mount in hundreds and thousands.

The estimates of patients themselves *during* analysis are scientifically unreliable. Statements of discovering vital, previously unconscious trends and experiences are usually valid, but this in itself is no index of the therapeutic value of the discovery. Sometimes enthusiasm while in treatment is in progress is based on ephemeral elements of the experience, and is no more valid a basis of objective appraisal than are adverse opinions during a period when a patient needs to discredit the analyst and his work. The retrospective conviction of presumably successful cases that later periods of their lives have been much happier and more successful as a result of analysis is a more valuable criterion, but not to be advanced as final. The basis of satisfaction is sometimes more apparent to the patient and those few closest to him than to casual friends, though not infrequently the external manner and appearance of people undergo a marked improvement which is obvious to all.

The confidence that the intimate friends of patients have in analysis perhaps does more to promote the most desirable type of partisanship for psychoanalysis than any other single agency. It is they who see most clearly, and at the same time objectively, the beneficial results. Nevertheless, the individual opinions of such intimates are also sometimes unreliable or unscientific. The alteration of some aspects of a personality which were previously very pleasing to a friend may produce a marked bias in the judgment, though the patient himself finds new friends and interests which he values more. A group of women who do not associate with men may severely criticize the "change" in an analysed friend because she is less responsive to their enthusiasms and hobbies since heterosexual life and prospects of a happy marriage and motherhood have come to dominate her preferences. A wife who had found a large measure of enjoyment in domineering in the home and "mothering" her husband may miss in some degree these pleasures and declare him worse after analysis, completely oblivious of the fact that the happiness she derives from his increased tenderness, reliability, and potency is also the result of his analysis. On the other hand, a wife's enthusiasm may, when carefully examined, have no more significant basis than that there are fewer visits to her mother-in-law.

If anything, the carefully intellectualized appraisals of medical colleagues are less often valid than circumstantial opinions and impressions.[3] In addition to the emotional sources of opposition common to all human beings, such as the violent pressure to deny the existence of infantile sexuality, physicians are often entrenched in professional tradition, idealize the study of organic diagnoses and researches to which they have consecrated their own lives, and sometimes bitterly resent the convictions of analysts that mastery of Freud's technique yields a vast amount of empirical data and an etiological therapy. If there be a bias, there is never a lack of opportunity to justify an adverse opinion of analytic therapy. No analyst has ever eliminated *all* personality defects and evidence of neurosis in a single case, and critics confirm their adverse criticisms by observing these as readily as a man discovers the faults of one he hates. But even the most impartial and objective critics are extremely handicapped in their appraisals by the fact that so many patients state that they have been "analysed" when no such procedure was

---

[3] But see Leo Kessel and H. T. Hyman: "Value of Psychoanalysis as a Therapeutic Procedure," *Journal of the American Medical Association*, Vol. 101, p. 1612 (1933); Editorial, ibid., p. 1643; H. T. Hyman: "Value of Psychoanalysis," ibid., Vol. 107, p. 326 (1936).

These practicing physicians reported their opinion of the. results of analysts with patients whom they had referred for treatment. Although their criteria of therapeutic success should be criticized because they are based upon what would seem consciously significant for the patient before analysis began (for example divorce or improved marital adjustment), not upon the nature of the neurosis as disclosed by analysis, it is a valuable study.

undertaken, or when it was undertaken by one who exploited the word "analyst" without understanding the science and technique of analysis at all. Other patients have had only a very short period of analysis and have discontinued it themselves or been advised that results would not repay them. The general conception of what is and what is not psychoanalysis is very confused, except among analysts themselves.

On the whole, it would seem to analysts that their own impressions are not the least valuable criteria. Most of them have been disciplined in medical science and have assimilated its heritage of scientific ratiocination and skeptical scrutiny. True, they have as natural an inclination to esteem their own work too highly as have other human beings, but the inclination and aptitude of their analyst colleagues in detecting flaws in their reasoning and over-estimation of their successes are quite on a par with those of any other group of specialists. Certainly they are in a position to appraise all aspects of therapy as no other critics are. They know the details of each patient's previous experience, even those which he has most scrupulously concealed from his intimates. The analyst does not need to compare the lives of his patients with some personal theory of what a man *should be*, for he can compare the actual lives of a series of patients before and after analysis in every detail.

The criteria of "cure" are also very difficult to establish. Cures of symptoms are not usually regarded by analysts as the most significant data, except occasionally symptoms which have been unrelieved by repeated therapies of other kinds. Absence of recurrences and of further need for psychotherapy after analysis is more valuable. The analyst's chief basis remains the general adjustment to life—the capacity for attaining reasonable happiness, for contributing to that of others, and for dealing with the strenuous problems of maturity in an adequate way. Very important criteria are the reduction of an unconscious, neurotic need for suffering, of neurotic inhibition, and of infantile dependency, and the increment in capacity for responsibility, for success in marriage, social friendships, and work, and for pleasurable sublimation and recreation, relative to the patient's potentialities prior to analysis. Most important of all criteria, and perhaps the most difficult to appraise with certainty, is the release of normal potentiality for further development and maturation which had been blocked by the basic neurosis. From this standpoint, psychoanalysis may well be regarded as a second chance at adolescence.

The first available summary of therapeutic results by a group of qualified analysts was that of the ambulatory clinic of the Berlin Psychoanalytic Institute over a ten-year period (1920–30).[4] "Cured" was defined in the psychoanalytic sense of an essential personality-change resulting from a fundamental redistribution of instinctual energy formerly exploited by the neurosis, and as far as possible the cure was checked by post-therapeutic follow-ups. "Much improved" denoted an essential and worth-while change, but with considerable evidence of neurosis persisting; some of these would be "cured" by a short second period of analysis. A symptomatic cure resulting, not from a fundamental change in the personality dynamics, but from the temporary effects of the therapeutic relationship on the symptoms was classified as "improved." Cases in which the analysis was "interrupted" were chiefly those doubtful ones where a short trial was made, and terminated by a negative recommendation as "uncurable" by the analyst. The compiler, Dr. Otto Fenichel, called attention to the fact that these results were somewhat less satisfactory than those of private practice, for the following reasons: first, nearly half of the treatments were given by students undertaking their first analyses, though their failures were much reduced by the instruction and careful clinical supervision obtained at the institute. Secondly, a larger number of cases involved novel problems than in private practice. Thirdly, economic and other practical considerations more often led to premature termination of treatment; for example, the practical necessity for patients from other cities to return home, and the imminent need of many of the patients to leave Berlin to earn a livelihood.

A second report of a ten-year period (1926–36), published by Dr. Ernest Jones, Director of the London Clinic of Psychoanalysis,

---

[4] See Tables, pages 244–5.

SUMMARIES OF DIAGNOSIS, DURATION OF TREATMENT, AND THERAPEUTIC RESULTS OF THE BERLIN, LONDON, AND CHICAGO PSYCHOANALYTIC INSTITUTES *

(Rearranged slightly and condensed)

BERLIN INSTITUTE

Diagnosis	Total	Incomplete Analyses	Complete Analyses	6	12	18	24	Longer	Cured	Much Improved	Improved	Unchanged
(PSYCHONEUROSES, etc.) Hysteria (symptomatic and character)	105 / 57	31 / 25	74 / 32	19 / 11	22 / 4	18 / 7	7 / 5	8 / 5	25 / 14	21 / 6	22 / 10	6 / 2
Anxiety hysteria	10	7	3	3	1	2	·	·	·	2	1	·
Neurasthenia and anxiety neuroses												
Compulsion neurosis and character	106 / 37	35 / 13	71 / 24	11 / 4	17 / 8	11 / 2	15 / 5	17 / 5	21 / 7	26 / 5	18 / 10	6 / 2
Neurotic depression	80	24	56	6	17	16	7	10	21	15	15	5
Neurotic inhibition (sexual, social, vocational)	8	4	4	1	3	3	·	·	1	1	1	1
Sexual perversions	8	4	4	2	1	1	·	·	2	·	3	1
Homosexuality	13	3	10	·	·	3	2	·	1	2	·	3
Stuttering	4	2	2	·	1	1	·	·	2	1	·	1
Tics												
Character disturbances	37	7	30	7	6	11	4	2	4	12	8	6
Enuresis												
Infantilism	12	5	7	·	3	1	·	·	2	·	5	1

LONDON INSTITUTE

Diagnosis	Total Analysed	Duration of analysis (in hours)	("Satisfactory") "a"	("Improved") "b"	("Failure") "c"	"a"	"b"	"c"
			Therapeutic Result			Scientific Result		
Hysterias	31	230–600	13	17	1	12	17	2
Obsessional neurosis	17	aver. 445	4	13	·	7	8	·
Sexual impotence (includes 1 paranoia and 3 homosexuals)	8	·	3	5	·	·	·	·

CHICAGO INSTITUTE

Diagnosis	Total	In analysis at present	Duration less than 6 months	Completed analyses	Apparently cured	Much improved	Improved	Unchanged	Aggravated
		Cases			Successful			Unsuccessful	
Hysterias (includes anxiety and character hysterias)	26 / 10	10	6	10	4	1	3	2	·
Unclassified anxiety state	1	·	·	1	1	·	·	·	·
Compulsion neurosis	13 / 14	5 / 4	1 / 1	7 / 9	1 / 3	3 / 4	3 / 2	·	· / 1
Neurotic depression									
Disturbance of sexual functions	14	2	4	8	3	1	2	1	1
Stammering	1	·	·	1	·	·	1	·	·
Character disturbances	66 / 14	14	13	39	5 / 23	·	9	2	·

BERLIN INSTITUTE

Diagnosis	Total	Incomplete Analyses	Complete Analyses	6	12	18	24	Longer	Cured	Much improved	Improved	Unchanged
(PSYCHOSES)												
Manic-depressive psychosis	14	5	9	1	3	2	2	2	1	2	4	2
Schizophrenia and schizoidism	45	26	19	4	7	2	2	2	1	2	8	8
Paranoia	22	1	1	1								
Psychopathy	23	18	5	3								
Hypochondria	4	4										4
(ORGANIC DISEASES)												
Organic neuroses	3	1	2	1							1	
Organic nerve disease	3	3								1	1	
Bronchial asthma	2	1	1			1					1	
Endocrine disease	3	3		1	1					1		
Epilepsy	6	5				1						
Traumatic neurosis	3	1	2	2	1				1	1	1	1
Süchtigkeit	5		3	1		1			1		1	
Undiagnosed	9											
Totals	604	241	363	70	108	74	51	60	111	89	116	47

LONDON INSTITUTE

Diagnosis	Total analysed	Duration of analysis (in hours)	("Satisfactory")	(,,Improved,,)	(,,Failure,,)	"a"	"b"	"c"
Manic-depressive Insanity	7		1	5	1			
Schizophrenia	7			6	1			
Children (includes 3 severe eating problems, 3 cases of mental deficiency, 3 of antisocial behaviour, 1 psycholepsy, 1 failure to learn to talk)	16	aver. 332	9	6	1			

CHICAGO INSTITUTE

Diagnosis	Total	In analysis at present	Duration less than 6 months	Completed analyses	Apparently cured	Much improved	Improved	Unchanged	Aggravated
Manic-depressive psychosis	10	3	4	3	1	1	1	2	
Schizophrenia	5	1	2	2	1	1	1	1	
Chronic alcoholism	13	6	2	5	4	1	3	1	
ORGANIC DISEASE AND ORGANIC CONDITIONS									
Peptic ulcer	6	1	1	5	1	1	1		
Gastric neurosis	5	8		4	2	1			
Colitis	19	2		5	1	3	6	1	1
Chronic psychogenic constipation	3	1		1	1	1			
Epilepsies	3			2	1	1			
Asthma	2								
Hay fever	1								
Skin condition									
Female disorders									
Endocrine disturbances	5	5		5		1	1	1	
Essential hypertension	4	1	1	4		1	1	1	
Cardiac neurosis	1	1		1			1		
Migraine	3	2	1	1	1	1		1	1

* Statistischer Bericht über die therapeutische Tätigkeit 1920–30: Zehn Jahre Berliner Psychoanalytisches Institut (Vienna: Internationaler Psychoanalytischer Verlag; 1930). "Report of Clinic Work," by Ernest Jones; Decennial Report, May 1926–May 1936 (The London Clinic of Psychoanalysis). Statistical Survey, Five Year Report (1932–1937) (The Institute for Psychoanalysis, Chicago).

differed in some respects from the Berlin report. There had been only 91 cases whose analyses were completed, because during the early years of the London clinic there was a small staff and a smaller student body than in Berlin. The report summarized only two definite diagnostic groups; these are quite comparable to the corresponding groups of the Berlin report. Of special interest is the double rating—one of "therapeutic results," the other of "analytic results," the latter indicating the analyst's scientific success in learning the major unconscious factors. As in medicine, there may be a discrepancy in many cases between practical achievement and technical success; but the report shows this has not been the usual experience.

A third report was that of the Institute for Psychoanalysis of Chicago. In this, 226 cases were reported, but the therapeutic results were given for only the 114 whose analyses were "finished," in the opinion of the analyst. In addition to summarizing tables, an appendix gives important information on each case, including the secondary neuroses of the patient, as well as the primary. Although it covers only a five-year period (1932–7), and the time elapsed since the completion of all analyses was brief (6 to 18 months), it has special interest as the only report which includes a number of organic cases.

Abbreviations of the reports of these three institutes are given on pages 244–5. The original publications contain statistical detail and discussion which must be omitted here. Perhaps the point of greatest interest in comparing them is that, even with full allowance for great differences among the institutes in organization, personnel, scientific points of view, and details of method, there is a general correspondence in duration and outcome of analyses in those categories large enough to have numerical significance. The classifications of results in the Berlin and Chicago reports are quite comparable though the terminology is slightly different. The London report is less detailed, but "a" therapeutic results are cases labeled "cured" in the other reports, and "b" cases correspond to the "much improved." In all reports the higher grades of success are based upon psychoanalytic criteria of a fundamental change in total function—a very different criterion from improvement in the presenting complaint.

These three reports are of more than historical interest. They represent a new professional era, in which the published cases of Freud and other individuals are supplemented by such studies of the work of a group of psychoanalysts. In recent years there have been increasing discussions, reports, and symposia on the enormously difficult problems of scientific evaluation of psychoanalytic therapy. This led the American Psychoanalytic Association itself to undertake a major study in 1953, initiated by Dr. Lawrence S. Kubie and carried out under the chairmanship of Dr. Harry Weinstock of New York. Its purpose was the evaluation by modern statistical methods of data concerning the therapeutic results of cases treated by 675 members of the Association and 1,000 senior students in training at approved institutes. Detailed data on 9,000 cases, 2,500 on completed cases, were assembled, but in 1958 the project was discontinued because of difficulties in statistical evaluation.

In this generation the requirements of science, especially the more exact sciences, and of research method are becoming increasingly rigorous. Their impact is felt by the less exact sciences, and there is some danger of a false effort to emulate exact methods which are not yet applicable to psychoanalytic data. It is easy to overlook the fact that mere imitation of a laboratory or statistical science would not itself be psychoanalytic science. For one of the essential reasons why psychoanalysis has added to our knowledge of the human species is the fact that it developed its own method for exploring a total personality in terms of the uncountable variables involved and the variety of factors in interpersonal relations. If it had instead used a method based on reduction of the variables involved to a minimum number, as is necessary for a laboratory experiment, it could not have made its own unique contribution to knowledge. Freud himself was a scientist of high reputation in embryologic and neurophysiologic research before he turned to psychologic study. But, instead of following methods well known to him for the investigation of laboratory problems, he developed a technique for the fullest possible demonstration of all the mental and emotional processes involved in human adaptation and inter-personal relationships. The analytic situation is itself a special laboratory where *all* simple and complex relationships between the patient and other human beings, past and present, are reduced to the standard conditions of the interactions of two persons during the analytic interview.

Similarly, exact quantitation is the ultimate goal of every science, but it is never achieved in the earlier history of any, and in this respect psychoanalysis is no exception. We have discussed (Chapters V and VI) the achievements of analysis in applying quantitative thinking to its data, especially by the creation and application of the libido theory. That hypothesis has not provided an infallible or exact instrument for the quantitation of emotional values, but it has served better than could the arbitrary application of standards of other sciences. Finally, the "control experiment" is the *sine qua non* of proof in many sciences, but analysis, quite like astronomy in this respect, must study the phenomena as they come its way. Astronomy cannot, like physics or physiology, arbitrarily decide what kind of star will be placed in the telescopic field; and psychoanalysis cannot set up in advance a plan for just what aspect of unconscious thinking shall be selected for any individual's analysis on any special day. At present we may well be quite satisfied that psychoanalysis has provided a new fund of knowledge about the most complex operations of the mind, as well as a new technique for exploring such phenomena, and has established an appropriate set of principles for their useful evaluation.

PART FOUR

THE
PSYCHOANALYTIC
MOVEMENT

PSYCHOANALYSIS AND DYNAMIC PSYCHIATRY

B E S I D E S the position which psychoanalysis has attained as a specialized science for research and therapy, its effect upon the thought and techniques of general psychiatry has been profound. There is perhaps no discussion today among progressive psychiatrists, involving the non-organic aspects of their patients' lives, which does not imply acceptance of some of Freud's discoveries. The "unconscious," "psychogenesis," "repression," "defense mechanisms," and "ego" have become almost as much a part of the useful everyday vocabulary of the psychiatrist, psychiatric social worker, and many clinical psychologists as of analysts themselves. And the fundamental significance of childhood experience, especially the psychological derivatives of family relationships of the past in the life of the adult, and the unreasoned tendency of a neurosis to create not only specific symptoms but life-situations which reduplicate emotional difficulties of childhood, are today also accepted as fundamental by these professions. Especially is this true in American psychiatry, where a primarily psychological orientation to psychiatric problems began in the first quarter of this century, and has now extended to the psychiatry of many (but not all) medical centers, psychiatric clinics, and hospitals. This approach to clinical psychiatry, with emphasis on the study of psychological determinants of normal and abnormal mental and social adjustment, is widely known today as "dynamic psychiatry." It is that department of psychiatry whose central focus is the study of ideas, emotions, phantasies, conflicts, interpersonal relations, and personality development, and the manifestations of these in the conscious and unconscious experience of the individual patient.

Not that this professional usage of "dynamic" is entirely recent. It was a word occasionally used by Freud himself in his early psychoanalytic papers. But it was also used technically here and there by non-analytic psychiatrists interested in psychogenesis, acquiring its general meaning and widespread application in modern psychiatry in the nineteen-thirties.

The development of dynamic psychiatry has been complex, and we shall first describe the specifically psychoanalytic contributions of Freud and other analysts to the understanding of psychoses, then the development of dynamic psychiatry in America, and finally the applications of psychoanalysis in modern dynamic psychiatry and in psychotherapy.

CONTRIBUTIONS OF PSYCHOANALYSIS TO THE STUDY OF PSYCHOSES[1]

As most psychoses are regarded in modern psychiatry as purposeful adaptions to functional disturbances of thought-processes, not as meaningless consequences of undemonstrated brain disease, it has been inevitable that what psychoanalysis learned about mental processes, originally by study of the neuroses and of dreams, should illuminate somewhat the psychology of mental diseases. For "psychotics" are people; they have minds, emotions, personalities, and they respond to the same primal need for adaptation according to the Pleasure Principle as do other human beings. Psychoanalytic knowledge of the unconscious, of conflict, of the emotional relation-

[1] See also: Ives Hendrick, 'Psychoanalytic Contributions to the Study of Psychosis": *Journal of the American Medical Association,* Sept. 2, 1939, Vol. 113, pp. 918–25.

ships of ideas, of sexuality, the Œdipus complex, infantile sexuality, and of the repressive process, has therefore been a major contribution to understanding human beings disabled by psychosis.

But psychoses and neuroses are different kinds of maladies, and it has been essential to understand the differences as well as the identities. The most basic principle underlying their investigation is that psychotic symptoms, such as delusions or bizarre behavior, are not just random accidents but are specifically determined. This is, indeed, an application of the principle established by the pre-psychoanalytic studies of hysteria by Breuer and Freud, who had shown before 1893 that a hysterical symptom is not a chance product of a weak constitution, but individually determined by specific events.[2]

Probably the most easily understood application of psychoanalysis to psychotic thinking, though not the first to be understood, is the meaning of mental *symbolism*. Phallic and other symbols occur profusely in the language and behavior of many psychotics, as they do in both primitive and civilized art. The psychotic person, however, not only often thinks in symbols but is much more conscious of what many of the symbols mean than are other people. Thus a psychotic boy of fourteen reported during the first week of treatment: "I like to go on hikes and camping trips. I like to find caves; they're cut from the side of a hill, with bushes on each side, and there's water trickling down." A year later, he said: "I think of what I said about camping a year ago; I told you that because I didn't think then you'd know what I meant [symbolic picture of female urination]."

Still more important is the fact that delusions and hallucinations are in many ways identical with dream-thoughts, except that in psychotics they occur in the waking state. This similarity had been clearly recognized and scientifically formulated by some ancient Greek physicians and philosophers. Yet for two thousand years the fact was neglected by physicians until Freud mentioned it in *The Interpretation of Dreams*, and Carl Jung, in 1907, made it the basis of his most important contribution to psychiatry, his ap-

[2] See page 12.

plication of Freud's principles of dream analysis to the delusions of psychotic patients. This principle is the key to scientific comprehension of delusions. For many delusions, like dreams, are wish fulfillments, either obvious or disguised. Of still greater importance is recognition that the laws of dream work demonstrated by Freud [3]—the transformation and disguise of emotionally charged phantasies and experiences by such unconscious processes as condensation and displacement—are as applicable to the psychoanalysis of delusions as to dreams of the sleeper. The Greeks had an inkling of this astounding fact, but had not worked out the basic laws which Freud discovered.

Besides this empirical contribution to the psychology of psychoses, psychoanalysis made major theoretical contributions to their comprehension, especially Freud's theory of narcissism.[4] For another important similarity between the waking mind of some psychotics and that of the normal person when asleep is the absence of mental responses to real people; one does not perceive during sleep the actual existence of beloved people, and in some forms of psychosis the patient does not fully respond while awake to the real attributes of those about him. Karl Abraham, when a young student of psychiatry at Zürich (1907), had already recognized this difference. Freud developed the idea further in theorizing that in schizophrenia, paranoia, and similar psychoses there occurs what he called a "return of the libido to the ego," or a "narcissistic regression." These technical phrases mean that the individual's sexuality no longer impels to full love of another person, not even the pain-producing need for unrequited, unfulfilled, or ambivalent love which are such painful consequences of object-love in neuroses. The libido instead is turned "inward" upon an image of oneself, in the sense of loving with pathological intensity one's own body, a body part, a personality trait, or an ideal of oneself. In consequence, a psychotic person tends to restore that infantile state of mind which existed before he had learned to distinguish himself from any other person. This theory of narcissism has helped us to understand the

[3] See pages 18–22.   [4] See pages 117–21.

psychoses and to explore them further, even though Freud himself extended the theory one step too far when he concluded that in psychoses narcissistic regression is so complete that the patient has not even the potentiality of object-love and consequently cannot respond with a therapeutically useful feeling for his doctor.

During the period when Freud was elaborating this theory of narcissistic libido, he was also developing his first concept of personality structure [5] and thus providing a view of the total personality which his successors, especially in America, would apply profitably to the psychoses. Freud himself had some prophetic recognition of this; he made several passing comments that further understanding of the ego would eventually be necessary for an adequate elucidation of psychotic processes, even though he himself never applied his genius intensively to this profitable approach.

In the 1930's the studies of defense mechanisms in the organization of personality structure and particularly in the determination of neurotic character problems largely occupied many analysts. One by-product of these studies was increased analytic understanding of some psychotic defenses, such as projection in paranoid psychoses, pathological denial of reality, and the "acting-out" of delusions in psychotic behavior. A quite different application of the concept of personality structure to the study of psychoses had been suggested by this author in 1931, namely, the question: why do many psychotics, particularly schizophrenics, manifest not only "symptoms," but a partial absence or defectiveness of some functions ("ego-defects") which are always present in the mental life of both neurotic and normal people? [6] A few other analysts—e.g., Drs. Thomas French of Chicago, Heinz Hartmann of Vienna (later New York), and Rudolph Loewenstein of Paris (later New York)—and I independently developed during the 1930's various contributions to ego psychology which had one basic idea in common: that the ego is much more than an aggregate of defense mechanisms for avoiding difficulties, that it also includes a highly organized system of "executant" mechanisms for effecting the individual's

---

[5] See pages 140–3.   [6] Loc. cit., footnote 1, page 252.

relations with his environment. There are, therefore, in psychoses and some similar personality disorders, not only abnormal defense mechanisms, but also a deficiency of certain executant functions for effecting either the normal or neurotic fulfillment of wishes.

Before these new applications of ego-psychology were developed, it had been assumed that repression was the primary cause of limited wish-fulfillment in schizophrenia as in neuroses. Yet in many ways the stream of consciousness of schizophrenics is notable for a pathologic absence of repression. Not only is there commonly a preternatural awareness of symbolic meanings, but also a tendency to protracted production of infantile sexual phantasies, consciousness of which would cause intolerable disgust, revulsion, shame, or inferiority-feeling in a non-psychotic person. There is similar evidence in such patients of abnormal awareness of primitive hatred and jealousy and need to annihilate or be annihilated. Who but certain psychotics or very little children could find pleasure in handling feces, in masturbating with indifference to the presence of observers, in acting their asocial wishes without thought of consequences? There is therefore in schizophrenia some basic difference from neuroses in the whole structure of guilt and in the lack of effective punishment phantasies, as well as in the presence of delusional thought and pathological failure of reality-testing. From the perspective of personality structure, therefore, it is apparent there is a failure to develop some of the organized components of the personality which are essential for repression and for avoidance of guilt in a normal personality; and there is consequent "flooding" of consciousness by infantile, symbolic, and narcissistic thought.

Today there is in American psychiatry widespread recognition of the dream-mechanisms which determine the content of delusions; of the dominance of the primary process ("autism") in psychotic thought, which makes this thinking sound "crazy" to normals; of the clinical evidence of narcissistic self-love and libidinal infantilism; and, above all, of the pathological absence in psychoses of some essential functions of the personality structure. Psychoanalysis and many modifications of analysis are widely practiced in the psychotherapy of patients who were formerly regarded by Freud as well as by most psychiatrists as untreatable [7] because of the erroneous assumption of European psychoanalysts that psychotic patients, whom they termed "narcissistic neuroses," could not, like psychoneuroses, react emotionally to their therapists. Thus Freud's contributions to psychosis were profound, though the actual study of the psychopathology and treatment of psychoses has been much more intensively pursued in America.

PSYCHOANALYSIS AND THE DEVELOPMENT OF DYNAMIC PSYCHIATRY

The facts and theories contributed by psychoanalysis to the understanding of psychoses, and the facts and theories resulting from the exploration of the neuroses, together constitute the backbone of contemporary dynamic psychiatry; this is so true that "dynamic psychiatry" and "psychoanalytic psychiatry" (or "psychoanalytically oriented psychiatry") are today not infrequently regarded as synonyms.

From a historical perspective, however, it would be erroneous to regard psychoanalysis as solely responsible for modern medical interest in psychological processes. More accurately, Freud emerged as the greatest scientist of a historical era in which here and there a scientific interest in psychologic data was awakening. Quite possibly this psychologic tide was itself an inevitable reaction to the scientific age of medicine, which, in its quest for empirical proof during the nineteenth century had produced pathology, bacteriology, physiology, and eventually biochemistry, and achieved the acceptance of these laboratory sciences as the basis of medical knowledge. But this century of progress had contributed little to the understanding of neurotic and psychotic symptoms of a multitude of patients who confronted every intellectually honest physician in practice with his own ignorance and frustration. Inevitably, it would seem, physicians were compelled to seek in the study of mental phenomena answers to medical questions not elucidated by medical knowl-

[7] See page 228.

edge of the body, its functions, and its neurological and chemical structures. And that is what happened in the twentieth century; a few physicians began to study psychological material and produced dynamic psychiatry.

There were already in the medical sky a few signs of the dawn when Freud himself first edged above the horizon. Since the days of Mesmer (who died in 1815) the dramatic effects of hypnotism on certain symptoms had intrigued a few physicians. The great Jean Charcot of Paris, to whom Freud had first gone in 1886 in his quest for psychological enlightenment, had demonstrated irrefutably the effect of mind on some somatic processes, and other physicians in France were studying more carefully than hitherto the effects of hypnotism, though more from the pragmatic and therapeutic than from the scientific point of view. Their contemporary Pierre Janet had demonstrated before 1900 the significance of phantasies, and particularly the dissociation of certain groups of phantasies in hysteria, with scientific results which might well have proved to be landmarks in the development of psychiatric knowledge if the greater contributions of Freud had never been made. Even in the 1890's there were physicians besides Freud in Vienna who were interested in the possibilities of psychotherapy, among them Freud's collaborator, Joseph Breuer. In England F. M. H. Myers and the psychologist Wilfred Trotter called Ernest Jones's attention to Freud (1903), and the views of the great iconoclast Havelock Ellis on sexual psychology were becoming known. In America there was also a group of able men who before 1910 had established the *Journal of Abnormal Psychology* and the American Psychopathological Association; this group included Dr. Morton Prince, whose studies of automatic writing had produced his theory of the "co-conscious" (closely resembling the unconscious), Dr. James Jackson Putnam, and other Boston associates, all of whom were actively and productively studying the neuroses from a psychological viewpoint.

Of still greater importance in building the foundations of modern dynamic psychiatry was the lifework of a dozen or so pioneers who regarded the non-organic psychoses as problems of personality adjustment. Dr. Adolf Meyer, who had come to America from

Switzerland at the age of twenty-six, was the greatest of these. Though at first a pathologist, he was already initiating a dynamic view of psychiatry at Worcester State Hospital in 1900, and continued this work from 1904 to 1910 at the Manhattan State Hospital ("Ward's Island") as Professor of Psychiatry at Cornell. He was a charter member of the American Psychoanalytic Association, and from 1910 to 1941 was Professor of Psychiatry at the new Phipps Clinic at Johns Hopkins Medical School. A parallel (though not identical) development was inaugurated at the Boston Psychopathic Hospital, established in 1912 by Dr. Elmer Ernest Southard, a man of amazing versatility and originality of mind. One indication of his new interest in the relationship of environmental stresses to mental breakdowns was his collaboration with Miss Mary C. Jarrett in creating the new profession of psychiatric social work and in founding the Smith School of Social Work. Another is the lifelong influence of Southard on the development of such students as Dr. Karl Menninger, creator, with his father and brothers, of the first center of dynamic psychiatry in the West; Dr. Marion Kenworthy, pre-eminent for a generation in the development of child psychiatry and social work; and Dr. Lawson Lowrey, Director of the New York Institute of Child Guidance (1927–33). Southard's dynamically oriented work at the Boston Psychopathic Hospital was brilliantly developed after his untimely death in 1920 by Dr. Charles Macfie Campbell, who had previously been associated with Adolf Meyer at Johns Hopkins. Similar developments transpired at the University of Pennsylvania under Dr. Earl Bond and at Columbia under Dr. George Kirby.

An equally dynamic, but more specifically psychoanalytic, approach was initiated by Dr. William Alanson White at St. Elizabeth's Hospital in Washington, D.C.; his most original work, the application of psychoanalytic technique as well as knowledge to the treatment of hospitalized psychotic patients, profoundly affected the development of psychoanalytic hospital psychiatry in America, especially at St. Elizabeth's, Sheppard Enoch Pratt Hospital (Baltimore), Chestnut Lodge (Rockville, Md.), and the development of psychoanalysts in the Washington-Baltimore area.

The work of these pioneer psychiatrists, their associates, and their students in a few Eastern clinics was dynamic and original in the specific sense of approaching etiological research in mental diseases by psychologic methods. They all had in common the conviction that many psychoses represented forms of adaptation to intolerable stresses of the personality, that mental symptoms were intimately related to the prepsychotic personality of the individual, and that study of childhood development, especially family relationships, should be the basis for understanding the development of major personality problems.

These developments during the first quarter of the century in a few hospitals and teaching centers laid the foundation for the remarkable development of dynamic psychiatry during the second quarter. They were not entirely a consequence of psychoanalytic science, but were likewise based on the principle of exploration of mental and social experience. As psychoanalysis developed, it was constantly discussed at these centers, where it engendered heated controversy between the "Freudians" and "non-Freudians." The major differences between dynamic psychiatrists who did not practice analysis and those who specialized in analysis was the distinction between the psychiatrist's study of conscious psychological data and the psychoanalyst's primary interest in the unconscious and his method for analysing its infantile and early childhood determinants. These were very important differences, which at times made the work of non-analysts appear to analysts like that of a doctor who had never studied anatomy or used a microscope. But there was still a common meeting-ground; the controversies, though sometimes explosive, did not usually end in irreconcilable hostility. The segregation of analysts, and the separation of psychoanalysts and university psychiatrists which characterized the European situation, did not happen here.

This new orientation in psychiatry also affected the development of psychoanalysis through its impact on individual students. For these pioneers in modern psychiatry were the teachers of young physicians who became interested in psychoanalysis at their clinics and sought out the new opportunities for complete training in the late 1920's. And it was a two-way tide because they then returned to teach psychiatry and to apply the techniques and knowledge of psychoanalysis to psychiatry. Today psychoanalysis is widely, though not universally, accepted as the basic science of modern psychiatry. The main division between the two groups, the psychoanalysts and the non-analysts practicing dynamic psychiatry, is between those who apply to psychiatry what can be learned of analysis without special training and those who contribute knowledge from their first-hand experience as trained and practicing analysts.

PSYCHOANALYSIS AND DYNAMIC PSYCHOTHERAPY

During the first generation of modern psychiatry—indeed until the Second World War, dynamic psychiatry and psychoanalysis held important principles in common, yet the methods were essentially different. In psychiatry a history was obtained by the systematic interrogation of relatives, and a systematic and skillful examination of definite categories of a patient's intellectual and psychopathological functions was made. These two principal methods of fact-finding were supplemented by thorough physical and neurological examinations, and often by laboratory studies and tests by a psychologist.

Of paramount significance to the most progressive psychiatrists of this period, roughly 1905–35, was the study of the "personality": the interests, abilities, traits, and patterns of social adjustment which characterize each patient as an individual. Special attention was paid to both similarities and differences of the sick patient under study and his former "pre-psychotic personality" and its development. As psychiatric social work developed during the twenties, thorough "field-work" studies by the social worker, who visited the home, the school, the employers of the patient, were considered essential supplements to what was learned directly by the psychiatrist from the patient and relatives. These initial examinations of the patient were extended, often over months or years.

Special emphasis was given to helping the patient to understand he was ill and in what way, and to understand the stress situation of his life which had produced the illness. Techniques varied a great deal according to the interests, talents, and experience of the psychiatrist, and were determined to some degree by his psychoanalytic orientation or its absence. But until recent years they rarely included such requirements of therapy by the psychoanalytic method as scheduled appointments of fixed duration and interpretation of the unconscious.

During these years when dynamic psychiatry was emerging, many psychiatrists specializing in psychoanalysis treated some of their patients by those more superficial methods which are known as "psychotherapy." Though this was not the subject of many publications or extensive discussion by analysts, the Report of the Berlin Institute [8] included 955 cases treated briefly, as well as 608 treated by analysis; there were 738 in the London Institute's Report, and 715 in Chicago's. Psychotherapy without thorough analysis was even more common in America, where analysts working as individuals gradually learned to apply analytic experience and to improve the earlier non-analytic techniques. This happened more or less inevitably to those engaged in a predominantly psychoanalytic practice, and, remarkably enough, was not considered a special discovery or invention or the occasion for special papers for many years. Nonetheless, the function of some American analysts as teachers of psychiatry in hospitals, clinics, and medical schools, and in psychiatric social-work agencies, naturally led to the application of what was known by analysts and profoundly influenced students of psychiatry and social work in the 1930's. More and more psychoanalysts rode the crest of the dynamic-psychiatry wave, and during the last twenty years the applications of analysis to psychotherapy consitute a voluminous technical literature.

Since the Second World War, psychotherapy which deliberately applies fundamental principles of psychoanalysis has become the usual practice, not only of a few analysts, but of most nonanalysts, whether they are friendly or hostile to the science of the

[8] See pages 244–5.

unconscious. Today there is usually only one choice, the "new" kind of psychotherapy, or else therapy by shock machines, brain surgery, or drugs. Though there are many variations in objectives and techniques, it has become useless to try to distinguish by definition "psychotherapy," "dynamic psychotherapy," and "analytically oriented therapy." This tidal wave of dynamic psychotherapy has in some centers produced new problems. Some practitioners are sailing the stormy seas of psychotherapy before they have learned to take a reef. And some are like the novice helmsman of a motor cruiser who, when far out of sight of land, was given his compass bearing by a sailor and responded: "Don't do that— point!"

The technique of dynamic psychotherapy today is usually based upon three principles adopted from the psychoanalytic method. The first and cardinal principle of modern therapy is almost always "free association" by the patient, and, as in analysis, the patient, whether in the hospital, in the out-patient clinic, or in the private office, is assigned a regular schedule of appointments, each of definite duration.

The second principle of psychoanalysis to be widely adopted and consciously applied in contemporary psychotherapy is appraisal of the "transference" of the patient, and, more recently still, the "counter-transference" of the psychiatrist when responding emotionally to the patient. For the existence of transference is one of the outstanding and most valuable discoveries of psychoanalysis. It is not indeed a phenomenon peculiar to a patient in analysis; it develops, as we have described,[9] in a great many interpersonal situations, especially those in which one person reacts to another who is invested with professional or technical authority, such as a physician, social worker, minister, teacher, even a politician. The unique contribution of psychoanalysis is the clear recognition of those emotional reactions of people in such situations which are determined by their phantasies and previous love-objects rather than by the real personality of the analyst. The psychoanalytic method has provided the best opportunity for exploration of these transfer-

[9] See pages 192–202.

ence phantasies, and especially their unconscious determinants, and modern psychotherapy applies this knowledge.

The third principle of psychoanalysis which has been adopted by contemporary psychotherapists is *interpretation*.[1] In fact, it is this feature which not infrequently is regarded by the inexperienced as the only effective element in psychotherapy, and it is this feature which is glamorously dramatized in magazines and movies. Striking incidents of cure and unexpected release of forgotten memories do occur in psychotherapy as well as in psychoanalysis, but they are exceptional; in actual practice, therapeutic success usually depends upon much more complex and less theatrical sustained work, and not upon a single dramatic interpretation.

In recent years, therefore, dynamic psychotherapy has come to resemble psychoanalysis more and more, especially in the deliberate application of the analyst's knowledge of free association, transference, and interpretation. It also utilizes factual psychoanalytic knowledge of the unconscious, phantasy life, adult and childhood sexuality, repression and other defense mechanisms, object relations, and personality development. Indeed, the resemblance of contemporary therapy and psychoanalysis has produced no little confusion, and at times the clear differentiation of the two methods is not easy. The most expert in analysis recognize that their work does differ fundamentally, but cannot always define this difference clearly for others. The intensiveness of psychoanalysis, the greater frequency of appointments, the longer duration of the treatment, the opportunity for skillful analysis of dreams are true distinctions but not the only basic differences. Certainly much more complete exploration of the unconscious and reconstruction of the individual's development and its relationship to adult symptoms are achieved by analysis, and most especially by the analysis of the infantile neurosis which has been perpetuated in the adult's unconscious.

Dynamic psychotherapy is therefore today a product of the complex interrelationship which has developed over two genera-

[1] See pages 210–13.

tions between psychoanalysis and dynamic psychiatry. Without Freud and his followers in psychoanalysis, dynamic psychiatry as we know it and teach it today could not have evolved; but without other contributors to dynamic psychiatry, psychoanalysis would probably still be restricted to a much smaller and more isolated group of specialists, as it was thirty and forty years ago. The leading teachers of psychiatry in America created the students of psychoanalysis, and today a majority of psychoanalysts in many medical centers are happily repaying this indebtedness by teaching psychiatry in medical schools and hospitals. And dynamic psychiatrists are today seeking complete training in psychoanalysis in numbers which exceed the facilities of America's seventeen institutes.

SUMMARY

The contributions of psychoanalysis to dynamic psychiatry are, therefore: the demonstration of primary factors in the etiology of psychoneurosis and character problems; a less complete but revolutionary elucidation of several aspects of psychosis; an important and integrated theory of instinctual dynamics; and a specialized technique for the effective treatment in many cases of the basic unconscious conflicts which are manifest as the symptoms and psychological problems of the patient. Another contribution, as yet inadequately realized, is the rational appraisal of the *unconscious* dynamics of other methods of psychotherapy. Whether one evaluates these or ignores them, they are always effective in the reaction of the human being to psychotherapy, as to other experiences of life. One cannot affect conscious psychology unless one influences unconscious psychology as well, and for this reason psychoanalysis remains the basic science of modern dynamic psychiatry.

XIII

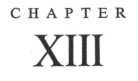

CHILD ANALYSIS AND CHILD PSYCHIATRY

T H E direct and modified clinical application of psychoanalytic principles to the psychoneuroses and personality problems of children also became an important specialty during the 1920's. For the discovery of the continuity of conflicts from the earliest childhood years until they culminate in the neurosis analyzed in the adult had made the treatment of these problems when they first appear in childhood inevitable. We can only wonder that the revelation of such fundamental determinants of childhood—the child's mental life and growth, his infantile sexuality, the Œdipus complex, the basic emotions producing family patterns, the meaning of phantasy and play to him—should have been first understood by the analysis of the unconscious of adults, and not until a generation later confirmed by analysis of children directly.

THE CASE OF LITTLE HANS

The development of this new branch of psychoanalysis had been anticipated by Freud himself when he published the first case of "child analysis" in 1909.[1] "Little Hans," as this famous patient is known in psychoanalytic history, had, when five years old, developed strong anxiety associated with an idea, that if he went outdoors a horse would bite him. The treatment of this "phobia," actually carried out by the boy's father, who consulted Freud frequently about it, was the first use of psychoanalysis for treatment of a child, and was the first occasion when the basic technique of child analysis, the use of play as well as verbalization, was attempted.

For several other reasons this case proved a landmark in psychoanalytic history. First, Little Hans's own phantasies fully confirmed Freud's induction from his analyses of adults of the significance of the Œdipus complex at the age of five. Secondly, the patient's phantasies confirmed directly Freud's earlier conclusion that a mother's pregnancy is well understood by so young a child. Thirdly, the boy's idea, after seeing his baby sister's genital, that she had been deprived of a penis and that all other females as well as males possess this organ, was one of the first clear empirical observations of what was later recognized as the "castration complex" of boys and girls. Finally, the case also provided direct evidence of the mechanism of anxiety hysteria which ten years later was to become the nuclear fact from which Freud's revolutionary anxiety theory of neurosis was derived.[2] In spite of these great achievements, Freud himself was inclined for many years to regard the successful therapy of this child as the fortunate consequence of an exceptional situation, especially the effective help of the parents, and he held the opinion that psychoanalysis of children was generally impractical since they had not the ego strength and conscious motivation to endure, as adults can, the painful stresses of etiologic treatment. But possibly Freud himself did not have that special talent for sustained therapeutic relationship with a child; for later work showed that he was over-cautious in this respect.

[1] Sigmund Freud, *Analysis of a Phobia in a Five-Year-Old Boy* (1909). English translation, *Collected Papers,* Vol. III; Standard Edition, Vol. X. Previous references in this volume to this case: pages 37, 72, 166, 170, 172–3, 267 n., 268–9, 280, 292.

[2] See Chapter IX.

ANNA FREUD AND MELANIE KLEIN

Child analysis as a specialty, therefore, has been definitely the
creation of the second generation of analysts, and especially of two
women: Anna Freud, daughter of Sigmund, and her pioneer group
of child analysts at both the Vienna Institute, including colleagues
in Budapest and Prague, and at the Berlin Institute during the
1920's; and Melanie Klein, at the London Institute during the same
period. The ideas and therapeutic techniques of these two leaders
and their students were both based upon the experience of adult
analysts and their methods, but they differed radically in some vital
principles, and the controversies engendered were agitated and have
not yet been fully reconciled.

Child analysis, as practiced by Anna Freud and her group,
was an application of the existing psychoanalytic knowledge of the
phantasies of childhood, especially those derived from infantile
sexuality and the Œdipus complex. But *play technique,* first used
with Little Hans, and further developed by Dr. Hermine von Hug-
Helmuth in Vienna, supplemented to a considerable extent the free-
association technique of adult analysis, especially in treating
younger children. Children were encouraged to reveal their phantasies in games they played, as well as expressing them in language.
Other basic modifications of the technique of adult analysis by the
Vienna and Berlin child analysts resulted from emphasis by Anna
Freud on the fact that the ego of the child, especially his capacity
for sustained tolerance of emotional frustration and realistic obstacles, is so relatively undeveloped. This was the same fact that for
fifteen years had made her father skeptical of repeating successfully
with other children the analytic treatment of Little Hans. Anna
Freud concluded from this premise that treatment of childhood
problems should involve education as well as analysis, because the
child necessarily has the difficult problem of immature resources
for controlling his primitive instincts and the problem of tolerating
repression and other mental controls. The child's unconscious, she
believed, is less decisive than the adult's in selecting and creating

his own environment, both its pleasant and its painful elements. The personality of the child is more the result than the cause of unsolvable environmental and personality problems, particularly those produced by his relations with other people.

A third principle of Anna Freud was that the child does not produce a typical "transference neurosis," [3] and therefore child analysis, if it is only a slightly modified adult analysis, cannot make use of this important phenomenon. The child is constantly reacting to the actual emotions of the people he meets, and does not inevitably reproduce the experiences of the past in his reaction to the therapist. In consequence, direct influence by the therapist plays a more active and real, a less passive and "transferred," role in the child's emotional life, and methods for treating him should take this difference into account. The child analysts in Vienna therefore originated methods for supplementing analysis by direct and educational control of the family and teachers. As there was in Europe no profession which duplicated the expert psychosocial study and supervision of environmental situations by the trained American psychiatric social worker of that day, the child analysts in Vienna recruited and trained teachers for a somewhat similar type of work in schools where progressive pedagogy and analytically oriented principles were interwoven.

Anna Freud also taught that in children with definite symptomatic psychoneuroses, like the phobia of Little Hans, child analysis is indicated, but this should be preceded by a lengthy period of preparatory treatment. The older the child and the more definite the neurosis, the more closely her method approached that of adult analysis. In adolescence, when the ego and super-ego are fully developed, mature sexuality is biologically established, and the essential structure of the personality is no longer altered by each change of environmental stresses, the therapeutic problem becomes essentially that of the adult. The main differences then are that the adolescent patient, though his neurosis is the same, has not yet the experience to recognize fully his own neurotic handicap in meeting

[3] See pages 203–5.

the problems of the adult world; it is rare for him to come for treatment on his own initiative, and hard for him to recognize the primary problem is himself and not just bad luck which won't recur or the cantankerousness of other people. For adolescence itself is at first a natural, biologically intensified re-awakening and re-experiencing of the repressed but crucial problems of the infantile period, a new opportunity for their solution. But it is often difficult or impossible for the professional observer to judge the ultimate outcome of adolescent conflicts and symptoms, to predict whether a good solution will be achieved as the patient matures or whether his unsolved problems will remain the basis of a repetitive neurotic problem of adult years.

The methods of Melanie Klein and her followers in London were like Anna Freud's in their use of play technique as an important supplement to free association. But Klein used play technique in a somewhat different way; she approached more closely than did Anna Freud the principle in adult analysis of relying chiefly upon work during treatment sessions. The little patients were given the opportunity to express their phantasies, and eventually their typical conflicts, in the spontaneous invention of games, and the role of the analyst was chiefly to interpret verbally the secret or unconscious significance of this play. Even more clearly than in adult analysis, this led to a freer expression of the revengeful aggressiveness of the thwarted child, and to a gradual diminution of the associated anxieties which are so intense in the child and so fundamental in his conflicts.

Not only Klein's technique of child analysis but her scientific conclusions precipitated intense controversies. Especially her description of the first three years of life clashed with views held in Vienna and Berlin. In the first place, she claimed that traces of an Œdipus complex can be observed even in the first year of life, and that it becomes an important determinant of phantasies and behavior during the second year, whereas Freud and his daughter considered that it becomes a crucial problem only in the fourth and fifth years of boys, and may occur at an even later age in girls. Secondly, Melanie Klein contributed new ideas about the source of primitive anxiety. In general, Sigmund Freud's conception was that the instinctual demands of infants culminate in real frustrations by adult prohibitions; that both the wishes and denial of them are elaborated in phantasies; that punishment phantasies are the chief occasion for excessive anxiety, and the ensuing frustrations of sexual needs reinforces the child's need for aggression. But Klein emphasized that the primitive aggressive phantasies of the first two or three years of infancy, as well as frustrations imposed by adults, are primary sources of intense anxiety. These primitive, aggressive phantasies of the earliest years, she contended, are quite different from the products of sexual rivalry in later infancy (Œdipus complex) which Freud had emphasized, and are earlier and more important determinants of both healthy and neurotic development. They especially represent desires to injure unpleasant objects whose existence within the body of the mother is vividly imagined, and the little child's anxiety is especially associated with phantasies of a retaliatory attack upon his own insides. By contributing such knowledge of early phantasy-life, Klein unquestionably made an original and important contribution. It was in the use of this knowledge by direct interpretation in the therapy of little children that she encountered strenuous criticism by analysts, except among her London students.

Not only did Klein's views produce a method of child analysis practiced chiefly at the London Institute; it also led in London to modifications of some principles of adult therapy and of the training of psychoanalysts. Her followers emphasized more than other analysts the need to analyze these primitive phantasies of the "internal object" (primitive phantasies about what is inside the mother's body), and the associated unconscious expectation of retaliation by the object according to the talion principle ("eye for eye, tooth for tooth"). This required longer analysis (four years being considered moderate) than is usual in other countries. My own observations have convinced me of the importance of the primitive unconscious phantasies described by Klein in certain types of cases, especially in the analysis of adults with inhibitions related to unusually primitive sexual wishes, and in some conditions allied to psychosis, but I do not feel that a method based primarily on this fact is necessary in the treatment of most neurotic and character problems of people for whom the everyday world has normal significance.

Destruction by the Nazis of the Berlin Institute in 1935 and the Vienna Institute in 1938 ended the geographical separation of these groups of child analysts from the followers of Klein. For Anna Freud and her students have since that time also worked in London. During the Second World War her efforts were concentrated on the study of problems of English children evacuated because of bombing, and the work of Anna Freud and her closest associate, Dorothy Burlingham, showed conclusively that the chief traumatic effect of war on little children was not the explosion of bombs but the grief and anxiety produced by separation of these children from mothers and other important people of their accustomed environment. In postwar years further development of child analysis and training of its practitioners has progressed in London under both Anna Freud and Melanie Klein. The controversies of the two schools of child analysis are less violent than in the twenties, but the essential differences of technique and ideas have survived the passing of the years.

CHILD ANALYSIS AND CHILD PSYCHIATRY IN AMERICA

In the United States child analysis also developed much later than adult analysis. It was scarcely represented during the 1920's. But in the early thirties American child psychiatrists who had studied with Anna Freud in Vienna introduced child analysis here, at first in Boston, New Haven, New York, Philadelphia, Chicago, and Topeka. Its development soon became a major interest of both analysts and child psychiatrists in America and was in the later 1930's accelerated by the arrival of Europeans from Vienna and Berlin.

Though the knowledge and techniques of child analysis were not used in the United States till the 1930's, the professional soil had been well prepared in the United States for a generation. What was later to be known as "child psychiatry" and "child guidance" originated in Chicago in 1909 under Dr. William Healy at the Juvenile Psychopathic Institute (later the Institute of Juvenile Research), and was developed by Dr. Healy and his associate in psychology, Dr. Augusta Bronner, at the Judge Baker Foundation in Boston, founded in 1917. The initial interest of these pioneers had been juvenile delinquency and court reform, but their work led to the early development of techniques in the new fields of child psychiatry and the closely related profession of psychiatric social work, to the training of early workers in these professions, and to the appreciation of the primary importance of dynamic psychiatry and eventually child analysis in comprehending the adjustment problems of children.

In 1918, the same year that the ideas of Dr. Southard and Miss Jarrett at the Boston Psychopathic Hospital had led to the founding of the Smith School of Social Work,[4] courses in mental hygiene under the psychoanalyst Dr. Bernard Glueck were inaugurated at The New York School of Social Work (originally the School of Philanthropy). After 1920 these were organized as a two-year curriculum for training in the new profession of psychiatric social work. Dr. Marion Kenworthy, as a young physician working with Southard at the Boston Psychopathic Hospital, had fully awakened to the possibilities of dynamic psychiatry, had studied children's work with Healy, and had in 1920 been the first American child psychiatrist to undertake psychoanalytic training. She joined Dr. Glueck at the New York School in 1920, succeeded him in 1924, and for a generation has been pre-eminent in the development of this school and of many other important developments in child psychiatry.

After 1921, "child-guidance" clinics were established in several cities, largely in consequence of the far-seeing policies and support of the Commonwealth Foundation, and the closely interrelated leadership of the National Committee of Mental Hygiene under Dr. Frankwood Williams (also an early associate of Dr.

---

[4] See page 259.

Southard and an analyst). In 1927 the New York Institute for Child Guidance opened under Dr. Lawson Lowrey, still another student of Southard, and Dr. David Levy, who had already in 1922 initiated part-time "mental hygiene" for children at the Michael Reese Hospital, Chicago. At the New York Institute the close integration of child psychiatrists, psychiatric social workers, and psychologists for therapy and research, as well as training in these specialties, was intensively developed. Though this pioneer center existed only seven years, its pattern of therapy and training rapidly extended to new clinics throughout the country, some closely, some remotely, related to the rapid development of psychoanalysis during the thirties.

Thus the orientation of American child psychiatry, like adult psychiatry, had from the first been "dynamic" in the sense that its basic principles were the psychological and environmental study of the non-medical problems of children. Treatment techniques varied greatly from simple advice to thorough exploration of the child's own conscious psychology and his emotional reactions to family members, school, neighborhood, and other social situations. Its methods were focused by the principle that treatment of children should involve the close professional co-operation of a child psychiatrist, a psychiatric social worker, and a psychologist (the "psychiatric team"). The new profession of psychiatric social work had become an especially important adjunct to investigation and to therapy, as study of family members by this profession produced a body of new knowledge about family relationships. Most important of all, child psychiatrists began to realize, were the extraordinary discrepancies between appraisal of a little patient's parents and siblings by adults and appraisal of those emotions, phantasies, and mental images of a parent which actually control the child's mind and adjustment. It became clear that the child's "subjective" impression often disclosed more of importance concerning his normal and abnormal development and his neurotic problems than the most perfectly "objective" description of the family members ever could.

This new definition of the essential problem of child psychiatry, the problems of understanding the child's mind (not merely his behavior, his social setting, his test scores, or abstract principles of education and training), was an indispensable basis for utilizing psychoanalysis itself. A few of the most gifted pioneers in child psychiatry had, between 1920 and 1930, already recognized the importance of adult psychoanalysis for work in child psychiatry and had themselves undertaken partial training in it. Thus psychoanalysis was influencing not only their own work, but that of students in this new field. Yet there were still only a few who approached these problems with expert psychoanalytic knowledge of the unconscious forces in parents, teachers, and foster-parents as well as in the child, and very few with training in the new technique of child analysis itself.

After 1930 an increasing number of American child psychiatrists felt that special training in child analysis as well as adult analysis was necessary. Some of these were most active in those clinics specializing in child psychiatry which we have discussed. Others contributed fundamentally to the development of a new field, "pediatric psychiatry," the applications of psychoanalytic (and non-psychoanalytic) psychiatry to pediatric services in medical schools. The first pediatric psychiatry had been developed at Johns Hopkins Hospital under Dr. Leo Kanner; though it made substantial contributions to the field, it was not influenced substantially by psychoanalysis. Dr. Margaret Ribble, after training with Anna Freud, began in 1932 to study the normal and abnormal psychology of nursing infants and its decisive role in development.[5] Dr. Grover Powers, Professor of Pediatrics at Yale, had already taken special interest in these new developments, and Dr. Marian Putnam, formerly a Yale pediatrician (and daughter of America's first psychoanalyst [6]), had been associated with his department as psychiatrist since 1930; when, in 1935, she returned from two years' psychoanalytic study in Vienna and attendance at Anna Freud's seminars, analytically oriented child psychiatry became an integral

[5] Margaret Ribble, *The Rights of Infants* (New York: Columbia University Press; 1943).
[6] See page 348.

part of the Department of Pediatrics at Yale. This example has since been followed by other medical schools of the country, especially those which have long been centers of dynamic psychiatry, and pediatric psychiatry has become not only a specialty for the treatment of psychologic and psychosomatic problems in children but a healthy influence in nursing and the hospital care of children.

Another very definite movement in the pediatric care of infants was deeply influenced in its early years by American analysts, in consequence of their knowledge of the importance of the earliest relationship of the baby and his mother on his later personality development, and the observations of a few exceptionally far-sighted pediatricians and obstetricians. This is the development of the "rooming-in" plan for the twenty-four-hour care of newborn babies by mothers, in a few American hospitals. The great victory of scientific medicine initiated a century before (1843) by the poet-doctor Oliver Wendell Holmes in protecting mothers against infection after delivery had led to universal separation of mothers and newborn infants for the first week or more of life in all modern hospitals. But in the achievement of this medical victory over infection the unnatural and harmful psychologic effects of depriving mothers of their babies had been forgotten or neglected. The principle of allowing mothers as much care of their newborn babies as they desired was envisioned at the Yale Medical School before 1938 by Dr. Putnam and her close associate and successor in psychoanalytic child psychiatry there, Dr. Edith Jackson, a pediatrician who had studied and worked with the child analysts in Vienna from 1930 to 1936. Administrative difficulties, the results of long-established hospital procedures, prevented the realization of this plan by Dr. Jackson at Yale till 1944, but not its ultimate effect upon professional thinking. Meanwhile, a small group of obstetrical, pediatric, and psychoanalytic specialists in Detroit had in 1942 organized a discussion group they called the "Cornelian Corner" under the Chairmanship of the analyst Dr. Leo Bartemeier, leading to highly successful rooming-in experiments in hospitals of Detroit and Washington, D.C. These Cornelian Corner and Yale rooming-in plans were thoroughly discussed, first at conferences organized by a Committee of the American Psychosomatic Society [7] and later at a series of Conferences on Infancy and Childhood (1947–54) of the Josiah Macy, Jr., Foundation,[8] a small group of analysts, pediatricians, obstetricians, and non-medical research workers. Similar plans in other cities in the last fifteen years have gone a long way in the reorientation of the medical and nursing professions to the basic mother-infant relationships.

Another new venture was the inauguration of the James Jackson Putnam Children's Center, Boston, in 1943 with Dr. Marian Putnam and Mrs. Beata Rank as Co-directors. This was supported by the Rockefeller Foundation, whose medical director, Dr. Alan Gregg, had taken an active interest in the modern development of psychoanalysis and psychiatry since his meeting with Freud, Jung, and America's first analysts as long ago as 1909. Dr. Putnam's original conception of the Children's Center had been a clinic providing twenty-four-hour care for babies under one year of age, and the opportunity for early treatment and analytically oriented study of their development. This, however, became impractical under wartime conditions, and the Children's Center became chiefly engaged in the development of new techniques for the daytime treatment of pre-school children, utilizing the co-ordinated skills of child analysts, psychiatrists, social workers, and specially trained nursery-school teachers. Research into the more difficult problems of this age group and their mothers and training in their treatment became a major contribution of Mrs. Beata Rank, Dr. Eleanor Pavenstedt, Dr. Gregory Rochlin, and many other staff members. The Children's Center has also been unique as a professional school for the applications of psychoanalytic psychiatry to treatment of the younger age group of children.

Not only has child analysis since 1935 been an important con-

[7] "Report of the Meeting of the Committee on Infancy and Early Childhood of the American Society for Research in Psychosomatic Medicine," Drs. Ives Hendrick and Marian Putnam, Co-chairmen, *Psychosomatic Medicine,* Vol. VII, p. 169 (May 1945).

[8] "Problems of Infancy and Childhood," Milton Senn, Editor (Packanack Lake, N.J.: Josiah Macy, Jr., Foundation Publications; 1947–54). Transactions of the First Conference, March 3–4, 1947.

tribution to therapy and to the exciting development of new facilities for child psychiatry; it has also, especially since the Second World War, made increasingly important contributions to the scientific problems of psychoanalysis, to its total knowledge of the unconscious and of the organization and early development of the personality. Psychoanalysis was already vitally interested in those more complex aspects of early development in which emotional factors and primitive identifications play a vital role. Recognition of pathological "ego-defects" [9] had led to important hypotheses by this author, Ernst Kris, Heinz Hartmann, and other analysts, concerning the early organization of the personality.[1] The science of normal development owes a great deal in more recent years to the empirical study of these difficult problems by child analysts. Dr. René Spitz, formerly of Berlin, initiated research in the infant's earliest visual responses to other people, in relation to development, and later to the pathology of the infant's dependence. Dr. Margaret Fries, of the New York Infirmary for Women and Children contributed studies of the relationship between the earliest behavior and the early development of definite neuroses in childhood. And the psychoanalytically trained psychologist Dr. Sybil Escalona of the Menninger Clinic (and later at the Yale Child Study Department) studied by direct observation the identification processes in the earlier stages of ego-development. The accumulation since World War II of knowledge from such psychoanalytic research by direct observation of infants and small children is rapidly providing a new basis for understanding the non-intellectual aspects of the "learning process," defined broadly as the acquisition during growth of new and

---

[9] Page 255. See also: Ives Hendrick, "Instinct and the Ego During Infancy," *Psychoanalytic Quarterly*, Vol. XI, p. 33 (1942).

[1] Useful contributions to the description and physiology of early personality development by non-analysts already provided an interesting substratum: the projects of Dr. Lester Sontag at Antioch College concerning neonatal physiology; of Dr. Alfred Hamlin Washburn at the University of Colorado in studying child development; of Dr. Arnold Gesell at Yale in measuring the development of mental and motor skills of little children; the epochal work of Jean Piaget of Geneva, Switzerland, on the speech and learning of pre-school children; and the studies of Charlotte Bühler on early child development (more closely related to analysis by their special attention to emotional factors).

effective techniques, mental and motor, for dealing with problems of the external world.

The fact that American analysts have been prepared by psychiatric training to make important contributions to the study of the psychoses is also apparent in a dominant scientific interest of American child analysts in this subject. Attention was originally focused on this problem of the psychoses of small children by a non-analyst, Dr. Leo Kanner, of Johns Hopkins Medical School, early in the 1930's. In recent years much productive study of the closely related problems of "the autistic child," "the psychotic child," and "the schizophrenic child" has been undertaken by analysts. These are all problems, under different names, of the pathology of little children who are abnormally unresponsive to the environment, especially other people, are preoccupied (like adult psychotics) with magical ideas, and are failing badly to learn about reality and to cope with its problems. Other major research by child analysts concerns depressions in childhood, asthma, and other important psychosomatic problems.

Since the beginnings of child analysis, the principle has been accepted in all approved training institutes in Europe and in America that complete training in adult analysis is an essential preparation for its specialized application with children. Recent studies [2] of standards for training in child analysis have shown that adequate facilities for full training exist in five of the American institutes, and that the development of such training is already well advanced in several others. This training is today increasingly in demand by many child psychiatrists as well as by future child analysts, partly because child psychiatry itself has now adopted basic analytic principles and is often taught by child analysts, and partly because some partial training in the problems and development of children by child analysts is being more and more recognized as a valuable contribution to full training in adult psychoanalysis.

In spite of this widespread recognition of child analysis today,

[2] Minutes of the Board on Professional Standards, American Psychoanalytic Association, Dec. 1955: *Report of Committee on Minimal Training Standards in Child Analysis,* Gregory Rochlin, M.D., Chairman.

and the rapidly increasing number of child psychiatrists who are studying it, there is considerable doubt that it may survive as a sub-specialty. For it is a paradoxical and startling fact that every year fewer child analysts are practicing child analysis. It is a strenuous occupation, and by middle age an analyst finds many cases a day fatiguing. And those who are qualified are in demand for work in child psychiatry, in teaching, and in administrative tasks. After years of postgraduate training—four in medical school, two or more in medical or pediatric internships, perhaps two years of training in general psychiatry and several in child psychiatry, and concurrently five part-time years training in both adult and child analysis—a highly skilled, no longer youthful, fully trained child analyst who has reached maturity rarely has time for this major specialty.

The situation in child analysis today is, therefore, that treatment by child analysis, the study of its techniques, and the training of its practitioners is highly developed at the clinics of Anna Freud and Melanie Klein in London, at five American psychoanalytic institutes, and in smaller groups in other cities in Europe and this country. The question of the future of child analysis as the most thorough technique of child psychiatry, involving treatment five times a week over a long period, is not even theoretically settled. But there is no question that the applications of dynamic psychiatry in child psychiatry, pediatric psychiatry, schools, and public health projects have stimulated not only interest but the desire of many young psychiatrists for training in child analysis; that, conversely, child analysis in America has made a profound contribution to child psychiatry, and to notable research in normal and abnormal child development. Play technique, discovered in the analysis of Little Hans and developed by Melanie Klein and Anna Freud, has been the most vital contribution of child analysis to modern therapy, and also to the exploration of the most subtle, complex, and often unverbalized phases of early personality development, the irrational aspects of learning, and the organization of social adaptability and the functions of the ego.

XIV

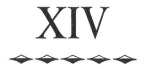

PSYCHOANALYSIS AND DISEASES OF THE BODY

T H E family doctor of former days is a figure whose passing is deplored, not only by those he served, but by the specialists who are replacing him. A sentiment enshrouds his memory, and, like all sentiments of distant things, it evokes to some extent a myth. Yet, though the sentiment does conceal his shortcomings, it also perpetuates the memory of what he really did for people, his ministrations of the best the medical knowledge of a former day provided, and deeds of the heart which cannot be learned in the laboratory or bought at a drugstore. Though he knew too little, by modern standards, of tissues and diseases, he did not overlook their relation to the "total man," to the way his patients lived and acted. He gave more attention to the whole life-course of his patients than to the test-tube and the microscope.

Some physicians honor psychiatrists with the opinion that it is upon them that the mantle of the family doctor has fallen. In actual fact, psychiatry cannot claim this tribute; it is itself too limited by the defects of this age of specialization. Yet psychiatry is at least the only modern specialty whose practitioners take hours (and often years) to learn how a patient looks at things, how he used to live and how he lives today, how his whole life is related to his illness, and how he reacts mentally to disease. It is the only medical specialty which takes full cognizance of unsophisticated words, phantasies, and emotions; it is not exclusively preoccupied with the machinery and the chemistry of the human body. Emotions, thought, and behavior, which are the primary objects of modern psychiatric study, are manifestations of the integrated total organism, not of an anatomical fragment. In this important respect psychiatry, and especially psychoanalysis, may justly claim that it is filling a scientific place which other specialties tend to ignore in practice, even when they protest sincerely against doing so in theory. It has contributed a new basic science to medicine, in the exact sense of a science based upon data, the psychologic, which are not expertly studied by other branches of medicine.

MEDICAL PRACTICE AND THE TOTALITY CONCEPT

What was called the "totality concept in medicine" by Dr. Karl Menninger, the "organismal concept" by Dr. Flanders Dunbar, the "holistic concept" by Drs. Stanley Cobb and Angya, is today emerging as a basic orientation in several departments of medicine. Dr. Adolf Meyer, the "father of modern psychiatry," had in fact already in 1915 defined "psychobiology" as "activity and behavior of the total organism." And Dr. William Alanson White, pioneer in the applications of analysis to therapy of the psychoses, had enunciated the principle with equal clarity in 1927 and in earlier reviews, while his associate, Dr. Nolan D. C. Lewis, worked at its application to the psycho-physical problems of hospital patients with psychoses. It is the fundamental premise of research and practice in today's "psychosomatic medicine." It is the idea that the total life experience of a person, especially his conflicts, frustrations, and other emotional difficulties, are causally important in producing some abnormalities of tissue structure and function. It is therefore a concept of the relation of the total organism to its parts. It serves as a junction-point for some important aspects of modern medical, physiologic, and psychiatric thinking and study.

This totality concept is especially relevant to important problems of clinical medicine. Practicing physicians have long known—though in scientific discussions it was until recent years usually disregarded—that emotional crises repeatedly initiate the diseases of some organs. As the relationships of emotions to clinical problems are most productively studied by psychologic data, it has been inevitable that the knowledge and technique of psychoanalysis should be made available for their deeper exploration.

These implications of the totality concept are well illustrated by their applications to Graves' disease, a serious disease of the thyroid gland, involving a swollen "goiter" of the gland in the neck, bulging eyes, quickening of emotional reactions, and an abnormal excitability of the heart which can sometimes lead to death. Explanation of its abnormal physiology is one of the achievements of modern chemistry. The substance which this gland produces, "thyroxin," has been chemically analyzed and artificially manufactured. Many lives are saved by medical and surgical application of this knowledge. But these valuable treatments are directed at the dangerous symptoms after the gland has become diseased. When the investigator searches for the cause, he encounters the fact that the symptoms of a large percentage of these cases began immediately after some situation, often trivial in itself, had produced an emotional storm. Thus the psychiatric exploration of one woman, admitted to the hospital for a third serious—indeed, life-threatening—attack of Graves' disease, disclosed what she herself had not recognized: that each medical episode had immediately followed the occurrence of extreme rage when she and her mother, both intense man-haters, discovered that a male neighbor had driven his car across their front lawn. This fact not only adds significant understanding of the etiology of the medical symptoms, but suggests the therapeutic possibility of analysing the reasons for repression of such violent hate.

The medical profession of America was dramatically challenged in regard to another disease twenty-five years ago by two of the world's greatest surgeons. They were Dr. Charles Mayo, who with his brother had built the greatest surgery clinic in America, the

Mayo Foundation; and Dr. Harvey Cushing, pioneer in operations on the brain and creator of a surgical specialty of pre-eminent importance. Both men declared at large medical meetings that stomach ulcers could be influenced by emotional tension. Dr. Cushing, who as early as 1913 had polemicized concerning the importance of emotions in the etiology of diseases, in 1932 reported his experimental evidence that an organ of the nervous system (hypothalmus) controlling much of the machinery of emotions could transmit currents which cause ulcer of the stomach, and concluded that emotional tribulation could therefore produce this physiologic effect.[1] The revolutionary impact of these words was not the novelty of the idea; it was its emphasis by men who had achieved greatness in the study of body-mechanics and surgical treatment, surgeons whose primary medical interests were directed not at all by the data of modern psychiatry or analysis, but by their own observations.

And there are many other diseases in which clinicians have long recognized a close relationship with emotional experience. Asthma is a classic example. Medicine has shown that many who suffer severely from the gasping, breath-restricting spasms of asthma are physically over-sensitive to one or more proteins which they breathe as dust into their lungs, ingest with their food, or touch with their skins. Medicine has devised tests to demonstrate the special sensitiveness ("allergy") of many of these individuals to a specific chemical (usually a protein). After its identification the dangerous substance may be avoided, if it is feasible; or the sensitiveness may be reduced by chemical "de-sensitization" of the body. In many cases these methods have sufficed to cure the distressing symptoms of asthma, but not in all. For it is also well known to physicians that the onset and recurrences of asthma often bear a close relationship to the emotional lives of many patients—whether or not their protein-sensitiveness is one of the causes. The first symptoms of asthma, for example, sometimes appear in conjunction with nightmares, especially in small children. Some people are asthmatic when married to one person and are relieved by divorce

[1] Harvey Cushing, M.D., "Peptic Ulcers and the Interbrain," *Journal of Surgery, Gynecology, and Obstetrics*, Vol. 55 (1932), No. 1.

and remarriage. In one classic case a patient's asthmatic attacks were shown to be due to a definite chemical reaction to the pollen of primroses; but it was also demonstrated that identical attacks could be induced under deep hypnosis by suggesting the idea of primroses to the patient's mind. In a case of this author's, a long search by a famous specialist in medicine for the chemical cause had finally shown that the patient was sensitive only to the fur of cats, and only to a special species of cat at that. In spite of this accurate medical analysis of his allergic sensitivity, it stll remained a mystery why the patient did not always have asthma when exposed to the fur of this breed, but only during a definite period of certain weeks each year, until it was discovered during psychoanalysis that his asthmatic sensitivity developed only when he was exposed to an individual cat of the species to which he was allergic. This cat belonged to an aunt whom he visited during these weeks each year, and, deeper analysis showed, he was threatened by the possibility of recalling the deep rejection by this aunt in his infancy and childhood, and the repression of his intense jealousy of her beloved animals.

PSYCHIATRY AND ORGANIC DISEASE

Dynamic psychiatrists as well as internists have accumulated a multitude of similar observations upon the relationship of emotional processes to activities of the body of an indubitably "organic" nature. A common observation has been that severe psychoses (schizophrenia, for example) frequently improve, even to the point of total recovery, when the patient is ill with a fever. Conversely, statistical studies have shown that a large percentage of patients with incurable psychoses tend to be much less susceptible to acute infectious diseases, more susceptible to tuberculosis. In more recent years, analysts investigating some organic diseases in whose etiology emotional problems have played a part have observed that when a patient is relieved of his organic symptoms, he may develop a definite mental disturbance. The nature of such reciprocal relationships is not by any means clear, but there is sufficient evidence to indicate that the inner tensions of some people alternately produce either physical or mental difficulty, one type of illness apparently protecting them against the other or making it unnecessary.

Of equal interest are the facts concerning actual organic disease revealed in medical histories taken by the psychiatrist in his everyday work. These are facts he shares with his medical colleagues, but they are appraised with a different perspective. In these and many other ways, some duplicating the experience of other specialists and some uniquely his own, the clinical experience of the psychiatrist, like that of the medical internist, is constantly forcing him to recognize that the interrelationships of the emotions and organic disease call for extensive research.

PHYSIOLOGY AND THE TOTALITY CONCEPT

Thus clinical medicine and modern psychiatry have tended to converge toward a "totality concept" of the human organism and its adaptation to severe stresses by either physical or psychological symptoms. At the same time, modern physiology has provided useful knowledge of the machinery essential for adaptations which involve the total human organism, including those subjectively experienced as mood and emotion. Harvey Cushing's announcement in 1932 of how disturbed emotions may be transmitted from the brain and cause ulcers of the stomach is an important example. An instrument called the "psychogalvanometer," physically testing resistance to an electric current passed through the skin, shows variations in resistance closely correlated with emotion. The first to use it for psycho-physiologic studies was the American Dr. Frederick Peterson of New York in Carl Jung's laboratory; it was demonstrated by him to medical audiences in England and America in 1907, and for a generation was a favorite instrument for hundreds of research studies on emotion. Another discovery, the recording of brain waves in 1929 by Hans Berger, has had a similar and more important effect. This technique was applied a few years later to the study of psycho-physiologic relations by the physiologist Dr. Hallowell Davis and the psychoanalyst Leon Saul, first at Harvard and soon after at the Chicago Psychoanalytic Institute. Still more famous has been the investigation of "conditioned reflexes" demonstrated by the Russian Nobel prize winning Ivan Pavlow. Some students more physiologically than psychologically minded have done excellent experimental work on the artificial production of neuroses in animals by using this technique, and have mistakenly felt that knowledge of conditioned reflexes consequently made knowledge and study of mental repression unnecessary. Of special interest to analysts, however, has been the corroborated demonstration by the researches of Howard Liddell, Professor of Psychobiology at Cornell, that the conditioned reflexes themselves vary according to the emotional relationship of the experimental animal to the experimenter—surprising experimental evidence of the effect on physiologic mechanisms of what analysts call "transference" in human beings.

But the most notable and comprehensive factual contributions of all by physiology to the totality concept have resulted from investigations of those two master systems chiefly responsible for the integration of all vital processes essential to life, the *autonomic nervous system* and the *hormones.*

The *nervous system* is an anatomical apparatus which transmits impulses (or "signals") through nerves from the cells of one organ to another so that widely separated units of the body are integrated. It has well been compared to a complicated telephonic network of central switchboard, trunks, and individual lines. But it is in fact two such networks, the central and the autonomic systems, and these differ greatly both in structure and in biological purpose.

The "central nervous system" includes the brain; the "afferent" or ingoing nerves, which carry impulses from the organs, especially those of sensation, to the brain; and the "efferent" or outgoing nerves, which carry impulses from the brain to the muscles and other organs. It may be roughly characterized as that nervous system concerned with three interrelated functions: the perception of stimuli from outside the body; the intellectual and other ideational processes; and the "voluntary," brain-directed exercise and inhibition of the muscles by which the environment is controlled. This central nervous system had, in past generations, been the chief object of investigation by students of brain and nerves. Its structure, mechanism, and diseases are far better understood than those of the autonomic system. Yet it is of secondary importance to the student of emotions, as it contributes much more fundamentally to conscious and rational mental experience, perceptual, cognitive, and conative, than to deeper functions of the mind.

The anatomy of the *autonomic system* had also long ago been described in great detail, but its full physiologic significance had been rarely surmised until after the First World War. Its central organs are less highly developed than those of the central nervous system. They include the inner portions of the brain and numerous ganglia (little primitive "brains" or "nests" of nerve cells) scattered throughout the body. The autonomic nerves, which ramify from these central organs, dominate the control and integration of those organs which are least under "voluntary" control and least part of conscious mental experience. Thus the autonomic nerves control the rate of the heart beat, the diameter of the smaller blood-vessels and therefore the supply of blood to various regions, the movements of stomach and intestines, the internal organs of excretion and reproduction, the pupils of the eye, the caliber of the smaller air-tubes of the lungs (bronchioles), and all secreting glands. All these are organ functions which are affected by various "psychosomatic" diseases.

The special importance of the autonomic system to psychoanalysis and its medical applications is that it controls the physiologic apparatus of which emotion is the mental representation. By and large, the central nervous system, controlling the senses, intelligence, and muscles, enables man to master the environment and to avoid external dangers. The autonomic system has a very different role in health and in disease: it controls those internal processes whose delicate adjustments are essential to the perpetuation of life. This differentiation of the function of the central and autonomic systems is then the anatomical basis of some "conflicts," as these are defined on a basis of psychologic data: a conscious, intelligent, self-preservative act whose execution involves central nervous system integration is antagonistic to a simultaneous reaction of the autonomic. Intelligence gives, for example, the command to run or fight; but the autonomic system's responses to the same situation are those mentally experienced as fright. The central and autonomic systems then are opposed and fail to supplement each other and function as a unit.

Normal activities of the autonomic nervous system are represented mentally by two kinds of experience: by "mood," feelings of satisfaction or dissatisfaction arising from what is physically going on inside; or by the more consciously specific mental excitement which we call "affect" or "emotion," experienced as a desire and associated with a wish to behave in a certain way. These important mental states differ, then, from those originating in the central nervous system by either absence or vagueness of intellectual content. We feel gay or sad whether we think we know why or not. With our minds, we refer love of another to the sight or thought of the sweetheart; and when love is consciously erotic, we ascribe its origin to our external sexual organs. Physiologically, however, though unromantically, it is more exact to say we "love with our guts" or "hate with our guts." For such moods or passions as love and hate are really a mental awareness of changes in the muscle tone and blood supply of our internal organs, produced by autonomic nerve stimulation, rather than primary stimulation of the external organs such as genitals or fists by which these tensions can ultimately be discharged.

Modern physiology, especially bio-chemistry, is also illuminating the complex phenomena of human life by its study of *hormones*. These are powerful, highly specific chemical substances secreted by "endocrine glands" and carried by the blood-stream from their source to distant organs. Many of them directly supplement or duplicate autonomic-nervous-system functions. For example, Dr. Walter B. Cannon (1873–1945), pioneer in these physiologic investigations, showed that a hormone "adrenalin" (identified in 1895 by Oliver Schäfer as the secretion of a small gland situated above the kidney) acts upon some organs in the same way as does a part of the autonomic nervous system, except that its effect is more slow to appear and lasts longer. When there is fear, not only does the individual mentally experience this special type of conscious emotion, but his body as well reacts in a specific way: his pupils dilate, his hair rises, he has gooseflesh and pallor and trembles, his heart rate is quickened, his stomach, intestines, and excretory organs may function abnormally, and some of the central-nervous-system functions, such as reasoning and co-ordinated muscle skills, may be inhibited.[2]

This major contribution of Walter Cannon was a milestone in the development of physiology, one indeed which was closely correlated by him with the emotions of fear and also rage. It was therefore an empirical demonstration of the physiologic substratum of some mental phenomena. Since this work of 1910–20, endocrinology has become a major field of medical research; many other hormones have been discovered and their effects analyzed. Yet, with the exception of a few extraordinary pioneers, such as the psychoanalyst Jelliffe, it has only begun to dawn upon the medical profession that the autonomic nervous system and the hormones constitute one meeting-ground of dynamic psychiatry and physiology. The psychoanalyst, who studies the emotional experience of his patients, and the students of the autonomic nervous system or hormones, who study the complex bodily reactions which are the physical machinery of these emotions, are studying two manifestations of the same phenomenon. Thus the mental and emotional experience of the individual provides evidence of bodily functions which otherwise are too complex to be evaluated by physiologic experiment. The autonomic system and some hormones are the machinery—the trunklines and pipelines—by which "instinct," as defined by Freud, is made effective; mood, affect, phantasy, and behavior are the most delicate indicators we yet can conceive of the most complex interreactions of the total organism with the environment. Psychoanalysis becomes important from this point of view because it provides

[2] Walter Cannon, *Bodily Changes in Pain, Hunger, Fear, and Rage* (London and New York: D. Appleton and Co.; revised edition, 1936).

the most adequate data obtainable about these highly integrated processes considered as totality reactions of the total organism. From this point of view, psychoanalysis can and should be regarded as a physiological technique: it is the science based on the study of unconscious as well as conscious *mental representations* of those total functions of the autonomic system and of the hormones, functions which are too subtle and too complex to be isolated and studied as a totality in the laboratory.

PSYCHOANALYSIS AND PSYCHOSOMATIC MEDICINE

Thus the physiologist's contribution to nerve and chemical integration, and also his technical limitations for achieving his ultimate goal; the medical practitioner's everyday experience; the psychoanalyst's understanding of mental representations and conflict, and the dynamic psychiatrist's use of this knowledge—all these are converging today on the scientific and therapeutic problems of psychosomatic integrations. They require a basic reorientation in the fundamental premises of medicine. The theological idea of "body and soul," the philosophical concept of "body and mind," had in the last century been incarnated in the medical dichotomy of "functional" (or "psychogenic") and "organic." This medical tradition, that emotional problems are entirely the province of the psychiatrist, and organic disease without mental abnormality entirely outside his field, is being discarded, and has already been replaced in many medical centers of America by the attitude that "psychosomatic medicine" is an important new area of research and treatment.

Though the philosophical dichotomy of "mind" and "body" has today no useful place as a basic premise in scientific thinking, psychiatric *technique* and mental *data* are becoming more important than ever before. They constitute an indirect method of studying functions far too complex and too delicate to be studied, even crudely, by simpler methods. Thus the role of adrenalin and the autonomic nerves in the physiology of fear could only be demonstrated by laboratory experiment on the bodies of animals, and it is often argued by organicists that this knowledge makes the study of mental data superfluous and even "unscientific." But only psychoanalysis, a psychologic method, could show why a child like Little Hans [3] felt anxiety *only* when he saw a horse; and only a psychologic method affecting his unconscious could cure him. Chemistry and pathology were essential to the study and treatment of changes in the patient's thyroid gland after a violent rage; allergy studies were necessary to demonstrate our asthmatic patient's sensitivity to cat fur, but psychoanalysis was essential to clarify his etiologic hatred of one individual cat. Chemistry and X rays revealed what changes had taken place in the stomach wall of a patient whose ulcers became serious whenever his wife went away from home; only a psychiatric method could demonstrate why this individual reacted to such emotional stresses in a physiologically abnormal way, and it showed that unremembered affects initiated these organic changes. The biologic principle involved is that the functions of all organs are related, both as causes and effects, to the functioning of the organism as a whole. And it is the mental representations of the organism as a whole which are studied by psychoanalysis.

It is because psychiatric investigation must be more closely coordinated with organic and medical technique in the study of psychosomatic problems that psychoanalysis has become indispensable. It is not the best instrument which could be imagined, and probably not the best which will ever be devised, but at present it possesses the same advantages in studying the psychology of organic disease that have been proved in the study of psychoneuroses.

This is a relatively new field for psychoanalysis. But as early as 1909 Dr. Smith Ely Jelliffe, American neurologist, psychoanalyst, and editor, had recognized and studied clinically the relationship of mental phenomena and somatic pathology. His remarkable

---

[3] Chapter XIII, pages 266, 270, 273.

Cannon studied the physiology of "fear" and Freud the psychology of "anxiety." Freud distinguished by definition anxiety (*Angst*), as a consequence of ideas, from fear (*Furcht*), a consequence of real external danger. There is, however, no reason to suppose that the quality of the affect and its physiology are different, or that Cannon's observations on fear do not apply to "anxiety," as analysts and psychiatrists use the term.

prescience was fortified by an unusual knowledge of the work of other scientists in botany, philosophy, and psychology, as well as in neurology, psychiatry, and most departments of medicine, laboratory and clinical. In 1911 he was lecturing to medical students on the relationship between the autonomic nervous system (rarely referred to at this period of medical history), emotional experience, and organic disease, and had published reports on the psychologic aspects of arthritis, kidney disease, and psoriasis (a skin disease).[4]

Here and there the interest of other analysts had been aroused in these problems. Freud himself, always, in the last analysis, seeking biologic answers, empirical or hypothetical, to his psychologic observations, compared the phenomena of organic and hypochondriacal pain. Asthma had been the first organic illness to be clearly recognized as having emotional determinants by analysts as well as by other modern physicians and to be studied from this viewpoint; Freud himself had mentioned it in his earliest analytic papers, and analyses of cases were reported by early students of Freud: Sadger in 1911, J. Marcinowski in 1913, and M. Wulff in 1913. The European contemporary of Jelliffe, George Groddeck, though not a physician, had also displayed remarkable intuition of the relations between psychologic, physiologic, and somatic experience, first in 1917 and later in *Das Buch vom Es* (*The Id*) (a term borrowed by Freud in his later ego psychology). But Groddeck had not, as Jelliffe had, technical knowledge of medicine to support his views. Freud's great Hungarian follower, Sandor Ferenczi, in 1916 and 1917 published important papers on the psychology of organic diseases, giving such illnesses a new technical name, "pathoneuroses." By 1922 a younger analyst, Dr. Felix Deutsch, up to that time a medical practitioner, was already attempting to define the problems of "psychosomatic" disease. Since then he has made the application of psychoanalytic principles to the study of organic disease his chief life work, at first in Vienna and after 1935 in Boston, an original—and, some believe, the most significant—psychoanalytic contribution to this new department of medicine.

---

[4] Smith Ely Jelliffe, *Sketches in Psychosomatic Medicine* (Nervous and Mental Disease Publishing Co., 1939).

These were the earliest studies of individual analysts responding to their unique perception of the deepest implications of mental conflict for psychosomatic medicine. Besides these psychoanalytic pioneers, the basic "totality concept" had also been perceived and expounded by several individual leaders in Germany and America. By 1919 Dr. George Draper, Associate in Medicine, Columbia University (then the College of Physicians and Surgeons), became vitally interested in the difference in physical type and personality type between patients who have ulcers of the stomach and those who have ulcers of the duodenum (a problem quite parallel to Freud's unanswered question: why does one patient "choose" a hysterical and another an obsessional neurosis for symptomatic resolution of his conflicts?). Dr. Draper's interest in a very few years convinced him of the unity of body structure, physiology, and personality, and led in 1922 to a "Constitution Clinic" at the Presbyterian Hospital in New York; this in turn engendered specific interest in the psychogenesis and in psychotherapy of somatic disease. Dr. Draper himself published a paper on the psychobiologic factor in stomach ulcer in 1927, and in 1928 a paper entitled "Disease, a Psychosomatic Reaction"; these showed both clinical and conceptual awareness of this new embryo of the medical family, now gestating in a few youthful minds. Early work of the analyst Dr. George Daniels of the psychiatric department at this hospital led to the first panel on the subject at a meeting of the American Psychiatric Association in 1932. The psychiatrist Agnes Conrad and the internist Dr. Cecil Murray on Dr. Draper's service were already engaged in applying their techniques to the study of medical cases. By 1931 a second group at the same hospital, at first encouraged by the elderly Dr. Frederick Peterson (the very man who had introduced the psychogalvanometer before 1907 and suggested psychoanalytic study abroad to Abraham Brill in 1908), and later supported by the Josiah Macy, Jr., Foundation (1934–8), was developing under the exceptionally productive Dr. Helen Flanders Dunbar. She more than any other person is responsible for permanently establishing the word "psychosomatic" in the medical lexicon (though it had been used previously). Her work led to the founding in 1939 of the journal *Psychosomatic Medicine* (then called *Psychosomatic Medicine: Experimental and Clinical Studies*), under Dr. Dunbar's editorship till 1947, subsequently Dr. Carl Binger's. The Editorial Board consisted of a group of leaders in various fields of medicine at various schools specially interested in the new field. In December 1942 they established the American Psychosomatic Society (till 1948 the Society for Research in Psychosomatic Medicine).

In the meantime another, entirely psychoanalytic, research study of several medical problems had been inaugurated in 1932 by a grant of the Rosenwald Foundation to the new Chicago Psychoanalytic Institute with Dr. Franz Alexander as Director, and a notable staff of analysts which eventually included Drs. Thomas French, George Wilson, Catherine Bacon, Helen McClean, Leon Saul, Therese Benedek, Gerhart Piers (now Director), Lucia E. Tower, and Joan Fleming. Besides Columbia and the Chicago Psychoanalytic Institute, active work in the applications of psychoanalysis, dynamic psychiatry, and physiology in this new medical field was appearing in other centers: the analyst Dr. Béla Mittelmann at the New York Postgraduate Hospital; Dr. Giles Thomas and Dr. Frank Fremont-Smith at Harvard, leading to a full psychiatric staff under Dr. Stanley Cobb at the Massachusetts General Hospital in 1953; Dr. Harold Wolff, originally a physiologist studying nervous diseases at New York Hospital (Cornell); the internist Dr. Edward Weiss and the analyst Dr. O. Spurgeon English at Temple Medical School in Philadelphia, and Dr. George Engel at Rochester Medical School.

This decade, the 1930's, witnessed the unfolding of the chrysalis, spun long before by the psychosomatic needs of patients, the psychologic curiosity of a few physicians, and the techniques of psychoanalysis and modern psychiatry. In the last twenty years units for research have been granted an important place at many other medical centers where dynamic psychiatry is also well developed. A new specialty, *psychosomatic medicine,* has thus been established and its basic concepts are now widely accepted by physicians. One problem understood by psychoanalysts has not, however, been clearly understood by many internists who now apply the theory of emotional etiology to some diseases. For the common statement to-day that "emotional problems" are etiologic factors in the medical illness of a certain patient is scientifically to be considered a jumping-off point for thorough psychoanalytic study, not an answer to the question of what caused this "psychosomatic" disease. It does not help the patient merely to be told: "You have no organic trouble"; "Your difficulty is emotional"; or even "Your ulcers get worse when your wife goes away." Such statements are abstract labels, and do not tap the emotional source of the patient's conflict. Nor do such statements advance our knowledge of body-mind relationships. Scientists in medicine not infrequently overlook this, and especially the fact that the exploration of the repressed mental conflicts responsible for a psychosomatic process is as difficult a task as any in medicine and requires expertness in psychiatric technique. Breuer and Freud did not just say: "We think the hysteria of our patients is due to psychologic traumata"; they demonstrated the exact mental experience which had been repressed by each patient, otherwise there would be no science of psychoanalysis today.

The best work in the application of skillful psychoanalytic technique to cases of psychosomatic disease has demonstrated that the theoretical diagnosis can be documented by the analysis of repressed unconscious events. Thus a young woman, who sought analysis for psychologic problems, had a medical history of recurrent attacks of very painful inflammation of the iris of one eye ("iritis"). These had been treated by the best specialists in diseases of the eye, without amelioration. During her analysis, though it was not undertaken for this disease, there was the opportunity to observe that, although there was no obvious correlation of the symptoms with conscious external events of her life, every attack of iritis did coincide with the repression of the same painful thought: that someone did not love her best. The first attack during analysis occurred when her analyst, the only person in whose interest she believed at that time, took a Christmas holiday; she had then repressed a profound belief that this proved he was indifferent, and so was unconscious of this pain-causing thought. At another time an acute attack was coincidental with a dream of a white lady, whose "latent content" proved to be the patient's belief in childhood that her mother (white lady) always went away when the patient most wanted her. This patient had suffered an unusually complete lack of romantic experience since early adolescence, but eventually she recalled the one forgotten exception to this, a love-affair for ten days on a boat to Europe; it was then discovered that she had fully believed the love of this man for her was lasting, and her first attack of severe iritis had occurred the day after he failed to keep a date back in America. This traumatic disappointment of her hope, like those which occurred during analysis, had been repressed. A possible clue, at least something interesting to think about, as to why the eye of this patient should be the organ attacked by somatic disease, was finally suggested after two and a half years of analysis when her repressed college experiences were "worked through." She had had not a single date during those four years, had preserved no belief in her attractions, but she did have an unfaltering belief that she had the most remarkable vision of any girl at college. When hope that she was loved was later so acutely disappointed, it was her eye which was somatically attacked. The scientific lesson of such data is that there is a consistency in the relation of a physical symptom to the repetition of a specific repressed experience which can only be demonstrated by analysis; there was in this case no recurrent experience in terms of external situations of her life which could have been discovered by questioning or introspection.

Though the "common cold" is often a consequence of infection regardless of psychologic events, some psychoanalytic data indicate that the mucous membrane lining the nose, like that of other organs, may become inflamed in consequence of a conflict peculiar to the individual. For example, acute symptoms of a cold always occurred in one woman when some incident threatened to undo the repression of the memory of a teen-age experience which had produced unbearable shame: she had discovered at a party that others had seen some menstrual spotting of her white dress. Another woman who had acute recurrent colds learned during analysis that they were always precipitated by repressed awareness that another woman appealed to men: once, walking in a park, she observed the sexual glances of men at her girl-friend; on a train, a feminine companion became acquainted with a man; on these and a dozen similar occasions when she repressed her envy she suddenly developed typical symptoms of a "cold." [5]

An opportunity for still more thorough exploration of the relations of unconscious mental and physiologic events in one patient was provided by the exposure of the lining of his stomach by an accidental wound.[6] Psychoanalysis was conducted over a long period, and concurrently direct physiologic examinations of the exposed interior of the stomach were made frequently. When the notes of psychoanalyst and physiologist were eventually compared, the remarkable fact was disclosed that a specific pattern of disturbed physiology, involving the gastric juices and the blood-supply of the stomach lining, always coincided with a specific emotional difficulty during psychoanalytic hours.[7]

These examples of psychosomatic research illustrate admirably the use of thorough psychoanalytic technique in contrast to mere statement of psychosomatic etiology in terms of conscious experience and coincidence. Similarly, the collaboration of the physiologist Dr. Boris B. Rubenstein and the psychoanalyst Dr. Therese Benedek at the Chicago Institute showed that microscopic evidence of changes in the lining of the female reproductive organs

[5] These data concerning colds are all the more intriguing when one recalls the well-known fact of "vicarious menstruation," the peculiar tendency of some women to have nosebleeds during menstruation or instead of it. Neither the psychology nor the physiology of this teleologically useless replacement of the uterus by the nose has been clarified, though Freud's chief confidant in the 1890's, Dr. Wilhelm Fliess, and many other physicians have taken a special interest in it.

[6] Sydney G. Margolin, "Psychophysiological Studies of Fistulous Opening into Gastrointestinal Tract," *Journal Mt. Sinai Hospital*, 1953.

[7] The use of this remarkable opportunity to study the exposed interior of the stomach recalls a great medical classic, the first scientific contribution to the relation of psychologic and physiologic events. This was a report in 1833 of the observations of a U.S. Army doctor, William Beaumont, a Vermonter without medical-school education, that the interior of a man's stomach, exposed by a gunshot wound, became active when the patient became emotional. Today we have physiologic apparatus and the psychoanalytic method, if not the genius, to analyze Dr. Beaumont's observations in more fundamental detail.

coincided with changes in the predominant phantasies of each woman at a definite phase of the menstrual cycle.[8]

PSYCHOANALYTIC TREATMENT
OF PSYCHOSOMATIC DISEASE

Medical history bears witness that each new discovery, as soon as it is generally known, creates an avalanche of panacea-seekers. But actually years of study and experience are essential to evaluate its efficacy. This is true of new forms of treatment for very specific diseases; it is far more true of so vast a field as psychosomatic medicine. The assumption would be ridiculous that psychoanalysis is, or ever can be, a successful or preferential treatment for every disease to whose development emotion and personality have contributed. The therapeutic possibilities in this field are not identical with those of personality disorders, where psychotherapy or psychoanalysis is usually indicated because there is no body disease. Judgment as to the choice of organic method or psychoanalysis, or a combined treatment, will for a long time depend upon the nature of each individual case, and the opinions of experienced internists and psychoanalysts in consultation.

At least one guiding principle in the selection of organic cases for psychoanalytic therapy has long been clearly formulated—the *reversibility* of some somatic processes. Definite psychoneurotic symptoms, which may involve bodily functions—for example, bedwetting—are clearly "reversible," in the sense that no alteration of the tissues has occurred; therefore, if the conflict of which bedwetting is a symptom is benefited therapeutically, the organs of urination can automatically readapt themselves. If, however, an individual has a neurotic conflict which has been resolved unconsciously by getting a finger amputated, psychoanalysis may well cure the neurosis, but it cannot restore the finger. Similarly, in some

---

[8] Therese Benedek, M.D., and Boris B. Rubenstein, Ph.D., "The Correlations Between Ovarian Activity and the Psychodynamic Processes: I. The Ovulative Phase," *Psychosomatic Medicine,* Vol. I, No. 2, April 1939.

cases of stomach ulcer, there may be no question in the mind of either internist or psychoanalyst that this particular patient has a severe neurosis; that crises in the neurotic conflict have been discharged through the autonomic nervous system; that altered nerve-stimulation has affected such physiologic functions of the stomach as blood-supply and acid-secretion; and that ulcers are the end result and produce distress, misery, and physical danger. Whether or not such a process is "reversible," like enuresis, depends upon the type and amount of tissue damage. Even though the abnormal nerve tension can be reduced, or can be discharged in other ways, by improved sexual and social relations and sublimated activities as a result of analysing the unconscious conflict, the stomach may have been so damaged that natural healing processes can no longer restore the normal tissue. If such "reversibility" is unlikely, will treatment prevent the continuation and recurrence of the process? This principle of reversibility is of prime importance, though actually it cannot be applied as a basis for certain prediction in many cases.

At present we must be satisfied with the fact that compelling theoretical and clinical considerations are focusing more and more study of psychosomatic disease by internists, physiologists, analysts, and dynamic psychiatrists; that already a sufficiently large number of cases have been helped to indicate its practical possibilities. The seed of these achievements was sown so long ago by the greatest of Greek doctors, Hippocrates (460–377 B.C.), who relieved the distressing symptoms of King Perdiccas of Macedonia by the analysis of a dream.[9] The seed found scant nourishment in the soil of mediæval scholasticism, and was uncultivated while nineteenth-century medicine concentrated on the microscope and test-tube. But it has been fertilized by medical and psychiatric leaders of this generation, and watered by the psychoanalytic contributions of Freud. It blooms today as a new major field of psychoanalytic research.

---

[9] Quoted by A. A. Brill, "Anticipations and Corroborations of the Freudian Concepts," *American Journal of Psychiatry*, Vol. XCII, p. 112 (1936).

APPLIED PSYCHOANALYSIS

T H E cornerstone of psychoanalysis was laid when Freud discovered the unconscious meaning of the hysterical symptom. Its foundations have been the analysis of neuroses, dreams, and character-development, and they bear a superstructure for which they were not originally designed. For the resulting facts and theories describe such fundamental human processes that they have applications, not only in psychiatry and medicine, but in all professions which deal with the effects produced by the human mind. These include those disciplines in which practical assistance to other human beings is the immediate purpose, such as social work, clinical psychology, criminology, and education, and also those whose purpose is primarily cultural or artistic.

EARLY APPLIED PSYCHOANALYSIS: THE ARTS, ANTHROPOLOGY, SOCIOLOGY, RELIGION

The important applications of psychoanalysis to cultural studies have, by usage, come to be known as *applied psychoanalysis*. The discovery of psychoanalysis, for example, that the perpetuation of infantile sexuality in the adult unconscious is a primary factor in the creation of dreams not only means that we can better understand the motivation of dreams. It means that, from the analysis of dreams, neuroses, and mistakes, Freud discovered fundamental facts which are reflected in one way or another in all the psychologic activities of all human beings. It means that some aspects of psychotic thought as well as dreams are now comprehensible.[1] It means that some rites and customs of primitive peoples can be better understood by analysis of features they have in common with the phantasies of civilized children. It also enables us to realize that the arts, in order to achieve and communicate an æsthetic experience, must create the means for evading infantile guilt while expressing more or less elaborately and unconsciously tabooed phantasies of a universal nature. "Originality" in art is the conscious disguise invented by the artist; but the emotional appeal of his creation is a universal phantasy, often unconscious, which it expresses and communicates.

The Œdipus complex itself derives its name from the fact that Sophocles in his classic drama told this universal story of the incestuous and patricidal son who also fulfilled his primal punishment-phantasy by being blinded. And the discoveries of Freud show that, however the external form and content of *Hamlet* may differ from *Œdipus Rex*, Hamlet is motivated by the same deep phantasy. Shakespeare's drama likewise tells this story of incest and patricide, but with a more complex disguise. For Hamlet consciously perceives his own infantile phantasy not as his own, but as the behavior of his stepfather, King Claudius, who killed Hamlet's father and made Hamlet's mother his bedmate. It is further made to appear that the fulfillment of Hamlet's patricidal phantasy was a failure, and that the elderly and "harmless" Polonius, not the guilty King, died through mischance. Thus the morality of Shakespeare's audience is appeased by the conscious emphasis of Claudius's real guilt; Hamlet's own incestuous phantasy is concealed, and his infantile rivalry with his own father as object is replaced by obedience to the Ghost and conscious hatred of the King. Yet in using the dramatic device of the players, Hamlet actually exposes Claudius to the identical "trauma" to which Claudius had mentally

[1] See pages 252–4.

exposed Hamlet, the "acting-out" of his own primal wishes before his very eyes.

As Hamlet's torments are unraveled, another primitive theme is added to the drama, that of Hamlet's rage at his mother, because her seduction of the King induced the crime. And at the same time, much as psychotics occasionally become fully conscious of what is normally repressed, he then recognizes fully how sexuality is at the root of these passions, for he accuses his mother of it. Hamlet is therefore victim not only of his terrible wishes but of his punishment phantasies too, as is apparent in his tragic failure to achieve the murder of Claudius, his sexual failure with Ophelia, his flight to England, and the tortured mental state of his soliloquies.

Thus Shakespeare's technique utilizes conscious disguises of unconscious wishes which are familiar to the analyst of the content of dreams. This psychoanalytic knowledge illuminates the greatness of the tragedy; it shows that *Hamlet* portrays a universal phantasy of mankind, cast by the genius of Shakespeare in a form which lulls the conscience of his audience while yet it rouses their inmost passions. The unconscious themes of these masterpieces of Sophocles and Shakespeare are identical. Yet it is not the use of these phantasies of patricide that proves the genius of either Sophocles or Shakespeare; it is the artistic form and the language by which these creative dramatists gave these phantasies expression.

The application of analysis in the psychologic study of literature and the other arts has especially appealed to some psychoanalysts of scholarship and culture. Freud himself contributed to applied analysis, analysing the story of Jensen's novel *Gradiva* in the book *Delusion and Dream*, first published in 1907. In the next few years he published other works of this kind: *The Relation of the Poet to Day-dreaming*, *The Theme of the Three Caskets*, *The Moses of Michelangelo*, and *The Prometheus Myth*. These works of applied analysis all reflect not only Freud's interest in the unconscious factors in mental life, but his voluminous reading in many fields; the works of Shakespeare were his favorites from his youth. He also took a special interest in sculpture; this too is reflected in his choice of several subjects for studies in applied analy-

sis. Especially notable was a work which Freud himself most es-
teemed, his book on *Lèonardo da Vinci* (1910), a scholarly
psychoanalytic biography based on Leonardo's only childhood
memory, that of an early phantasy of a bird, perhaps a vulture, flying with its tail in its mouth.

As his maturity advanced, the study of archæology became
Freud's most passionate avocation. He devoted many vacations to
its pursuit; and he would have been the first to recognize the deep
identity of this insatiable curiosity aroused by the buried clues to
history and his curiosity about the hidden regions of the individual
mind which was motivation of the science he gave to the world.

A number of other psychoanalysts have from time to time indulged in similar essays. Among these none have applied their talents more productively to the study of literature and mythology
than two lay analysts, Hanns Sachs and Otto Rank, both men of extensive culture and both among the first group of Freud's students
in Vienna. Sachs's work in the applied analysis of Shakespeare's
Tempest, his interpretation of the character of the Roman Emperor
Caligula in his book *Bubi*, and his long editorship of the German
journal of applied psychoanalysis, *Imago*, were invaluable contributions to this field.

No one has surpassed Rank's skill and scholarship in his
working out of the theorem that what day-dreams are for the individual, myths are for the human race. For, in myths are those
phantasies which are common to a multitude of individuals and are
crystallized as the folklore of a tribe or race. The infantile phantasies of individuals are disguised and repeated as the life story of
the founders of their nation and these myths, like the phantasies of
the child about his parents, are constantly being altered in little details, combined, and multiplied, as they are retold, until finally they
are fixed in a written form. It is therefore no simple coincidence that
the analysis of dreams frequently reveals an unconscious phantasy
of birth which is likewise to be found in Greek mythology. In his
masterpiece, *The Myth of the Birth of a Hero* (1909), Rank illustrated these principles, showing that different forms of one basic
phantasy existed among many different races—the story of a royal

child who is removed from his parents, reared by a foster-mother, and later achieves greatness and wins back his birthright. The stories of Moses in the bulrushes, Romulus and Remus, Siegfried, Lohengrin, Sargon, and many other myths are all alike in this respect; though the details of each myth are different, they are variations of the same unconscious phantasy: if we get away from our bad mamas and papas, we shall find better ones, who will treat us as princes and gods should be treated, and we shall eventually be recognized as of royal birth.

Freud himself was the first contributor to applied analysis of a work on anthropology, *Totem and Taboo* (1912). In this he sought to apply his own knowledge, gleaned at first hand from the analysis of the unconscious of patients, to the interpretation of a universal feature of the social customs of primitive people. This is the worship of the "totem," practiced in one form or another by all clans. The details of these customs vary greatly, but their fundamental characteristics are always the same. The totem is that animal—a different one for each clan—which is regarded by the clan members as the carrier of the spirits of dead ancestors and is therefore sacred. In every culture a system of prohibitions, called "taboos," in respect to the totem animal is instituted and their violation is feared and punished. For example, it is taboo to eat the totem, it may be taboo to mention its name. A great number of other "superstitions," rituals, and devices for the protection of the totem from the supposed magical effects of violated taboos are practiced. On the other hand, there are certain special conditions, such as the celebration of the death of a clansman, when the totem is treated as an enemy and is then eaten at a ceremonial feast. Traces of primitive totem-worship survive and may be identified in higher civilizations: in the taboo on pork of the Jews; in the representation of Christ's body and blood as wafer and wine to be eaten and drunk in the Christian Communion service. Freud, in this first book on psychoanalysis applied to anthropology, argued that ambivalence of feeling, which he had discovered was a feature of all infantile wishes, can explain this dual attitude of love and hate of the totem animal of primitive tribes; and that the totem itself, consciously representing the ancestor, unconsciously means to each individual an infantile image of his actual father.

Freud concluded this anthropological study with a theory: that totems and taboos and dreams all show traces of a state of human society, lost in prehistoric time, still more primitive than those we know some facts about. Following Charles Darwin, he called this hypothetical earliest human group the "primal horde." Reasoning inductively from his knowledge of primitive phantasies, he concluded that this "primal horde" must have had a social organization which in many respects is identical with the "harems" of dominant male apes, actually observed and described by Zuckermann [2] twenty years later. This society would consist of a dominant male who appropriates a group of females and keeps the weaker males at bay, preventing incestuous activity of his male offspring by means of his power. According to this theory, the beginning of a higher social order, and therefore of culture, was repeated many times in the early history of our race, when the sons of the primal horde learned that by banding together they could overthrow the father and divide the females among themselves. This was presumed to be the earliest form of a society in which individuals agreed to gain for themselves certain ends by the mutual renunciation of others.

Besides initiating the interest of social scientists in the applications of psychoanalysis to anthropology, *Totem and Taboo* has also proved to be the original inspiration of the later appreciation by psychoanalysts of the vital relationship of primitive culture to the mental life of abnormal adults, and of both normal and problem children.

The applications of psychoanalysis to *sociology* have also interested both analysts and sociologists. For sociology seeks to elucidate the structure and dynamics of groups and institutions. A society is composed of human beings; the motives of these human beings determine its culture, even though it is also doubtless true that a highly integrated culture is definitely something more than

[2] Solly Zuckermann, *Functional Affinities of Man, Monkeys, and Apes* (New York: Harcourt, Brace and Company; 1933).

the sum of the individuals who compose it. Thus sociology can assist the analyst to understand that environment to which his patients are reacting; while analytic knowledge can point the way to the unconscious motivation of human conduct, as manifested by groups as well as individuals.

Freud's own first contribution to applied psychoanalysis in the field of sociology was his book *Group Psychology and the Analysis of the Ego* (1922). His point of departure was the studies in mob psychology of the Frenchman Gustave LeBon, and the English-born American psychologist William McDougall. His major conclusions were that the integration of mobs, and the existence of every stable social group, are maintained by the identification by each member of the group with the deep unconscious love of a father felt by each other member, whether this father be represented by an actually existing leader or by a psychological ideal. According to this theory (an application of his theory of the origin of the individual's superego by the child's identification with his parent [3]), the raw material of societal organization is this emotional bond which brothers in a family find in their mutual love of father and their fear of his real and imagined power. Presumably Freud would not have disputed the existence of families ruled by mothers, nor the existence of matriarchal as well as patriarchal societies. In a later book, *Civilization and Its Discontents* (1930), Freud argued that the phenomenon of war is made possible by two psychological occurrences: first, the liberation of biologically determined needs to destroy or kill, the repression of which is a determinant of each individual's neurosis; and, secondly, the basic subordination of the individual's impulses to those fraternal and patriarchal bonds whose function in producing group solidarity Freud had originally discussed in *Group Psychology and the Analysis of the Ego*.

In applying psychoanalysis to the study of *religion*, Freud took two approaches, the understanding of specifically clinical material, and the philosophical discussion of religious faith. His original discussion in 1907 of the striking similarity between the rituals

[3] See pages 160 ff.

of patients suffering from compulsion neurosis and the ceremonies of a religious group had revealed an important psychological fact. The need of many sufferers from compulsion neurosis to wash their hands, repeated many times a day, is subjectively an atonement for a feeling of sin produced by unconscious punishment phantasies. The symptom is therefore similar to religious purification (such as Christian baptism or ablution by the Mohammedans), even though the sin whose punishment is feared by the neurotic is, without analysis, unconscious. A minor compulsion often experienced by practically normal people, such as that of avoiding stepping on cracks in the sidewalk, is determined by a similar half-conscious idea that an evil will be deflected; that is a superstition, and a superstition is a type of phantasy. The essential difference between these and the atonement rights enforced by religious dogmas and obeyed by the devout is that the neurotic ritual is personal and individual; it distinguishes the patient from his "normal" fellows and makes him peculiar in their eyes and his own, while the ritual of a religion is shared by many others and is, therefore, a normal, socially accepted practice of society.

In Civilization and Its Discontents Freud discussed another aspect of religion, the conscious feeling that one is immortal, which many people experience. He argued that this is not rational proof of theological premises, for the subjective experience of immortality is a regression to an infantile mode of thought. The actuality, or certainty, of an after-life, or of a personal Father in Heaven who hears and heeds our prayers, is not a problem which psychology can decide. But the ideas that human beings have upon the matter, and the emotional needs it satisfies in this life, are proper fields of psychologic inquiry. That adults satisfy in their religious beliefs needs which were once satisfied by the parents—their unquestioned power for good and evil, the certain refuge from helplessness they provide, their answers to a cry—seems beyond reasonable question. A little girl of three, unhappy when she goes to bed, murmurs as she drops to sleep: "Sal' go [to] Aunt Mary—swim—play—sleep." Aunt Mary lives in a distant city. The child had been blissfully happy there at the beach a week before. Her wish to return when unhappy is as elemental a prayer to go to a heaven of which she had not yet learned from adults as could be devised. But it is also a prayer she is helpless at three years to achieve without the will of the adult powers who can take her from her family world to the fairyland at Aunty's.

In his major essay on religion, however, *The Future of an Illusion*, Freud seems to me to have indulged in a tirade and to have arrived nowhere. In this single book he departed from his life-long analysis of unconscious motivation and attacked theology. Theology is the rationalization of religious needs and practices, but Freud here ignored the human need which gives rise to faith, as-sailed the logic by which it is justified, and argued that science, the supremacy of intellect, can some day take its place. When he said: ". . . in the long run nothing can withstand reason and experience, and the contradiction religion offers to both is only too palpable," the very man who had done most to demonstrate the irrational in human life showed that even his mind had its peculiar inconsisten-cies. Yet, three years before the publication of *Totem and Taboo*, Freud had written in a letter: "[Religion's] ultimate basis is the in-fantile helplessness of mankind. . . . But I don't intend to elabo-rate it." But he did, in early pages of *Civilization and Its Discon-tents*, and in his last book, *Moses and Monotheism*.

LATER DEVELOPMENT OF APPLIED PSYCHOANALYSIS: THE SOCIAL SCIENCES

Original and fascinating as the best of these early applications of psychoanalysis are, they do not have the empirical foundation that clinical analysis of the individual's unconscious does; they are applications of a new science, not the science. Though the greatest of them, *Totem and Taboo*, was no mere flight of an inspired imagination but was based upon extensive study of anthropological literature, some professional anthropologists have questioned the validity of data which Freud discussed. A still more cogent criti-cism is that the data of applied psychoanalysis are always second-hand; they cannot be amplified and further explored as can those of clinical analysis. For, with analytic patients, additional associations may be obtained, and interpretations by the analyst are from time to time either confirmed, amplified, corrected, or modified by the patient's response with unpredicted mental content. Leonardo da Vinci himself, for example, cannot, like a patient on the couch, rise up and report new material when Freud interprets his infantile memory of imagining a bird with its tail in its mouth. Nor can Hamlet "protest too much" that he has no "Œdipal" phantasies or memories, and angrily assert that the analyst is an illogical fool obsessed with his theories, and "work through" in subsequent weeks or months new phantasies and memories of his childhood.

In contrast to clinical analysis, therefore, these works are literally the *applications* to art and biography and social sciences of knowledge obtained by the use of the psychoanalytic method with living individual patients. Nonetheless, no matter how censorial one may be of the validity of works of applied analysis, one cannot escape the important fact that they do represent recognition of a very basic truth: that the unconscious functions in creative work, and in the integration of social groups and institutions, as surely as it functions in the production of the neuroses and dreams of patients. It is this which largely accounts for the change in the character of applied analysis and the increasing importance of analysis in the social sciences during the last twenty-five years.

These new developments were initiated by the great Polish anthropologist Bronislaw Malinowski, who gave serious consideration to Freud's major conclusions and undertook to test them with anthropological data. During the 1920's he confirmed Freud's views of the existence and characteristics of infantile sexuality throughout the human race with observations from his field studies of the primitive culture of the Trobriand Islanders.[4] He disputed, however, Freud's conclusion in *Totem and Taboo* that the male Œdipus complex is the central determinant of all cultures, and promulgated the important thesis that the fixed customs of a culture

---

[4] Bronislaw Malinowski, *The Sexual Life of Savages* (New York: Horace Liveright; 1929).

determine how the individual's early development is affected by his society's attitude to his wishes and behavior in infancy. During this same decade the Hungarian lay analyst Géza Róheim in his field studies adapted the actual technique of clinical analysis, studying the dreams and free associations of individual Australian bushmen. In this way Róheim tested the applicability of Freud's anthropological views to members of an aboriginal culture.[5]

In the early thirties the Yale psychologist John Dollard demonstrated a similar direct application of psychoanalytic technique in a sociologic study, "analyzing" the unconscious mental reactions of individual lower-class Negroes to the caste conditions imposed upon them in a Mississippi town.[6] A somewhat similar application of psychoanalytic methods, as well as clinical knowledge, was made by the talented Danish-American child analyst Erik Erikson in his studies of the Sioux and Navaho Indians, demonstrating, for example, how the Sioux's cultural pattern of training a boy to be a hunter affected his personality development. From facts of this kind he drew a conclusion much the same as Malinowski's: that the kind of culture determines what skills and acceptable attitudes are learned by a child responding to needs and phantasies which are universal for his age and sex and not themselves products of his culture. Phantasies identical with an Indian boy's, for example, motivate an American boy's interest in school achievement, story-reading, or baseball, and play an important role in the development of a personality which is adaptable to his own society.[7]

These early applications of analytic technique were contemporaneous with the increasing influence of psychoanalysis in the new discipline of cultural anthropology, which developed in this century. It was natural—or inevitable—that cultural anthropology should be the first of the social sciences to make good use of Freud's

[5] Géza Róheim, "Psycho-Analysis of Primitive Cultural Types," *International Journal of Psychoanalysis*, Vol. XIII, Numbers 1–2 (1932). And G. Róheim, *Psychoanalysis and Anthropology* (International Universities Press; 1950).

[6] John Dollard, *Caste and Class in a Southern Town* (New Haven: Yale University Press; 137).

[7] Erik H. Erikson, *Childhood and Society* (New York: W. W. Norton; 1950).

ideas. For, as Gardner Lindzey has emphasized, the great propo-
nents of early cultural anthropology were themselves imaginative
rather than doctrinaire, and their objectives resembled those of
psychoanalysis in one vital respect: the primary interest in the experience of individual members of a society. Franz Boas of Columbia, creator of this school in America, had recognized Freud as
significant in his contributions to this new and primarily empirical
approach to the science of man, though he had not tested his ideas
as Malinowski had. His follower Ruth Benedict also introduced
ideas some of which were closely related to, and some derived directly from, psychoanalysis. The most notable anthropological field
work, from the standpoint of psychoanalysis, has been that of
Margaret Mead, continuing that of Malinowski. Though her earlier
studies were oriented in part by ideas opposed to those of analysis
(especially her thesis that psychological sex differentiation is primarily culture-determined), her empirical contributions over the
years dealt increasingly with observations of early individual development in various primitive cultures. The data she has offered
are, in consequence, of even more immediate interest to analysis
than her generalizations. One example of her extensive field work is
that of reporting the customs which govern the rearing of infants
in Bali, the tolerance of adult natives to the enjoyment by children
in that culture of nursing, weaning, and other sensual pleasures,
and the relationship of this child-training to the development of personality among the natives.[8] Clyde Kluckhohn, in his anthropological studies of the Navaho Indians and much other work, and
Florence Kluckhohn, in her studies of the characteristics of Spanish
American societies, have also given recognition to the importance
of psychoanalysis for their fields.

Psychoanalysis during this century has had a quite similar influence on another branch of the social sciences, social psychology.
Several contemporaries of Freud took more than casual interest in
his work—William James, who in 1909 had said to Freud: "The
future of psychology belongs to your work," and Malinowski, who

[8] Margaret Mead, *From the South Seas* (New York: Morrow; 1939).

influenced the beginnings of social psychology as well as cultural anthropology. The leading American in this new field, William McDougall (English born), was especially active in the discussion of Freud. His own views, indeed, were closer to Freud's than most successors in his field in one respect, in basing his psychology on mentally experienced biologic needs. These McDougall classified as several dozen "sentiments," while Freud hypothesized two basic groups of "instincts." Many of the present generation who have specialized in the psychology of personality—to mention only a few, Robert R. Sears, Gordon W. Allport, Floyd Allport, Gardner and Lois Murphy, J. McVeigh Hunt, John Dollard—have fully acknowledged the importance of Freud's innovations for the social sciences.

The second of those two main areas of social psychology delineated by its great founder, Wilhelm Wundt (1832–1920), that of laboratory experimentation, reached its first zenith in the work of Kurt Lewin (1890–1947).[9] Eminent psychologists have said that Lewin and Freud are the two sources of all contemporary social psychology, defined as the relations of the individual to a social group. Lewin himself used some of the mechanisms discovered by Freud, such as displacement, repression, and conflict, in interpreting his own experimental results. There is also a fundamental similarity, almost an identity, in Lewin's primary concept of the "social field," used by him for the interpretation of the reaction of one individual to another in an experimental situation, and the controlled, standardized patient-doctor situation of clinical analysis. It is more than an extravagant play with words to say psychoanalysis might actually be called a "transference field" studied in terms of a patient's spontaneous phantasies. While Lewin studied by objective observations what a person does in the experimental field, Freud explored why a patient *needs* to act that way.

Social psychology has advanced even more rapidly in the last ten years. Some of this work is primarily based on psychoanalytic

[9] Kurt Lewin, *A Dynamic Theory of Personality* (New York: McGraw. Hill; 1935).

conclusions, such as experiments designed to test Freud's interpretation of dreams, unconscious sexuality, and other data and theories of analysis. Experimental studies (Jerome S. Bruner, D. Krech, L. S. Cottrell, and others) are especially designed for the deeper empirical exploration of perception and cognition, taking more fully into account than their predecessors early, non-rational mechanisms adumbrated by the modern study of ego development by analysts and child analysts, as well as by such genetic psychologists as Charlotte Bühler and Jean Piaget.

The third group of modern social sciences, sociology—in so far as we can distinguish its main objectives as the structure and function of society as a whole and of social groups from those of anthropology and psychology—has found much in psychoanalysis that is useful. Harold Laswell, now Professor of Law and Political Science at Yale, in the early 1930's pioneered in applying psychoanalysis to the study of politics and politicians. An analyst, Robert Wälder, studied the application of analytic knowledge to the social theory of racial strife. Erich Fromm was productive in the comparison of mediaeval, Reformation, and Nazi cultures, though he went so far in this direction as to be no longer considered a psychoanalyst by this profession.

An increasing number of modern sociologists, like their professional cousins, are tending to regard psychoanalysis as a basic contribution to their department of the science of man. Sociology itself, however, is primarily occupied with the description and structure of social institutions and large groups. There consequently has been less of a common basis than there is among anthropologists and psychologists for understanding the clinical foundation of analysis, and a greater trend to apply analytic theory and generalizations to their own abstractions. Sociologic preoccupation with the interpretation of society in terms of the "role" of the individual in various social groups, and the overemphasis of "status" and prestige as motivations, have not invited familiarity with other important determinants of the individual's adjustment. Some sociologists are themselves trying to come to closer grips with this problem by the study of smaller social units than they used to. Thus Parsons and Bales [1] have attempted to utilize the empirical contributions of psychoanalysis in formulating their theory of the roles of mother, father, and child within the family group. It is indeed in various studies of the family, theoretical and empirical, that sociologists in recent years approach closest to the analyst's primary interest in what human beings think and feel, as well as what they do when well integrated in a social unit. Several "interdisciplinary" research projects by analysts and dynamic psychiatrists themselves—for example, Dr. John Spiegel's at Michael Reese Hospital (Chicago) and at Harvard,[2] and that of Drs. Theodore Lidz and Stephen Fleck at Yale—have as their main purpose the exploration of the sociologic implications of family units as a base for better psychiatric understanding of individuals within the family structure.

The impact of analysis on these social sciences is, therefore, of accelerating importance. During the first generation of psychoanalysis, it was an occasional social scientist who was blazing hitherto unexplored regions—a Malinowski, a William James, a Trotter, a McDougall, a Boas, a Laswell—who glimpsed the importance of Freud to the evolution of man's knowledge of himself. Paralleling the emergence of psychoanalysis itself from organic medicine, these new social sciences were sprouting from seedlings implanted in the soil of eighteenth- and nineteenth-century philosophy and untested speculation. In the last generation they have sunk their roots deeper in the empiricism of the scientific age. This is true not only of field studies in cultural anthropology; it is true also of the increased efforts of social psychology to achieve factual proof by experimental methods, and of the trend of sociology to define the specific by statistics or to approach the interests of anthropologists and psychiatrists by investigating smaller social units. Individual social scientists have for a generation recognized that Freud's work is relevant to theirs. They have especially recognized

[1] Talcott Parsons and Robert F. Bales, *Family Socialization, and Interaction Process* (Glencoe, Ill.: The Free Press; 1955).

[2] *Integration and Conflict in Family Behavior,* Florence Kluckhohn, Ph.D., and John Spiegel, M.D., Editors (Topeka, Kans.: Group for Advancement in Psychiatry, Published Reports, No. 27).

that the non-logical components of mind are determinants of the behavior, the culture, and the interactions of societies and groups as truly as they are determinants of the individual's neuroses and dreams.

Nevertheless, an accurate estimate of what Freud has contributed to these social sciences, and how it is utilized, presents some special difficulties. One fundamental problem always arises in the critical evaluation of each social scientist's use of psychoanalysis: has he been primarily stimulated by Freud's most abstract concepts, hypotheses, and generalizations, or has he recognized the decisiveness of clinical data obtained by the analytic method and the difficulties of studying and testing them by other techniques? A psychoanalyst can, for example, take great interest in the sociologist's exact definition of the "role" a boy or girl or mother or father is *expected* to assume in the American family, or in very different types of family described by the comparative anthropologist. But, more often than not, when a sociologist attempts to apply his knowledge of role to the description of an individual's personality, this sounds to the analyst as though peaches and pears can be distinguished only by reading the labels on the wrappers. For the social scientist too often regards these culturally defined actions of a member within the family as ultimately rendering unnecessary the analyst's emphasis on "instincts" as biologic determinants of mental life and its development. This essential difference is especially clear in a rather new emphasis by sociologists on social "transactions" between individuals in a group, an emphasis which renders the idea of innate emotional needs of the individual scientifically unnecessary.[3]

On the other hand, the interaction of social sciences and analysis has already crystallized a few sound premises which seem beyond reasonable controversy. First, the facts of clinical analysis had made clear what the Italian sociologist Vilfredo Pareto had

---

[3] It should be noted that the same fundamental abrogation of the basic psychoanalytic hypothesis of biologically created "instincts" and the facts on which it is founded is also characteristic of most of the psychoanalytic "deviationists"—Jung, Horney, Sullivan, etc. (see Chapter XVI, pp. 331–46).

independently recognized by the study of history.[4] Inventing his own terminology for his own ideas, he duplicated a few of Freud's fundamental conclusions: that the logical explanations used to account for human institutions were rationalizations, that the real determinants of human history were emotional and unconscious, and that this was clearly shown in all social structures. Psychoanalysis has made still clearer that cultures and social institutions are not perpetuated from generation to generation by what is consciously taught the child by parents and teachers, or taught the adult by the precepts of religious, governmental, and other authoritative institutions. Cultural ideologies are the more conscious elements that one shares with one's group, and belief in them depends upon their appropriateness in formulating and enforcing the rationalizations of phantasies, myths, and beliefs which are perhaps only dimly perceived. Thus the best meetings of minds during the Second World War pretty much agreed that militaristic Nazism could not have become the compelling ideology of Germany if Germany had not been historically prepared by the survival since feudalism of a system of values determined by status and titles which was unique among the civilized nations of modern Europe. Again, a belief that an individual is "created" by his father or by his mother cannot, of course, be logically argued and is biologically absurd. Nonetheless, the ancient Greeks tended to think of the mother as merely the repository of the father's creative potency, whereas our civilization thinks of the mother as the life-giver and the father as essentially an adjunct. Such beliefs are without logical foundation, yet they play a vital role in the thought of each civilization, in the sentiments, phantasies, and ideals of its population, and also in its mythology, drama, and art. Similarly, our European emphasis on toilet-training and our disgust at excretions is minimal in Chinese culture, and consequently the anal-erotic components of infantile pleasures in excretion have a very different effect upon personality development in China.

[4] Lawrence J. Henderson, *Pareto's General Sociology* (Cambridge, Mass.: Harvard University Press; 1935); and Vilfredo Pareto: *The Mind and Society* (1916; translation, New York: Harcourt, Brace; 1935).

A second psychoanalytic postulate, too often not understood by "interdisciplinary" leaders in the behavioral sciences, is that in-dividuals, their personalities, their successes and failures, cannot be defined in terms of the most accurate statistics of a society's char-acteristics. Even such a statistically well-established fact as that Jews are less frequently alcoholic than members of other European races, or the fact that the suicide rate always diminishes when a na-tion is at war, do not help us to determine whether a certain indi-vidual is an alcoholic or imminently suicidal. Psychoanalytic knowledge of the individual's phantasies, conflicts, and infantile love-relationships does help to answer such a clinical question, however fallibly.

Thirdly, the most incontestable meeting-point of social scien-tists and psychoanalysts is the conclusion that basic cultural influ-ences are emotionally transmitted by the mother or other rearers in their care of infants and young children. The special contribu-tion of psychoanalytic knowledge, rather than quasi-analytic specu-lation, is therefore its understanding of some of the deep and com-plex processes whereby a child becomes like his mother, or his fa-ther, or his nurse, in his basic orientation to life experiences and behavior—in the way he later in his life satisfies, controls, or modi-fies his instinctual responses. These fundamental components of personality later determine his conformity or non-conformity, so-cialization or deviance, and, in multi-dimensional cultures such as ours, the subculture in which he finds his most comfortable adjust-ment. Before the direct, or infiltrated, effect of analysis upon them, sociologists tended to think of the individual's adaptation to society as entirely motivated by such factors as the power of the group, or the status the individual enjoys within it. But psychoanalysis showed that this capacity of the individual for a role in the com-munity is a consequence of early adaptation to family members and a complex series of unconscious identifications with parents, sib-lings, and their surrogates. A clear example of this preparation in infancy for later socialization is the child's acquisition of the mother tongue by a world-wide process entirely different from that of de-liberately learning a language later in life; once acquired, the mother tongue will determine much of how the adult thinks, and therefore what modes of ideation he can share and what modes his mind is alien to. It is a mutual understanding of this basic premise, that the psychoanalyst studies the mental functions determining the individual's response to a social group, which underlies the best interdisciplinary work and discussion.

APPLIED PSYCHOANALYSIS: THE CLINICAL PROFESSIONS; CONCLUSION

The facts and theories of psychoanalysis also have immediate applications to the practical work of those professions offering various forms of help to people. These include not only dynamic psychiatry, its subspecialty, child psychiatry, and medicine,[5] but such related professions as social work, clinical psychology, child psychology, pedagogy, nursing, and criminology. All of these may accurately be called the "parent-surrogate professions." For their work is derived from the technical development of some phase of the parental instincts—feeding the hungry, protecting the helpless, giving to the needy, training the mind and character, providing relief from suffering. These professional tasks involve more than the intellectual execution of their duties; they involve personal relationships of this special kind with pupils, clients, and patients. Thus some pupils seek in a teacher approval they miss at home, develop anxiety reactions which the teacher's attitude does not justify, or reject discipline they know how to evade in other situations. Similarly, a social worker encounters stresses and emotional disturbances which her routine has not invited. A nurse takes the place for a sick adult patient that his mother did years ago. Because the emotional relations of both client and professional worker are, like those of patient and therapist, derived from childhood and often basically unconscious, the knowledge of psychoanalysis in this domain is a professional asset. These professions have also

[5] See Chapters XII, XIII, and XIV.

found, through studying the analytic method, improved interviewing techniques for their own professions. And by applying analytic knowledge of the unconscious and neuroses, they have become aware of the limitations of traditional methods of conscious persuasion and ethical instruction in influencing many human problems.

The first of these clinical professions to develop a fully conscious use of analysis was psychiatric social work, both in child guidance and in its other applications.[6] By the early thirties a considerable number of leaders and students were seeking personal psychoanalysis as a means of understanding the unconscious elements in clinical work with their cases. This has led to the modern type of case-work supervision and case-work technique, closely paralleling developments in the collaboration of psychiatric social work and dynamic psychiatry.

Modern *clinical psychology* has, in more recent years, also applied analytic knowledge and theories extensively. The Rorschach test was originally conceived as a research technique for the impersonal, statistical evaluation of personality and psychopathology. Dr. Henry Murray's thematic apperception test was devised as a laboratory method for obtaining the thoughts of people responding to standardized visual stimuli. As both were based upon imaginative and unreasoned mental responses of test-subjects, they invited the application of psychoanalytic knowledge and theory by some psychologists. In more recent years some clinical psychologists have tended more and more to supplement the original statistical evaluation of these tests by elaborate interpretations of the patient's reactions to the interview during which tests were given. In doing so, they have more directly employed free-association technique in a manner closely resembling the clinical techniques of analytically oriented dynamic psychiatry. Other psychologists have found the analytic knowledge of dreams an important foundation for research into the psychology of perception, and still others have found knowledge of identification vital in the further exploration of learning. Even more direct use has been made of

[6] See Chapter XII, pages 259, 261, 274.

analytic principles of therapy among those clinical psychologists who have made therapy or "counseling" their chief interest.

The applications of psychoanalysis to the arts and humanities, to the social sciences, and to professions whose practical work involves psychologic research and helpful influence are thus permeating more and more widely the basic methods and purposes of these professions. Many regard Freud as not only one of the great doctors who have made new and important contributions to our scientific understanding of human life and its ailments, but also as a major influence on the contemporary evolution of our civilization and its ideology. It is hard, indeed impossible, to judge how much Freud has initiated some social transformations of our era, or to what extent he is a pre-eminent example of the inevitable currents determining the scientific and cultural history of our day. Beyond doubt the impact of his work and ideas has extended far beyond the immediate facts and theories derived from psychoanalyses of the individual.

XVI

❖ ❖ ❖ ❖

PSYCHOANALYSIS:
A NEW PROFESSION

BEGINNINGS

O N E evening in May 1896, Freud addressed the Vienna Medical Society. His collaboration with Josef Breuer had ended three years before. In the meantime he had discovered that one could in the long run work more effectively, though more slowly, with patients awake and unhypnotized; he had learned the elementary principle of psychoanalytic technique, free association, and had been pursuing his pioneer investigations by its use. On this evening he was prepared to offer some of his discoveries to the scientific world. The response of the members of the Vienna Medical Society was the bitterest disappointment of his career. Instead of enthusiasm for the new light on human maladies which had hitherto baffled the medical world, or even skeptical interest, Freud's announcement was received with coldness. "I understood that from now onwards I belonged to those who have troubled the sleep of the world," he later wrote.

Freud had discovered and reported that sexual conflict is a cause of psychoneuroses. The profession his audience represented took a generation to confirm the facts on which he had based his statement. But he himself learned in this one evening what he had not previously been prepared for: that he who first discloses facts about the sexuality which one normally represses will be ridiculed at best, more often reviled; that scientific objectivity can be drowned by the subjective protest that scientists share with others who are human.

In 1896 it was not mere controversy that Freud was obliged to face; it was isolation. He never returned to the medical society which rejected his work that evening, and, after 1904, never addressed any other medical society in Vienna, though he continued his lectures at the University. He could pay the price of professional solitude in order to pursue truths that had not been scientifically studied before. For almost ten years, Freud worked alone. During this decade he amassed his observations, drew his conclusions, and prepared a series of publications which stand today as the foundations of analysis: some short papers (*Collected Papers*, Vol. I), which constitute our basic knowledge of the unconscious psychology of neuroses; his first long case-history (Vol. III); the monograph *Three Contributions to the Theory of Sex*, the fundamental statement of the facts of psychosexuality and the libido theory, comprising his conclusions of the interrelationship between repressed sexual phantasies, normal forepleasure, infantile sexuality, psychoneuroses, and perversions; *Wit and the Unconscious*; and, finally, the monumental *Interpretation of Dreams*, his masterpiece. Only in 1951, long after his death, was it revealed that, besides these works for publication, there had also been in existence for fifty years one of the most significant of all Freud's contributions to his knowledge of the unconscious, and ours.[1] This was the manuscript of Freud's letters to his great friend Dr. Wilhelm Fliess, of Berlin, describing details of his own severe neurosis, his psychoanalysis of himself (approximately 1897–1900), the discovery of repressed phantasies he could not ignore proving his own Œdipus complex, much of the material on which *Interpretation of Dreams*

---

[1] *The Origins of Psychoanalysis: Letters to Wilhelm Fliess*, by Sigmund Freud. Edited by M. Bonaparte, A. Freud, Ernst Kris (1954). See also Ernest Jones, *Life and Work of Sigmund Freud*, Vol. I, Chap. 14.

had been based, and details of his concurrent struggle to regain his own health and to formulate a satisfactory description of the mind, taking these new psychoanalytic facts fully into account.

THE INTERNATIONAL PSYCHOANALYTIC ASSOCIATION

During these early years of psychoanalysis there had been occasional reviews and references to Freud's psychological work in both German and English literature, most of them unfavorable. When the *Interpretation of Dreams* was published, he was in the fifth decade of his life, and renowned as a neurologist and physiologist. But only 228 copies were sold during the first two years. By 1902 a few random students had begun to work with Freud in Vienna. In the autumn of that year four of these, Wilhelm Stekel, Alfred Adler, Max Kahane, and Rudolph Reither, had formed with Freud the Psychological Wednesday Evening Society, a small group which was to become the Vienna Psychoanalytical Society with twenty-two members in 1908. Of even more immediate importance had been the active interest in Freud's writings of several psychiatrists associated with Professor Eugen Bleuler at the famous Burghölzi Clinic in Zürich. Dr. Carl Jung, Bleuler's assistant, was soon concentrating his efforts on the applications of analysis to psychotic thought, and made a revolutionary contribution to this subject.[2] This was the first great extension of Freud's work by another analyst; it led in 1907 to personal visits to Freud, to formal collaboration for several years by Jung and Binswanger, and to the interest in psychoanalysis of two students at Zürich, Max Eitingon and Karl Abraham, both younger men who later collaborated in establishing the Berlin Psychoanalytic Institute.

During the next few years psychoanalysis became the activity of other small but enthusiastic groups whose members felt the im-

---

[2] Carl Jung, *The Psychology of Dementia Præcox*, translated by Frederick Peterson and A. A. Brill (New York: Nervous and Mental Disease Publishing Company, Monograph Series, No. 3; 1914).

petus of an exchange of knowledge and ideas. In 1908 the first international congress of psychoanalysts was held at Salzburg, in an informal manner without officers. Forty-three people, from Austria, England, Germany, Switzerland, Hungary, and the United States attended. In 1909 the first journal of psychoanalysis (*Jahrbuch für psychoanalytische und psychologische Forschungen*) was published. In 1910 the International Psychoanalytic Association was formally organized, with branch societies in Vienna, Zürich, and Berlin. Except for inactivity during both World Wars, the International Psychoanalytic Association has subsequently met every one or two years. By 1938, when European societies were disintegrated by the heels of dictators, it comprised 560 members, and the national branches included societies in America, Austria, Hungary, Holland, England, France, Switzerland, India, Palestine, Denmark-Norway, Sweden-Finland, Czechoslovakia, Italy, Japan, Russia, and Israel.

PSYCHOANALYTIC EDUCATION

Before the disruption of European societies, one development of outstanding importance to psychoanalysis had occurred: the recognition of the special training necessary for its skilled practice, and the organization of such training by the chief societies. The pioneer analysts, some of them men of exceptional gifts, of necessity traveled only the rocky roads through unexplored lands; there were no signposts, except those set up from time to time by laboriously acquired experience, to show how to avoid the errors to which uninstructed beginners are blind. Their only recourse was informal discussion of personal material with their sparse colleagues. Thus Freud and Ferenczi, on shipboard in 1909 on their way to the famous Clark University Lectures, had analyzed each other's dreams, and similar brief and informal searchings of one's own unconscious were not uncommon among the first explorers of analysis. As late as 1914 Freud had published the opinion that some self-analysis, such as he himself had achieved in 1897, should suffice for able analysts with only minor abnormalities. But as their science advanced, analysts became aware of how much more vast and decisive than they themselves or even Freud at first had realized was the unconscious as a source of human ignorance, as well as of human activities and symptoms. They became more and more aware how subtle and complex were many of the mechanisms for concealing one's motives from oneself, and fully convinced that even the most gifted in intuitive introspection could not achieve this task alone. The first step toward a formal education for the psychoanalyst's work came when the fundamental importance of the future analyst's undergoing a complete psychoanalysis of himself was fully recognized. In 1918 Hermann Nunberg had proposed at an international congress that this be required in the future; and soon thereafter it was generally considered an essential preparation by analytic societies in both Europe and America.

The purpose of such a "didactic (training) analysis" is, primarily, to ensure the practitioner of psychoanalysis against two tendencies which are common to him, his patients, and all other human beings. First, there is always the unconscious tendency to overvalue those personality problems from which one suffers oneself and to overlook what is subjectively less interesting but objectively more important for the individual patient. This tendency is most conspicuous and deleterious when it leads, during the study of others, to concentration on those conflicts in oneself which have been repressed and are unrecognized. Secondly, there is the tendency to err by ascribing to others (through "projection") a predominance of those very traits which one dislikes so much in oneself as to deny their presence. These two sources of error must inevitably impair any analyst's ability to appraise his patient's problems, unless they are very carefully controlled and reduced as far as possible by didactic analysis.

The didactic analysis is of pedagogic importance in other ways. For the future analyst will attain first-hand familiarity with the unconscious functions of the mind most readily, and far more rapidly, if less completely, by this method than by study of others. Didactic analysis is the dissecting-room of analytic education, the course in which the future analyst is first exposed to the empirical facts of mental "anatomy." Subsequently the student is in a position to confirm, correct, and amplify his observations of the unconscious in analyses of his own patients with more studious objectivity. And, finally, didactic analysis is the optimal way of learning by constant contact with an expert the principles and actual practice of technique.

In 1920 a new era in psychoanalytic education was inaugurated by the opening of the Berlin Psychoanalytic Institute. This was the culmination of the work of Karl Abraham, whose qualities as scientist and man had appeared early as a student in Zürich, and of Max Eitingon, who inspired and administered this project. Their new undertaking became pre-eminent not only for the quality of its work and its faculty, but also because here for the first time a psychoanalytic group was organized to provide clinical facilities for the psychoanalytic treatment of patients of small means and to provide, in addition to didactic analysis, a systematic and thorough course of instruction to students in psychoanalysis.

In 1925 it was proposed at a Congress of the International Psychoanalytic Association that all societies organize their training of students. The example of Berlin was then followed by Vienna, London, and Budapest. Within a few years several American societies had established similar training; and, prior to their disruption by the Nazis and the war, the Societies at Paris, The Hague, Jerusalem, Calcutta, Sweden-Finland, and Prague had all begun the systematic training of professional psychoanalysts. The major policies and functions of these various institutes were identical. They recognized that not everyone whose inclination is to become a psychoanalyst is well qualified. A high standard of personal character, maturity, and special aptitude for psychological investigation, as well as thorough preliminary scientific training, were expected before matriculation. The curriculum consisted of three portions whose completion took several years' study: first, a "didactic analysis" of the candidate himself by a "training analyst" approved by the institute; secondly, a group of "didactic courses" in the theory of psychoanalysis; thirdly, "supervised (or control) analysis," the conduct by the candidate himself of several therapeutic analyses, under the direct supervision of a senior teacher.

Each institute delegated its educational functions to an "educational committee," which took over the former responsibilities, sometimes poorly met, of the individual analyst who accepted students as apprentices entirely on his own initiative. These committees supervised the admission of candidates, the educational program, and the appointment of instructors ("training analysts"), and pronounced on the final fitness of a student to engage in the independent practice of psychoanalysis. The election of members to the constituent branches of the International and American Psychoanalytic Associations has, ever since institutes were first established, largely depended on the satisfactory completion of such an educational program.

These developments in organized psychoanalytic education during the past thirty years have resulted not only in serving the science of psychoanalysis and the students themselves, but in serving medicine and the general public as well. Previously a patient seeking a therapeutic analysis was necessarily at a loss as to whether a particular individual who termed himself a "psychoanalyst" was properly qualified. Psychoanalysis is still so recent an addition to the medical therapies that it has lacked that solidarity of tradition and authority which enables the medical profession, through its societies and schools and licensing boards, to offer the public a certain minimum guarantee of the fitness of its practitioners. Similar standards and authority are essential for the most effective safeguarding of the psychoanalytic clientele. These developments in standards of education and membership have reached their fullest development in the United States.

EUROPEAN CATASTROPHE AND PSYCHOANALYSIS

By 1930, psychoanalysis had become an established if small and highly controversial profession. Its early esotericism and its most violent controversies were receding into history, and the component societies of the International Psychoanalytic Association in Europe and America had become centers of active practice, scientific exploration of the unconscious, and organized post-graduate education for this new profession. Then the sulfurous elements of history began to smoke again. The recovered optimism of the world was proved ill-founded. At first insidiously, then with increasing violence, the academic life in some European institutes was proved unsafe and new political agencies sought out the principles of analysis and its teachers for destruction. In 1933 the advent of Hitler as Chancellor led in Berlin to the public burning of Freud's books to propagandize the Führer's concept of Aryan supremacy. In the next few years an increasingly large number of leading members (Jewish and some democratic gentiles) of the German Society and Berlin Institute of Psychoanalysis departed for other lands. In 1936 it was helped by the political patronage of a cousin of Hermann Göring to become officially a separate department of the new General German Medical Society for Psychotherapy; in this way a few former members cautiously carried on under censorship some of its scientific and educational activities.

In Vienna, the birthplace of analysis, the Psychoanalytic Society was immediately demolished when Austria was annexed in March 1938 by Nazi Germany. Its professional activities and its 102 members were dispersed. Professor Freud and his family, including Anna Freud, were welcomed by the President of the London Society and the British Government in June 1938. After the last of many operations for a cancer, whose pain he had withstood while he worked for sixteen years, Freud died in London, September 23, 1939. All except four of his Vienna colleagues also settled in London, in America, and in other countries. The dissolution of the important Hungarian Society, of the branch in Prague of the Vienna Society, and of the society which was forming in Rome soon followed, while small groups in Russia and Japan were no longer heard from. In the democratic countries, only in Sweden had serious governmental obstacles been encountered.

The devastation inflicted by the Nazis in their own countries, and by the Second World War throughout the world, has consequently altered but not paralyzed the development of psychoanalysis. The work of the British Society, founded in 1913 by Ernest Jones, and its Institute, was continued throughout the London bombings, and its continuity and postwar development were therefore ruptured but not disastrously affected; it now has three small branches, in Melbourne (1940), Sydney (1951), and Canada (1955). Of all Continental societies, only the Dutch, some of whose analysts continued underground training activities even throughout the German military occupation, survived the war as a vigorous major analytic group. A mere handful of survivors in Vienna, under the leadership of August Aichhorn, famed pioneer of the twenties in applying analysis to delinquents, re-established the Vienna Institute in 1946; it is now a tiny enterprise when contrasted with its pre-Nazi eminence. The Berlin Institute, though much reduced in size, has been functioning since 1951 under the direction of Dr. Muller-Braunschweig, a pre-Nazi teacher there. The Swiss Society continues its work with a loosely organized training program. The French Psycho-analytical Society, though sundered during and after the War by internal problems of its own, and disintegrated by German occupation, has been revived. The Italian Society has been re-established (1949). The Hungarian Psycho-analytic Society resumed activities in 1945, but was officially dissolved again in 1949 by the Communists. There are new, smaller groups of analysts in Sweden, Denmark, and Belgium.

On other continents, the most important development, besides those in the United States, has been the Argentina Psychoanalytic Society, started in 1943 by Dr. Angel Garma of Spain; its leadership in Latin America has favorably affected the development of two Brazilian societies and the beginning of smaller analytic groups in Chile and several other Spanish-speaking countries. The Israel Society, founded before war broke out by Dr. Max Eitingon, the first of the Zürich psychiatrists to visit Freud in 1907, and former director of the Berlin Institute, continues its leadership in the Middle East, a haven for some of the displaced analysts of Europe. Small psychoanalytic groups in Japan and India survived the War. Assistance to these demolished societies and to new centers has been a major interest of the venerable International Psychoanalytic Association at the biennial scientific Congresses since the war.[3]

PSYCHOANALYTIC CONTROVERSIES

EARLY CONTROVERSIES: STEKEL, ADLER, AND JUNG

This amazing development of the first generation of a science was based upon a principle, the empirical investigation of the unconscious, which was as new as the isolation of oxygen by Lavoisier a century before. It had, within forty years, achieved scientific recognition by others, been selected as a lifetime work by increasing numbers in many lands, inspired by the rapid discoveries of new facts and ideas by so youthful a branch of knowledge. It had well established international and national professional societies, a dozen scientific journals, and institutes for the professional training of analysts in Europe and America.

At the same time this new profession had, like a precocious and gifted problem child, been torn by inner controversies which at times threatened its destruction. By the time of the second International Congress in 1910, a very few years after Freud had acquired his first followers, there were serious personal and scientific cleavages, some of which would shortly prove irreconcilable.

The first of these was between Freud and Dr. Wilhelm Stekel of Vienna, the early follower from whom Freud had learned most about symbolism in dreams. Still more widely known and protracted was the controversy with Dr. Alfred Adler, who, after several years' association with the earliest analysts in Vienna, had resigned from the group in 1911 and founded a "school" of his own called "Individual Psychology." The clarity of his later exposition of "inferiority complex" furnished the languages of Europe with a

[3] Inquiry as to details of non-American societies may be addressed to Dr. Ruth S. Eissler, Honorary Secretary, International Psychoanalytic Association, 265 Central Park West, New York 24, N.Y.

useful term for describing this prevalent phenomenon, and his description of the "will to power" and the "masculine protest," the impetus which human beings feel to prove their feelings of inferiority unjustified, was important. Psychoanalysts criticized Adler, not because his views were false, but because they were superficial, and because it is absurd to define all emotional reactions in this one formula. Adler accounted for all aspects of conduct, character, and neurosis as varieties of "masculine protest," the wish to deny weakness or inferority. But psychoanalysis had shown that the "inferiority complex" is one of the commonest ways by which unconscious guilt produces conscious suffering, that both scientific research and therapy require dynamic analysis of the unconscious sources of this conscious symptom, that repressed wishes must be fully recognized, and that passive impulses are as important in human motivation as conscious desires for dominance. In short, the therapy of Adler became in practice chiefly a therapy of the secondary gains and not of the *primary* causes of neurosis.[4]

A still more famous and disruptive controversy, and the one to cause Freud most personal pain, was that with Carl Jung, the first editor of a psychoanalytic journal and, in accordance with Freud's expressed wish, first president of the International Psychoanalytic Association. But by that time, 1910, the personal and scientific breach was unhealable; in 1912 a Congress was called off in consequence of the acceptance by Jung, the president, of an invitation to lecture at Fordham University in New York, and two years later Jung resigned from the Association. A psychiatrist of profound intellectual gifts and unusual erudition, Jung had been Freud's leading follower and made major psychoanalytic contributions to experimental free association, the psychology of schizophrenia, and dream psychology. Unquestionably the irreconcilability of the disagreements between Freud and Jung was in part personal, in part scientific. There were many intense jealousies and temperamental outbursts among the pioneers in analysis; there were also strong feelings of solidarity among the Viennese associates of Freud and sometimes an attitude of regarding the Swiss as inter-

4 See pages 235–7.

lopers; and letters recently published have shown that pro-Jewish and anti-Jewish prejudices both unquestionably intensified professional discord.[5]

At the time of his resignation, Jung had declared he could no longer share Freud's views on the differentiation of sexual libido from other types of psychic energy. Unquestionably, Jung's still earlier inclination to avoid the facts of psychosexuality had been a more fundamental breach. For the views of Freud and Jung concerning the definition of libido, as well as other theories, were seldom irreconcilable. Freud's final theory, that sexual instincts and ego instincts are derived from the same fundamental source (Eros [6]), is indeed in harmony with this part of the theory of Jung which Freud had previously contested, though the more basic difference remained between Jung's "monistic" view that all psychic energy is from one source and Freud's "dualistic" concept of opposed instinct groups. Jung had also strongly emphasized the "collective unconscious"—those symbols and phantasies and religious beliefs which are common to many racial groups. But Freud, who had always in therapy focused especially on the personal experiences of each individual, had, nevertheless, been the first to show, and had never disclaimed, that besides the repressed memories of the individual's experience there is a vast realm of the unconscious which is common to mankind. He had emphasized it especially in his book *Totem and Taboo* (1912), where he discussed the unconscious determination of tribal rituals and taboo. Jung's still later description of the various "introvert" and "extrovert" types was an unimpeachable classification of personalities for any who find it useful, though without a thorough investigation of the unconscious ontogenetic factors which produce the subtypes its value to the analyst was limited.

---

[5] Jung himself in 1934 demonstrated in an unexpected way how his prejudice transcended the usual kinds. After the National Socialists of Germany had reorganized a professional journal, Jung became Editor and immediately announced in its pages that Aryan psychology must replace the "immoral" Jewish psychology of Freud. *Zentralblatt für Psychotherapie*, Vol. VII, page 7 (1934).

[6] See "Eros and the Death Instincts," pages 125–7.

The therapeutic practices of Jung diverged far more from those of Freud than did his theories. Though Freud did not dispute the "collective unconscious," he did not consider its existence justified the therapist in neglecting the investigation of that portion of the unconscious which psychoanalysis had shown to be the reservoir of the individual's own experience and the chief source of his neurotic conflicts. And though Jung still used free association to a considerable extent, his therapeutic principles and his methods were in other essentials very different from psychoanalysis. For Jung took special interest in the more symbolic elements of the patient's phantasy life, and in studying its similarities with those found in art, various religions, and mythologies. Psychoanalysts, however, did not favor the use of Jung's methods because they appeared far more an exciting academic tutorship than an etiologic therapy, providing the neurotic individual with a new philosophy with which to cloak his suffering rather than effecting a dynamic personality change and capacity for more mature development. Jung repeatedly stated that he still regarded Freud's psychoanalytic method as the therapy of choice for many psychoneuroses, except in elderly people. Yet he himself no longer practiced it, his students were not encouraged to study it, and somehow the misconception has always been widespread that Jung believed his own method should supplant psychoanalysis as a psychotherapeutic procedure.[7]

[7] A twenty-six-month detailed investigation of psychoanalysis by a committee of the British Medical Association reported in May 1929 that psychoanalysts should not be held responsible for other schools of psychotherapy, that there were many misconceptions of psychoanalysis, that other schools, such as those of Jung, Adler, Rank, Stekel, do not deal like analysts with resistances, and concluded: *"There is in the medical and general public, a tendency to use the term 'psychoanalysis' in a very loose and wide sense. This term can legitimately be applied only to the method evolved by Freud and to the theories derived from the use of this method. A psychoanalyst is therefore a person who uses Freud's technic, and anyone who does not use this technic should not, whatever he may employ, be called a psychoanalyst."* (Report of the British Medical Association on Psychoanalysis, Special Supplement, Appendix II.: *British Medical Journal,* June 29, 1929; abstracted by Isador Coriat, M.D., *Psychoanalytic Review,* Vol. XVII., January 1930.) Unhappily, no such authoritative distinction between "psychoanalysis" and other therapeutic methods exists in America.

POSTWAR CONTROVERSIES: FERENCZI AND RANK

After the zenith of these early dissensions (1910–12), psychoanalysis continued its own natural growth and accretion of supporters, and the former Freudians, Stekel, Adler, and Jung, founded psychological schools of their own. A relative lull in violent controversy ensued, possibly fostered by interruption of scientific communications during the First World War. But after the war there were again some important dissensions by a few former students of Freud. Dr. Sandor Ferenczi, founder of the Budapest Society, and throughout the years probably the closest personally to Freud of all his early psychoanalytic colleagues, deviated notably in the twenties, chiefly in regard to principles of technique. He proposed that a primary goal of all psychoanalytic technique should be active efforts by the therapist throughout the analysis to show the patient he was loved; he also advocated a technique which encouraged the patient to behavior during the treatment hour as a substitute at times for free association—a procedure somewhat resembling play technique in child analysis. Though the art of analysis has always allowed for similar expedients for dealing with exceptional problems, their adoption as standard modifications of therapeutic technique was a contradiction of the fundamental analytic principle that the analyst maintain a maximal impersonality. Ferenczi's last years before his death in 1933 were unhappy because Freud did not adopt his new ways. The fact that Ferenczi himself, more than any other of Freud's closest associates, had severe hypochondriacal and other neurotic symptoms throughout his life, and received more therapeutic help from Freud, may not be irrelevant to this overemphasis of the need of every patient—indeed, of every human being—for evidence of love by his therapist at all times.

The other dissensions by former analysts in later years produced particularly prominent but temporary effects in America. The most important of these dissenters was Otto Rank, a nonmedical analyst and one of Freud's earliest students in Vienna. Endowed with artistic as well as intellectual gifts, he was a man of exhaustive erudition, and had played a notable part in the application of psychoanalytic principles to the arts and to the study of the relation of myths of various cultures to the daydreams of individuals.[8] In December 1923 he published a new book, *The Trauma of Birth and Its Importance in Psychoanalytic Therapy*, in which he claimed that the anxiety of neurotics is always a repetition of the psychological experience of being born, and that later manifestations of anxiety are secondary.

This ill-founded idea soon led to a totally new theory of therapy by Rank. The effectiveness of psychoanalytic therapy, he now argued, is due, not to the ideas which emerge from the unconscious, but entirely to the emotional experience during the treatment. Freud's discovery that the source of neurotic conflict is to be found in the repression of infantile experience is valid, but it is only the present experience that is of therapeutic importance; the past experience of the individual cannot be treated and should be disregarded. Therefore, he concluded, let us revise Freud's technique, treat only the resistance to the emotional relationships with the therapist and make no special effort to resolve the resistances to recollection of past experience. Thus we may reasonably expect to achieve a cure in much shorter periods of analysis (two or three months) than is necessary with Freud's technique and find a solution to the problem which has baffled all analysts—the long duration of each individual patient's treatment. For three years (1923–6) Freud hoped that Rank's new attitude was curable, and attempted to cope tolerantly with the personal dissensions both he and Ferenczi had evoked. By 1926 Freud could no longer doubt that Rank's ideas were as incompatible with psychoanalysis as those of Jung had been, an inevitable conclusion which Abraham, Jones, Sachs, Brill, and others had long before accepted.

Rank had introduced his new views in New York in 1924, and in 1926 he came to live in America permanently. The controversies of American analysts with Adler and Jung and their proselytes were at that time still unsettled, and America became

8 See pages 304–5.

the chief battleground of this new controversy too. Rank's theory seemed to some based on logical hypotheses, and therefore justified experiment. In 1926 several of the foremost analysts of New York themselves tried out his novel principles. But they soon withdrew this support, partly because of the new theoretical concepts which Rank now advanced with increased vehemence. At any rate, there seemed to be no reason for ascribing all neurotic phenomena to a single cause, and that an entirely theoretical one. But the main occasion for the consistent disavowal of Rank by his former psychoanalytic colleagues was that, though the theoretical grounds for his experiments had at first made sense, the experiments were not usually successful.[9]

SECOND-GENERATION CONTROVERSIES

Rejection of some if not all of Freud's chief conclusions by a few followers has not been limited to these among his first students who founded anti-Freudian schools. There have been later similar deviations, provocative of strenuous controversies by analysts of the second generation. Probably the most important has been that of Melanie Klein and her followers in London, resulting from her different ideas of childhood development,[1] and particularly from the profound effect of these on adult analysis and the professional training of analysts. This has produced no major controversies in America; indeed, she is rightly considered to have made important additions to psychoanalytic knowledge of the little child. But in England it led to two groups within the Faculty of the London Institute, differing fundamentally in their concepts and techniques.

[9] During the subsequent two or three years Rank's revolt against Freud went still further. He renounced his effort to modify psychoanalytic technique and in a succession of publications offered a new "psychology" which he believed made Freud's work obsolete. With each new publication he departed further from the empiricism and determinism of Freud and finally repudiated scientific methodology. His final views appeared to analysts to be based on a philosophical concept of freedom of the will and the volitional control of neurotic wishes. If it were true that neurotic tendencies could be cured by will-power, there never would have been occasion for psychoanalysis at all.

[1] See pages 270–2.

American psychoanalysis also had its own difficult episodes during the 1930's and early 1940's, a few temporarily threatening the development of the still small American Psychoanalytic Association. Dr. Karen Horney, originally a "Freudian" training analyst of the Berlin Institute during its great decade in the twenties, was generally regarded by analysts as a specially gifted clinician and teacher. Shortly after coming to America in 1932, she surprised other analysts by the increasing vehemence of her attacks upon Freud's views. In her early diatribes and first books, she focused especially on the contention that Freud's views of the Œdipus complex and the "masculine-protest" of females were unjustified, and proposed that "self-analysis" of the unconscious was possible for many patients. In 1941 Dr. Horney and a small number of former Freudian analysts, after several years of increasing disagreement with their fellow members, resigned from the New York Psychoanalytic Society (as well as the American and International Associations), establishing a new society of their own in New York (The Association for the Advancement of Psychoanalysis), a new journal, and a new school of training.

Horney's views were much elaborated during the next decade, and in the opinion of most other analysts were totally irreconcilable with the science created by Freud. She proclaimed the primary determinant of personality development and health to be "self-realization," described as the need for the "real self" to be successfully experienced. She considered that all neurosis resulted from "basic anxiety," understood as the revival of the aloneness and helplessness of the infant when not protected by love. "Basic anxiety" and "basic hostility" result from insufficient love, making "self-realization" impossible. All agree that such problems are important in the lives of many children; but Horney differed by insisting they are chiefly the result of a patient's inability to deal with contradictory demands made by the culture—the cultural demand to love others and the simultaneous demand to compete with others successfully, for example. There ensues a "basic conflict" in interpersonal relations, manifested by the neurotic need to comply, attack, or withdraw in relations with other people. In her last book

(1950) Horney stressed even more a "central inner conflict" as the source of destructiveness, suffering, and neurotic defenses; this type of "intrapsychic" conflict results from the abnormal replacement of the drive to experience the "real self" by an unattainable image of a glorified, prideful "ideal-self."

Some of Freud's ideas, such as the unconscious, the defense processes, the interpretation of anxiety as "the dynamic center of the neurosis," and free-association technique are still acknowledged by Horney's followers. But the occasional allusions by this group to Freud have been chiefly in terms of his historical position. They consider ideas of other analysts outmoded, their own a sounder basis for therapy, yet continue to use the word "psychoanalysis" in the titles of their society, journal, and institute. As with the early deviations of Adler and Jung, most other psychoanalysts objected not so much to what Horney affirmed as to what she denied or treated as of little importance. The need to feel a complete and adequate person, which is the core of her theory, is unquestionably the healthy state for which everyone strives. But Horney regarded this "self-realization" as the primary "dynamic" determinant of health and growth, and she therefore explicitly repudiated the instinct theories and with them the whole mass of psychoanalytic knowledge from which they were induced. Freud regarded such a healthy state of mind as the end result of solving a complicated sequence of conflicts produced by biologic (instinctual) needs and other tensions, rather than the primary motivation. "Basic anxiety," or infantile helplessness, is also a fundamental experience and recognized by all as decisive in some personality problems, but its place in Horney's theory leaves out of account psychoanalytic knowledge of many other needs of child and adult which also evoke anxiety. Similarly, she regarded the enormous subjective importance of sexuality for human beings as itself a consequence of its over-evaluation by our culture rather than biologically inevitable. She also at times considered a personality "disturbance a neurosis only if it *deviates* from the pattern common to the particular culture"—a definition popular among some sociologists too, but just not clinically applicable to the unconsciously self-induced suffering of many patients.

And finally, from the beginning of Horney's quarrel with other analysts, an entirely different kind of protest against Freud has constantly been proclaimed. For she and her followers have never ceased asserting that the premises of their therapeutic method are superior, not merely because these ideas appear to them factually more sound, but because Horney regarded "self-realization" as an "optimistic" attitude toward human experience, and therefore a "moral" concept. They disclaim what they call the "instinctivistic" and "genetic" views of Freud because these are considered "pessimistic" and therefore "immoral" and a poor basis for therapy. In the last of Horney's books,[2] published two years before her death, she again unambiguously contended, as she had throughout the years, that only a pessimistic view of life is possible if one's morality is based on "instinctivistic" belief that "man is by nature sinful or ridden by primitive instincts." Horney's quasi-religious thesis is of course attractive to many. But to most analysts it seems not unlike arguing that a physician who is repelled by the sight of internal organs or blood should therefore not study or describe such unpleasant things. Perhaps the emphasis of this ethical thesis by Horney may help us to understand how a person of truly exceptional aptitude for work with patients could disclaim so much of Freud's reasoning. It certainly makes clear how Horney's deviance from psychoanalysis was not merely an attack upon facts and theories which Freud considered important, but more fundamentally a failure to appreciate and fully share his primary orientation as a scientist.

The views of the American psychiatrist Dr. Harry Stack Sullivan somewhat resemble Horney's, especially his emphasis on cultural factors in molding personality and on anxiety resulting from inadequate emotional situations in early years. Though Sullivan was a member of the American Psychoanalytic Association, it is probably not quite accurate to think of him as like those who after years of work in psychoanalysis set up a deviant school. But as Sullivan is quite widely spoken of as a "deviationist," and because a number of

[2] Karen Horney, *Neurosis and Human Growth* (New York: W. W. Norton; 1950).

students and associates most directly influenced by him were analysts, he has played a role in the analytic controversies of his generation. The fact is that his own primary interests and experience differed from Freud's to an extent that the true deviationist's had not. Trained in psychiatry under William Alanson White, pioneer in applying psychoanalysis to the therapy of psychoses, Dr. Sullivan for nearly a decade concentrated what might be called his genius for understanding the thought and language of psychotics on the study and treatment of schizophrenia at Sheppard Enoch Pratt Hospital, Baltimore. It was in the extension of his original interests after 1931 to the obsessional neuroses and to the processes of normal development and socialization that he elaborated his own system of "interpersonal dynamisms" which, though highly original and exciting, avowedly denied fundamental principles of analysis.[3] He was hyperindividualistic and both gifted and idiosyncratic in the use of words; he had a unique need to formulate his own "postulates," to think things out his own way and in his own language, or he might have found a larger part of Freud's contribution valuable. He agreed with Freud about the factuality of the unconscious and he accepted the core of Freud's anxiety theory of neurosis: that avoidance of this affect is at the root of neurotic processes. He did not, however, find the libido theory helpful to him, though in his own way he did utilize clinical knowledge of infantile sexuality. Like Horney, he placed great emphasis on cultural forces, but he went further and deeper, especially in his application of linguistics and of the work of Kurt Lewin and other social psychologists to his conceptions of "interpersonal dynamisms," and to his conception of therapy as a two-person "field" in which the psychiatrist was a reciprocal "participant." Since his death in 1949, Sullivan's surviving influence is most apparent among some psychiatrists and analysts closely associated with him over the years, among some psychiatrists specializing in the therapy of the psychoses, and most of all among social scientists who are interested in the applications of Sullivan's

---

[3] Harry Stack Sullivan, M.D., *The Interpersonal Theory of Psychiatry*, edited by Helen Swick Perry and Mary Ladd Gawell, introduction by Mabel Cohen, M.D. (New York: W. W. Norton; 1953).

theories to their field.

There have therefore been two sets of psychoanalysts who have quarreled with their colleagues and established schools of their own based on different psychological principles: those among the first generation of Freud's students, notably Jung and Adler, and at a later period Ferenczi (without complete separation) and Rank; and those of the second professional generation. Horney set up an entirely separate school, but still clutched tightly the name "psychoanalysis." There have been other prominent analysts of the second generation whose ideas have also produced serious controversies that did not, however, reach the point of complete disavowal of psychoanalysis as understood by most of their colleagues and the creation of entirely separate schools. A few prominent individuals in America also incited serious controversies concerning professional education which took years to resolve. And there are still a few individuals and small groups whose scientific and training principles cannot be endorsed by the American Psychoanalytic Association, although they refer to themselves as "psychoanalysts" and to their schools as "psychoanalytic" institutes.

CRITIQUE OF THE CONTROVERSIES

From the present vantage point of one or two professional generations since these two periods of rebellion by prominent students of Freud, certain objective conclusions seem today justified. The most obvious is that the breadth as well as the depth of Freud's genius has been proved by the survival of his basic conclusions and the accelerated attraction of scientifically trained psychiatrists to the psychoanalytic profession, while the influence of Jung and Adler and Rank, and later Horney, Rado, and Sullivan, and the agitated controversies they engendered, have proved themselves quite transitory.

A second conclusion is that all these scientific deviations were productive of intense personal rancor and were not entirely intellectual. How crucial was Freud's patriarchal intolerance of devia-

tion by his first followers? Or, to use his own professional language, to what extent was Freud himself unable to cope with his
anxiety lest the "sons" unite to slay the "primal father?" He knew
his own Œdipus complex, but was he too acutely sensitive to that
of his followers? Certainly he had a prescient consciousness in his
youth that he would achieve something more than ordinary men,
an appropriate ambitiousness, and in maturity a full awareness of
his own greatness. He also possessed much of the time the tolerance
of the seer, and a capacity within limits to comprehend and forgive
men of lesser wisdom. And finally, in appraisals of Freud's personal
contribution to the earlier quarrels, we should not overlook that
both bickerings and bitter controversies continued in the second
professional generation, under circumstances in which Freud himself was not directly in contact with the storm center, especially in
America in the thirties and early forties.

Still more decisive were the characters of those first followers
who turned against Freud. Not only were these adherents of the
small early groups of analysts men of special talents, but some were
of driven, non-conformist temperaments, and were inflamed by
having learned human secrets previously hidden from other people.
And some of them were exceptionally egocentric, as attested by the
need of several to form their own "schools," dominate groups of
proselytes, and create new professional vocabularies totally different from that of Freud. Not only was this true of the first deviationists in Europe; it is also conspicuous in producing some later
American disputes. Even within the small group of analysts during
the first fifteen years of analysis in America, severe dissension and
eventual separation was enacted by such pioneers as Trigant Bur-
row and Pierce Clark—names now forgotten. But most, not all,
of the explosive deviations and consequent controversy in this
country were produced by individual European leaders and a small
number of American followers. The schools of Adler and Jung had
been developed in Europe and were carried over here; the later
ones, those led by Rank, Horney, and Rado especially, were indige-
nous to America. Why some analysts, held in the highest respect by
their colleagues while they worked in Europe, were driven to de-

velop schools of their own after they came to this country is an interesting question, involving their personalities, their backgrounds, and American susceptibility to what purports to be new from Europe.

More important than the human faults and egoistic traits of these individuals is the lamentable fact that the early groups of analysts, especially in Vienna, did conduct their scientific affairs in some respects as a "cult," and justified in some degree the aspersions of their enemies. Though quite a number of the first generation of analysts were men of unusual ability and true scientific initiative, there was but one leader, one final authority in matters scientific and matters personal until analytic societies in other countries were highly developed. And he was leader of a group psychologically isolated to a considerable extent from medical and psychiatric colleagues by the hostility of "outsiders" to the new science. His followers regarded Freud with personal reverence as well as scientific awe, and they were culturally habituated to think in terms of loyalty or betrayal of a patriarchy, and of hierarchal allegiance to the "Herr Professor" tradition in German universities.

The most striking historical evidence of this is the now famous "Committee," [4] a personal compact whose existence was known to only a few "insiders" till after Freud's death. The "Committee" was formed in June 1912, at the suggestion of Ernest Jones, after the defection of Stekel, Adler, and Jung had almost destroyed the little group of Freud's colleagues. It was composed of six of Freud's most gifted first followers: Abraham, Ferenczi, Jones, Rank, Sachs, and later Eitingon; for a short time after 1925, Anna Freud was added. The primary intent was idealistic—to prevent the recurrence of the more disastrous consequences of disrupted scientific identity by a mutual agreement that, whereas none of the Committee should be deprived of the scientific prerogative of change of opinion, such an occurrence must be discussed with the other members of the Committee before it was publicly proclaimed. This purpose it

---

[4] C. P. Oberndorf, A *History of Psychoanalysis in America;* Ernest Jones, *The Life and Work of Sigmund Freud,* Volume II, Chapter 6, and Volume III, Chapter 2.

achieved to a considerable degree, especially in its discussion over several years of the merits and demerits of Ferenczi's and Rank's deviations. In 1927 the Committee was disbanded. The undesirable consequence of this Committee, other than the existence of a vow of secrecy by its members, was chiefly the spirit of an "inner circle" which permeated the first generation of European analysts and which permeated the psychoanalytic movement for many years. It was most apparent in the significance attached to approval in Vienna of analytic leaders in other countries. In the United States, for example, a few European teachers who had come to this country during the twenties and thirties repeatedly produced serious frictions by maintaining a right to ignore the authority of an American society in its own policies while accepting the authority of the International Psychoanalytic Association and its "International Training Commission." There are still some residuals of the factional politics induced in this way, though most of these effects of a former philosophy have at last become past history.[5]

Some other conclusions can be reasonably drawn from the history of the deviationists. It is most noteworthy that these individuals were not only psychoanalysts who eventually disavowed Freud's work, but individuals each of whom, in his own right, had made a creditable and original contribution to the analyst's total knowledge of the human mind and personality. Stekel made the major contribution to the psychology of symbolism. Adler focused attention upon the importance of self-depreciation in motivating human conduct, a contribution whose value is attested by his addition of an apparently permanent phrase to all European languages —"inferiority complex." Jung taught us much about the "collective unconscious," about dreams and delusions, and about the relationship of the phantasies of European individuals to the myths of primitive peoples. Karen Horney gave us a clearer clinical view in

[5] One of the major advances of American professional education— though it took several decades of strife to achieve—has been the replacement of an "apprenticeship" attitude (in which an individual analyst was chief sponsor of each student he analysed) by the principle that the Faculties of Institutes, rather than an individual, have full authority in educational policy and administration.

some ways of the exploitation of adolescent sexuality by some patients for neurotic gratification of infantile needs. Sullivan gave us deeper understanding of psychotic modes of thought. Rank's contribution after renouncing analysis was indeed more negative, but was important as the most dramatic demonstration of the limitations of efforts by himself and others to achieve the ardent wish of most analysts: to find a shorter road to accomplishing all that thorough analysis can. Appraisal of Stekel, Adler, Jung, Rank, Sullivan, and Horney involves, therefore, not so much a refutation of their positive ideas, as an answer to the thorny question: why did each of these prefer leadership of a "school" of proselytes of his own, with consequent denial of much of what Freud had discovered, to making a modest contribution of his own while maintaining coexistence with other analysts?

In every one of these cases careful study shows that the inevitable cause of cleavage was not that its instigator's chief scientific ideas could not be tolerated and included in scientific discussion by psychoanalysts, but that the deviationist's promotion of his own chief ideas invoked his denial of most other important and well-proven empirical discoveries by Freud, and the theories resulting from these facts. Each of these deviationists ultimately denied those facts of psychosexuality discovered by analysis: their biological inevitability, their role in determining important phases of infantile development, and the repression of sexual phantasies and memories. This observation makes even more significant the fact, not published at the time but well documented today, that the termination in 1893 of Freud's very first partnership in psychological investigation had really been a consequence of Breuer's refusal to recognize the importance of the sexual phantasies of some of his hysterical patients. Among all the later deviationists, there were likewise various degrees of abrogation of analytic data concerning unconscious sexuality, from complete revocation of their existence to various modifications of the significance ascribed to them by Freud. In all cases, denial of these facts led to rejection of the libido theory and a consequent redefinition of biologic forces in development, and of therapeutic goals and techniques. And with the repudiation of sexuality and the libido theory, as defined by other analysts, went the erection of a new vocabulary by each deviant, in several cases including new words for what were essentially Freud's own well-known ideas.

One more retrospective observation may be made: each of the first-generation deviationists appealed chiefly to a different professional group, at least in America. Thus the ideas of Alfred Adler in the twenties, when he was most influential here, appealed most to professional psychologists, and especially to educational psychologists and counsellors. Otto Rank, whose early influence in America was among a few psychoanalysts and psychiatrists, eventually affected only a small minority of psychiatric social workers. Carl Jung, though a few American psychiatrists have adopted his methods, has chiefly perpetuated his fame in the United States among academic professions whose ideas have not been primarily based on clinical experience with patients. In contrast, though Freud has to a still greater degree influenced such non-medical professions as social work, psychology, anthropology, and sociology, the momentum of his work has been particularly its impact on medicine and dynamic psychiatry, and the clinical professions closely associated with them.

It can fairly be said, in conclusion, that each of these deviates contributed something important to our total understanding of human personality, but that the "school" founded by each, with a new vocabulary for both its unique ideas and ideas it shared with analysis, was limited by its bellicose denial of many of Freud's most important discoveries and in consequence has been proved by history to have only a transient influence and existence as a professional entity at war with psychoanalysis.

PSYCHOANALYSIS IN THE UNITED STATES

BEGINNINGS

In these postwar years, while one gazes upon the ruins and rubble of world-known centers of psychoanalytic activity and their determined efforts at restoration, one also witnesses the unpredicted pre-eminence of the American Association, its seventeen affiliate societies, and seventeen accredited training institutes.

Already, when Freud's first small gatherings of students were meeting in Vienna and Zürich, the serious interest of a few Americans had developed in three cities of the United States. In Boston, as early as 1894, William James had referred to Freud in his lectures at Harvard. In 1906 Dr. James Jackson Putnam, who at sixty retained the capacity for new vistas which had made him in his professional youth first president of the American Neurological Association and later first professor of Neurology at Harvard, was attempting the new psychoanalytic technique and had published the first paper on analysis in English (other than reviews). He was later referred to by Freud as "the first American to interest himself in analysis." Within the next few years there were others in Boston, distinguished men in their professions, who met occasionally to discuss Freud's work among themselves. Among them were Morton Prince, editor of *The Journal of Abnormal Psychology*, first American journal to welcome papers on analysis, Boris Sidis, Hugo Münsterberg, G. M. Waterman, and Willis Taylor. Especially notable, in view of his later achievement, were the visits to this Boston group of the youthful Dr. Ernest Jones, then professor at Toronto; he had been made aware of Freud's work in 1903 by the psychologist Wilfred Trotter in England, and started psychoanalytic practice in 1905. A few years later he returned to England, established the British Society in 1913, and today is the last survivor of the first great students of Freud, and his biographer.

Meanwhile a group of progressive New York psychiatrists, including Dr. Adolf Meyer and Dr. August Hoch, were actively discussing analysis. Another New Yorker, Frederick Peterson, Professor of Neurology at Columbia, encouraged the youthful Dr. Abraham Brill to accompany him, in November 1907, on a visit to Bleuler and Jung in Zürich. During this first pilgrimage of Americans to Europe for the study of analysis, Brill became well acquainted with Ernest Jones at Zürich; together these pioneers attended the first gathering of European analysts at the Salzburg

Congress, and visited Freud in Vienna in May 1908. At a third center of American psychiatry, the Binghamton State Hospital, discussion of Freud by Dr. Richard Hutchings awakened the interest of young doctors in American analysis. One of these was Dr. William Alanson White, who later initiated the therapeutic applications of analysis to psychoses.[6] White became closely associated a few years later with Dr. Smith Ely Jelliffe, who visited Zurich in 1907, founded the first psychoanalytic journal in English, and made very early psychosomatic observations.

Dr. Abraham Brill, the most famous of the first American analysts, was in many ways the opposite of the philosophical, Boston-born-and-bred Dr. James Jackson Putnam. The child of poor Jewish parents, Brill came to America at fifteen, and throughout his life he remained eager to express his gratitude to America for his opportunity. Of volatile, garrulous, and indefatigable temperament, this furious warrior fought the enemies of psychoanalysis for thirty years, often in verbal single combat which reverberated from the staid walls of scientific forums. At times he was, like so many of the first generation of analysts, belligerent, jealous of rivals in leadership, and excessively insistent upon first place beyond dispute, as the appointed envoy of Freud and the first translator of his works into English. But he had in common with the much older Dr. Putnam the quality of intrepidity in publicly professing his new scientific convictions. They soon became acquainted, and together with Dr. Ernest Jones attended a Congress on Psychotherapy at Yale in December 1908, when the first formal presentations of psychoanalytic views in English were made by Putnam and Jones.

Meanwhile, psychoanalytic interest in Boston had led to an invitation by the psychologist Stanley Hall, author of a classic work, *Adolescence*, and president of Clark University, to both Freud and Carl Jung to lecture at that university. Though Freud had considerable reluctance to accepting this first acknowledgment by a university of his work, it remains a landmark in the history of analysis; as he remarked in accepting his honorary degree of Doctor of Letters on this occasion: "This is the first official recognition of

[6] See page 259.

our endeavors." The five *Lectures* were given in September 1909 without written preparation; but, thanks to Freud's almost photographic memory, were later published and remain today a standard text.

THE AMERICAN PSYCHOANALYTIC ASSOCIATION
AND PROFESSIONAL TRAINING

On February 12, 1911, the New York Psychoanalytic Society was established with Brill as president. Three months later, May 9, 1911, the American Psychoanalytic Association was founded in Baltimore with James Jackson Putnam as first president and Ernest Jones as secretary, and with eight charter members present. The further progress of American analysis was achieved both in its informal discussion among analysts and psychiatrists, and by the more formal regular meetings of the young societies. For the first twenty years after its establishment the New York Society was preeminent as a group of physicians who had dedicated most of their efforts to the new science; in view of the unflagging zeal and productivity of this group, as well as its influence in psychiatry, it seems unreal today to learn that for a decade most meetings were attended by only six or seven zealot members. Active, though small societies had also developed after 1914 in Baltimore, Boston, and Washington, and after 1931 in Chicago.

During its first twenty years the American Psychoanalytic Association, like these local societies, had been chiefly a forum for scientific papers and the exchange of ideas. Of great historical interest is its list of charter members, which includes not only analysts but such important leaders in modern psychiatry as Adolf Meyer, C. Macfie Campbell (who had visited Freud as early as 1907), August Hoch, and George Kirby, though not all of these were present at the first meeting. As they grew, both the national and local psychoanalytic societies felt an increasing need to restrict membership to physicians who specialized in psychoanalysis, and two new functions became increasingly important: the formulation of definite standards for membership, to distinguish between qualified practitioners of this medical specialty and swarming "wild analysts"; and, of even more importance, the formulation of principles for the development of professional education. In consequence, the American Psychoanalytic Association was reorganized in 1932 as a Federation of those four local societies which had already become active in training and were recognized by the International Psychoanalytic Association—New York, Baltimore-Washington, Chicago, and Boston. It also established a Council on Professional Training for the definition of standards of membership, and of standards agreed upon among the constituent societies for training at the new institutes. In 1946 the amazing growth of the American Psychoanalytic Association again required its reorganization. The 1932 Federation, granting final powers to individual societies, was replaced by a truly national organization of members granting rights and recognition to local (affiliate) societies; and the Council on Professional Training was replaced by the Board on Professional Standards, responsible for the standards for membership and the accreditation of teaching institutes which it approved.

These standards and the fulfillment of psychoanalytic education in America have been the achievement chiefly of the second generation of psychoanalysts here—of those who were young professionally twenty-five years ago—in contrast to the pre-war institutes of Europe which were created by the earliest of Freud's followers—Eitingon and Abraham in Berlin, Ernest Jones in London, the leaders of analysis in Vienna in 1925, Ferenczi in Budapest. Even before the institutes in Europe were founded, occasional New York analysts had already gone to Vienna for "training analysis," usually brief, with Freud or his more famous students. Then, in the late 1920's, a dozen or so young American psychiatrists availed themselves of the new opportunities for complete psychoanalytic training in Berlin, Vienna, and London. Learning there the imperative necessity of such training by organized faculties, these young Americans eagerly promoted this new development on returning home, often against strenuous opposition at first from some leaders of the older generation. Later developments had indeed been foreshadowed when the New York Society in 1922 resolved to require a medical degree for membership, and in 1923 established an Educational Committee, with Dr. Clarence P. Oberndorf as chairman. A few years later the activities of analysts recently trained in Europe, Bertram Lewin, Dorian Feigenbaum, Monroe A. Myer, Abram Kardiner, Gregory Zilboorg, assisted by older members of the Committee, culminated in 1929 in the planning of a complete educational program; and in 1931 the New York Psychoanalytic Institute was opened.

A similar development was soon initiated in Boston, through the activity of this author, M. Ralph Kaufman, and John Milne Murray, all recently trained in Europe. This led to didactic seminars and supervision of cases in 1930, under teachers from New York; the reorganization of the existing Boston Psychoanalytic Society in 1931 (founded in 1914, and revived by Dr. Isador Coriat in 1928); provision for training analysis by inviting Franz Alexander, well-known training analyst at the Berlin Institute and visiting professor at the University of Chicago (1930–1), to Boston in 1931 and Hanns Sachs of Berlin in 1932; participation in the reorganization of the American Psychoanalytic Association in 1932, and full endorsement by it and the International in 1933. A few analysts in Chicago had also begun to train students, in the late twenties, under the leadership of Drs. Ralph C. Hamill and Lionel Blitzten, and in 1932 the Chicago Psychoanalytic Institute, the first and only analytic institute supported by foundation funds, was established with a salaried faculty under the directorship of Franz Alexander. The Washington-Baltimore Society, the fourth constituent member of the reorganized American Psychoanalytic Association in 1932, was also beginning to develop training based on the same principles. Soon the *avant-garde* Philadelphia psychiatrists, who had long had analytic interests, had invited Dr. Herman Nunberg in 1933 to initiate training in that city; their society was recognized in 1939, and their institute in 1948. In Topeka, Kansas, the pioneer clinic of the Middle West in modern psychiatry and analysis, under the inspiration of Dr. Karl Menninger, his father, and his brothers, led to the founding of an institute in 1938.

Since this initial period of formal analytic education in America, a series of other institutes has been established in accordance with the standards of the American Psychoanalytic Association: Detroit; a second institute in New York City under the auspices of the Columbia Medical School; San Francisco; Los Angeles; a third in New York by the State University of New York (formerly Long Island Medical School), and the Western New England (New Haven, Hartford, and Stockbridge); the Washington-Baltimore Institute has divided into two institutes, one in each city; and second institutes have been recognized in Philadelphia and in Los Angeles. "Training centers," accredited progenitors of completely staffed institutes, have been established at Seattle, New Orleans, and Cleveland, and groups at the University of North Carolina and in St. Louis have begun development of accredited training.[7]

This on-surging of psychoanalysis in America, and its effects on dynamic psychiatry and other professions, has been a quite unpredicted development. By the 1920's the new science was widely recognized as an important contribution to psychiatry, but was still the inevitable focus of the most heated professional controversies. Yet, in spite of its prominence, there were still only sixty-five members of the American Psychoanalytic Association in 1930. The most optimistic enthusiasts among them could not have conceived that in 1957 there would be nearly seven hundred members, and that this number would represent not merely physicians with sufficient interest in analysis to join and pay their dues, but seven hundred men and women, all of whom, except seventeen who had been members before 1925, had completed medical, psychiatric, and specialized training according to the minimal standards adopted in 1932, and formally published in 1938. Even this number, however, is an insufficient indication of the immediate future of the psychoanalytic profession, as there are in addition almost a thousand psychiatrists who are already students at the seventeen ac-

---

[7] Inquiries regarding professional standards and training approved by the American Psychoanalytic Association may be addressed: Executive Secretary, American Psychoanalytic Association, 36 West 44th Street, New York 36. N.Y.

credited institutes and training centers of America, not to mention physicians and laymen who are associated with small "psychoanalytic" groups which will not or cannot accept these standards. The members and students have over six thousand patients in psychoanalytic treatment, and in addition most are intensively engaged in other therapeutic, educational, and psychiatric activities.

This numerical phenomenon reflects aspects of American psychoanalysis which are fundamental in its history. The most important is the organic relation of analysis with general psychiatry and medicine.[8] In Europe, from the earliest years of analysis when Freud had explored dreams, discovered infantile and unconscious sexuality, and been rebuffed by University medicine in Vienna, analysis had a basically hostile attitude to psychiatry. The single exception had been the collaboration of Freud's first supporters, Drs. Bleuler and Jung in Zürich; but this had lasted only a few years and led to the first of Freud's bitter quarrels with his earliest supporter. To a considerable extent the different history of analysis in America was a consequence of the teaching of a notable group of psychiatrists in a few clinics during the first quarter of this century.[9] Their new dynamic views of the psychoses—that they were patterns of adaptation to personal problems and not merely degenerative organic processes of the brain; that delusions and hallucinations were meaningful and their content could be profitably studied; that psychoses were resultants of developmental processes—were a stimulation to their students which had no parallel in Europe. Several of these psychiatrists had been charter members of the American Psychoanalytic Association, and almost all the second generation of American psychoanalysts, those who studied at the new institutes in Europe and then initiated the development of full training programs in America, were young physicians whose interest in analysis had been aroused by those early teachers of dynamic psychiatry.

These facts also explain, at least in part, the history of lay analysis in America. Since 1923 the official policy of the American

8 See Chapters XII, XIII, and XIV.
9 See Chapter XII, pages 258–61.

Psychoanalytic Association, and of all local societies and training institutes approved by it, has been to require a medical degree and psychiatric training as prerequisites for training in psychoanalytic therapy and for full membership.[1] Freud himself had formally favored lay analysis; but his experience had been different from that of Americans. In Vienna and elsewhere he had encountered a wall of medical hostility, especially from the universities. Moreover, several of Freud's earliest and most gifted followers had been laymen— Hanns Sachs, Otto Rank, the Swiss clergyman Otto Pfister, and a little later his own daughter, Anna, and others, especially in Vienna and London. There can be no question that these individuals were talented as analysts and made outstanding contributions to both clinical and applied analysis. But unqualified acknowledgment of this fact has not seemed to most Americans sufficient reason to justify a policy of training a whole new profession of dozens or hundreds of lay analysts. There is too great a responsibility, as compelling as the responsibility of physicians for medical patients; and "wild analysis" in America has been more than once a serious threat to professional integrity. American analysts have also felt from their own experience that medicine and psychiatry were important if not indispensable foundations for their science and its practice. The problem still arouses controversy by a minority who believe the advantages of lay analysis are too great to be sacrificed.

Though esteeming the work of his lay followers, Freud himself, not only in training and his early work, but in the essential premises of his thinking about psychologic data, was a physician and biologically oriented. His compelling scientific motivation was a need to discover true laws of mental functioning; his first major effort had been an application of the new "neurone theory" to mental processes, and only because this theory proved inadequate

---

[1] Between 1932 and 1938 a few lay Europeans, who had been fully trained and were members in good standing of European societies before emigrating to the United States, were admitted to full membership, the most distinguished and creative, Ernst Kris, to honorary membership. There are still five of these non-medical members of the American Psychoanalytic Association. Also, a few European lay analysts who emigrated to the United States after 1938 are special members of a few local "affiliate societies."

did he turn to those concepts, especially the libido theory, which have become the basic ideas for the scientific integration of psychoanalytic data.

The basic principles of psychoanalysis, empirical, theoretical, technical, and therapeutic, are the creation of one man, from a period of his life work remembered by people still living. The profession of psychoanalysis is the product of only two generations of followers, who also pioneered. Thus the European example of organized training, the development of a new generation of analysts for all of whom this has been available, the founding of American institutes with excellent faculties, teaching programs and standards, the tragic fate of this science in Germany, Austria, Hungary, and Czechoslovakia, the migration of European analysts to this country, the greater opportunities here for the collaboration of analysts with general psychiatry and medicine—all contributed to the remarkable development of American analysis during the last thirty years. America rapidly and inevitably attained pre-eminence, challenged only by the London Institute, in perpetuating the scientific work of Freud's lifetime and in extending it to new territories which had been blazed but not explored.

"Even today it is, of course, impossible for me to foresee the final judgment of posterity upon the value of psychoanalysis for psychiatry, psychology, and the mental sciences in general," wrote Freud in *An Autobiographical Study* (1927); [2] and he concluded: "Looking back, then, over the patchwork of my life's labours, I can say that I have made many beginnings and thrown out many suggestions. Something will come of them in the future. But I cannot tell myself whether it will be much or little."

This is the outlook of all sciences. How the future may show we are in error, what new and startling vision of the processes of human life the next genius may reveal, no one can foretell. At best we can survey the knowledge at hand and judge as best we can

[2] Published in German, 1925. Translated by James Strachey, and published with *The Problem of Lay Analysis* (New York: Coward-McCann; 1935).

from that. As Galileo shattered our faith that our earth was the universe, and Darwin our belief in the special creation of man, so Freud has proved that man's intellect is not supreme, that it is rather a unique instrument for utilizing and restraining the more primitive and fundamental impulses at work deep within us. This new knowledge wounds us deeply, especially those whose pride and life are consecrated to rational thought. Only the next generation can accept unemotionally what the great scientists of previous eras have proved; but Freud's demonstration of unconscious mental processes appears today to mark a revolution in the human being's scientific knowledge of himself.

SUGGESTIONS FOR FURTHER READING

HISTORY OF PSYCHOANALYSIS

Ernest Jones: *The Life and Work of Sigmund Freud* (New York: Basic Books; Vol. I, 1953, Vol. II, 1956, Vol. III, 1957). A definitive biography of Freud the man, Freud the scientist, and Freud the founder of psychoanalysis; a great and scholarly work.

Sigmund Freud: *The Origins of Psychoanalysis: Letters to Wilhelm Fliess*. Edited by Marie Bonaparte, Anna Freud, Ernst Kris (1950). Translation by Eric Mosbacher and James Strachey (New York: Basic Books, 1954). Freud's personal letters to his closest scientific friend, from the earliest and most fertile period of psychoanalysis, describing its early development.

Sigmund Freud: "On the History of the Psychoanalytic Movement" (1914; translation in *Collected Papers*, Vol. I, and in Standard Edition, Vol. XIV, London: Hogarth Press, 1957), colored by the violent professional controversies of the period when it was written; and "An Autobiographical Study" (translation by James Strachey in the volume entitled *The Problem of Lay-Analysis* [New York: Coward-McCann, 1935]). These are "autobiographical" essays, actually devoted largely to parts of the history of psychoanalysis.

C. P. Oberndorf: *A History of Psychoanalysis in America* (New York: Grune and Stratton, 1953). A highly personalized and interesting account by one who played an active and valuable role in the first forty years of analysis in this country, but with many factual inaccuracies in regard to dates, etc.

R. P. Knight: "The Present Status of Psychoanalysis in the United States," *Journal of the American Psychoanalytic Association*, Vol. I, page 197 (1953).

Ives Hendrick: "Professional Standards of the American Psychoanalytic Association," *Journal of the American Psychoanalytic Association*, Vol. III, pages 561–99 (1955).

OTHER WORKS OF SIGMUND FREUD
(partial bibliography)

Gesammelte Schriften, 12 volumes (Vienna: Internationaler Psychoanalytischer Verlag, 1925–34). Freud's technical papers, complete.

Gesammelte Werke, 18 volumes (London: Imago, 1940–52). Freud's papers and books, complete.

Collected Papers, 5 volumes (New York: International Psychoanalytic Press, 1924, 1950). For those who wish to read extensively, these shorter papers are as important as his books. The *Case Histories* (Vol. III) contain the original exposition of many of his most important conclusions.

The Standard Edition of the Complete Works of Sigmund Freud. Translated from the German, James Strachey, Editor (London: The Hogarth Press, 1953–   ). A scholarly complete edition of Freud's books and papers, now in preparation, nine volumes already published; translations of all are superior, and editing and editorial prefaces are superbly accurate and complete. (References to Standard Edition in these Suggestions for Reading are made only to those volumes already published, 1953–7.)

The Basic Writings of Sigmund Freud (New York: The Modern Library, 1938). A best-seller selection in one volume from six important books. Some of the translations are poor.

Studies on Hysteria (in collaboration with Josef Breuer, 1895). Translation by James Strachey (New York: Basic Books, 1957; Standard Edition, Vol. II, London: Hogarth Press, 1955). Today this is still the great, easily readable classic presentation of the empirical basis of our first knowledge of repression and the psychological mechanisms of psychoneurosis.

Three Essays on Sexuality. Translation by James Strachey (Standard Edition, Vol. VII, London: Hogarth Press, 1953). Original exposition (1905), with important additions in later German and English editions, of Freud's most revolutionary insight.

Five Introductory Lectures on Psychoanalysis (1910), Standard Edition, Vol. XI (London: Hogarth Press, 1957). Freud's own comprehensive and less technical résumé of psychoanalysis. The *New Introductory Lectures* (translated by W. J. H. Sprott, New York: W. W. Norton, 1933) are an important supplement.

An Outline of Psycho-analysis (1940). Translation by James Strachey (London: Hogarth Press; New York: W. W. Norton, 1949). A shorter and simpler introduction to psychoanalysis.

The Problem of Anxiety (1926). Translation by Henry Alden Bunker (New York: The Psychoanalytic Press and W. W. Norton, 1936). Freud's fundamental revision of his previous theory of neurosis; it is today almost universally accepted as the basic etiologic theory of psychoneurosis in psychoanalysis and in modern dynamic psychiatry.

Totem and Taboo (1912). Translation by James Strachey (London: Routledge; New York: W. W. Norton, 1952). The pioneer contribution of psychoanalysis to anthropology, and still the greatest work on the non-medical applications of psychoanalysis.

The Ego and the Id (1923). Translation by Joan Rivière (London: Hogarth Press, 1927). The original presentation of the final concept of personality structure, and Freud's most important contribution to ego-psychology.

Beyond the Pleasure Principle (1920). Translation by C. J. M. H. Hubback (New York: Boni and Liveright, 1924). Translation by James Strachey (Standard Edition, Vol. XVIII, London: Hogarth Press, 1955). This difficult and abstract work should be read by those particularly interested in the more speculative and biological aspects of Freud's final instinct theory, the repetition compulsion, and destructiveness.

Civilization and Its Discontents (1930). Translation by Joan Rivière (New York: Cape and Smith, 1930). Freud's view of problems of European culture, also containing important contributions to the theory of aggression and the psychology of unconscious guilt.

Moses and Monotheism (1939). Translation by Katherine Jones (London: Hogarth Press; New York: Alfred A. Knopf, 1939). The last book of Freud's lifetime, a psychoanalytic contribution to the Jewish religion.

The Interpretation of Dreams (1900; enlarged and revised in later editions). Translations by A. A. Brill and others (London: George Allen and Unwin; New York: The Macmillan Company). Translation by James Strachey (New York: Basic Books, 1955; Standard Edition, Vol. IV–V, London: Hogarth Press). As the years go by, psychoanalysts themselves more and more appreciate that *The Interpretation of Dreams* is the scientific masterpiece of Freud; it contains the germ of almost every empirical and theoretical contribution to psychoanalysis. It is, however, probably the most difficult to evaluate without clinical experience with the empirical basis of this subject.

GENERAL BOOKS BY OTHER AUTHORS

Anna Freud: *Psychoanalysis for Teachers and Parents.* (Translation by Barbara Low (New York: Emerson, 1952). The simplest, briefest, and clearest of all authoritative non-technical expositions; especially valuable for its clear presentation of the facts of infantile sexuality.

Lawrence S. Kubie: *Practical Aspects of Psychoanalysis* (New York: W. W. Norton, 1936). A brief orientation to some practical questions of psychoanalytic patients.

Otto Fenichel: *Outline of Clinical Psychoanalysis* (1932). Translation by Bertram Lewin and Gregory Zilboorg (New York: The Psychoanalytic Quarterly Press and W. W. Norton, 1934). An authoritative and comprehensive, clearly written technical presentation of the dynamics of psychoneurosis, with clinical material of special interest.

Otto Fenichel: *The Psychoanalytic Theory of the Neuroses* (New York: W. W. Norton, 1945). An exhaustive, scholarly survey of knowledge and theory for psychoanalytic students.

Helene Deutsch: *Psycho-analysis of the Neuroses*. Translation by W. D. Robson-Scott (London: Hogarth Press and the Institute of Psychoanalysis, 1933; New York: Anglo-Books, 1952). Lectures to students at the Vienna Institute, less comprehensive than Fenichel's book, but less technical; an excellent introduction to clinical correlations of conscious experiences of the present and repressed experiences of the past.

Jacob A. Arlow: *The Legacy of Freud* (New York: The International Universities Press, 1956). A small book of delightful vignettes about a variety of Freud's contributions, written for the American Psychoanalytic Association's centenary celebration of Freud's birth.

Charles Brenner: *An Elementary Textbook of Psychoanalysis* (New York: International Universities Press, 1935). A well-written and fairly elementary orientation to psychoanalytic hypotheses.

For the student making a thorough study of technical literature, the chief papers of the greatest of Freud's first students, Abraham, Ferenczi, and Jones, are indispensable supplements to the works of Freud.

Karl Abraham: *Selected Papers* (New York: Basic Books, 1953). The most important supplement to Freud.

Sandor Ferenczi: *Contributions to Psychoanalysis* (translation by Ernest Jones; Boston: Richard G. Badger, 1916). And *Further Contributions to the Theory and Techniques of Psychoanalysis* (London: Hogarth Press, 1926).

Ernest Jones: *Papers on Psychoanalysis*. Fifth Edition (Baltimore: Williams and Wilkins, 1949).

SPECIAL ASPECTS OF PSYCHOANALYSIS

Anna Freud: *The Ego and the Mechanisms of Defense* (1936). Translation by Cecil Baines (New York: The International Universities Press; 1946). The most inclusive account of the early work on defense-mechanisms of the ego, especially their manifestations in childhood and adolescence.

Anna Freud: *The Psycho-analytical Treatment of Children* (Parts I and II, 1927 and 1929, translation by Nancy Proctor-Gregg, Part III, 1946; London: Imago Publishing Company, 1946). A brief, lucid introduction to child analysis.

Melanie Klein: *The Psycho-analysis of Children* (New York: W. W. Norton, 1932). An early exposition of Klein's principles and ideas about child analysis.

Franz Alexander: *Psychoanalysis of the Total Personality* (1927). Translation by Bernard Glueck and Bertram Lewin (Washington, D.C.: Nervous and Mental Disease Publishing Co., 1930). A lucid introduction to the psychology of guilt and super-ego dynamics, of equal interest to psychoanalysts and laymen.

Karl Menninger: *The Human Mind* (New York: Alfred A. Knopf, 1930; Third Edition, 1945). An up-to-date rewriting of this classic text on dynamic psychiatry, psychoanalytically oriented.

O. Spurgeon English and Gerald H. J. Pearson: *Emotional Problems of Living* (New York: W. W. Norton, 1945). An excellent, readable account of Freud's contribution to dynamic psychiatry.

Maurice Levine: *Psychotherapy in Medical Practice* (New York: Macmillan, 1942). The clearest technical guide to the applications of psychoanalysis to psychotherapy.

Felix Deutsch and William F. Murphy: *The Clinical Interview*, 2 volumes (New York: International Universities Press, 1955). An interesting orientation to the practical use of free association for diagnosis and psychotherapy.

Edward Weiss and O. S. English: *Psychosomatic Medicine* (Philadelphia. W. B. Saunders, 1943). Clearly written introduction to analytically oriented psychosomatic medicine.

H. Flanders Dunbar: *Psychosomatic Diagnosis* (New York, London: Paul B. Hoeber, 1948). A classic professional compendium of psychosomatic literature, classified by syndromes.

Franz Alexander and Thomas M. French: *Studies in Psychosomatic Medicine* (New York: Ronald Press, 1948). One of the best of many volumes by senior contributors to these fields.

Phyllis Greenacre: *Trauma, Growth, and Personality* (New York: W. W. Norton, 1952). A gifted, scientific psychoanalyst's contribution, based on clinical knowledge, to some unconscious factors in development.

Lewis Hill: *Psychotherapeutic Intervention in Schizophrenia* (Chicago: University of Chicago Press, 1955). The best introduction to the clinical application of dynamic psychiatry to work with psychotics.

Bertram Lewin: *The Psychoanalysis of Elation* (New York: W. W.

Norton, 1950). The chief psychoanalytic contribution to the problem of moods and affects, a creative interpretation of clinical data.

Karl A. Menninger: *Man Against Himself* (New York: Harcourt, Brace, 1938). One analyst's attack on such problems resulting from human ambivalence as suicide, psychoneurosis, and organic disease, interpreted in terms of the death-instinct theory.

Annette Garrett: *Interviewing: Its Principles and Methods* (New York: Family Welfare Association of America, 1942). A lucid adaptation of technical principles of modern psychotherapy to psychiatric social case-work.

Otto Rank: *The Myth of the Birth of the Hero* (1913). Translation by R. F. Robbins and Smith Ely Jelliffe (New York: Robert Brunner, 1952). The classic application of psychoanalytic psychology to the study of a myth recurring in many cultures.

Margaret A. Ribble: *The Rights of Infants* (New York: Columbia University Press, 1943). Readable presentation of the author's chief professional interest.

Erik Erikson: *Childhood and Society* (New York: W. W. Norton, 1950). The exploration by a talented child analyst of the effect of cultural influences on early development.

Carl Binger: *The Doctor's Job* (New York: W. W. Norton, 1945). A delightfully written account of applications of dynamic psychiatry to the everyday clinical work of the internist with psychological aptitude.

Psychiatry and Medical Education, edited by John Whitehorn, Carl Jacobson, Maurice Levine, and Vernon W. Lippard (1951); and *The Psychiatrist: His Training and Development,* edited by John Whitehorn, Francis B. Braceland, Vernon W. Lippard, William Malamud (American Psychiatric Association, 1953). Reports of the two "Ithaca Conferences," landmarks in the development of professional education in dynamic psychiatry.

Problems of Infancy and Childhood, Milton Senn, Editor (Packanack Lake, N.J.: Josiah Macy, Jr., Foundation Publications, 1947–54). Transactions of seven conferences of a small group of psychoanalysts and members of allied professions, medical and academic, on the psychology of early motherhood, its psychological and medical management, its cultural determinants, and several allied topics.

Reports of the Group for the Advancement of Psychiatry: Vol. I, Nos. 1–20 (1947–51); Vol. II, Nos. 21–34 (1952–6); Publication Office, Topeka, Kansas. Reports on a variety of topics carefully edited by committees of a group of dynamic psychiatrists, many of whom are psychoanalysts, and consultants in allied professions.

Ruth L. Munroe: *Schools of Psychoanalytic Thought* (New York: The Dryden Press, 1955). A lengthy, source-documented discussion by a psychologist of the scientific principles of psychoanalysis and of the main founders of deviant schools.

TECHNICAL JOURNALS IN GERMAN AND ENGLISH

Jahrbuch für Psychoanalytische und Psychopathalogische Forschungen (1909–14); *Zentralblatt für Psychoanalyse* (1910–12); *Imago* (Applied Analysis) (1912–38); *Internationale Zeitschrift für Psychoanalyse* (first six volumes: *für ärztliche Psychoanalyse*) (1913–   ); *Psychoanalytische Almanak* (1926–38); *Zeitschrift für Psychoanalytische Pädagogik* (1927–38); *Psychoanalytische Bewegung* (1929–33).

Psychoanalytic Review (1913–57); *International Journal of Psychoanalysis* (1920–   ); *Psychoanalytic Quarterly* (1932–   ); *Journal of the American Psychoanalytic Association* (1953–   ); *The Psychoanalytic Study of the Child* (I–XI, 1946–56); *American Imago* (1944–   ).

GLOSSARY

[ABBREVIATIONS. M.: *medical definition*. Pa.: *psychoanalytic definition*. Py.: *psychiatric definition*. Syn.: *synonym*.]

Abreaction (Pa.): the therapeutically effective discharge of emotion associated with recall of a repressed idea or memory; especially that which occurs when a repressed traumatic experience is recalled under hypnosis. Syn., catharsis.

Acting-out (Pa.).: the neurotic gratification of a repressed wish by compulsive behavior, especially in reacting to another person; used chiefly for the acting-out of transference phantasies during psychoanalysis or psychotherapy.

Activity (Pa.): those instinctual aims whose gratification requires initiative in one's behavior toward an object.

Actual Neuroses (Pa.): anxiety neurosis, neurasthenia, and hypochondriasis. According to Freud, the symptoms of these neuroses, in contrast to the symptoms of psychoneuroses, are the result of a physiologic toxemia caused by either excessive prohibition or abuse of the erotic functions.

Adrenal Gland (M.): an endocrine gland, located above the kidney, and secreting "adrenalin" and other hormones into the bloodstream.

Affect (Py.): the subjective aspect of emotion; instinct-tension perceived as mood, sentiment, passion, or need to act.

Afferent Nerve (M.): a nerve carrying sensory and other stimuli toward the brain.

Aim, Instinctual (Pa.): a need for that specific act or experience which is productive of pleasure by reduction of instinctual tension; especially, for the sexual instincts, need for stimulation of a specific erotogenic zone.

Aim-inhibited Wish (Pa.): a wish which can be normally gratified by the substitution of an incomplete act for the original aim, usually unconscious—for example, a handshake for an embrace, "friendship" for erotic love, "latent" for "overt" homosexuality. (Cf. "Sublimation.")

Allergy (M.): an abnormal somatic reaction to specific chemicals which are eaten, inhaled, or touched; a biochemical cause of asthma, hay fever, hives, and other diseases.

Ambivalence (Pa.): bipolarity of an instinct; the need to satisfy both of a pair of antagonistic desires; especially the bipolarity of love and hate, activtity and passivity, masculinity and femininity, masochism and sadism.

Amnesia (Py.): inability to recollect consciously a specific idea, event, or period of one's life.

Amnesia, Infantile (Pa.): the normal inability to recall most of the experiences of the first five and one-half years of life (approximately), especially infantile sexual thoughts and observations.

Anabolism (M.): that phase of metabolism in which cells and tissues are built.

Anaclitic (Pa.): the narcissistic need to be taken care of, derived from dominant needs of early infancy.

Anaclitic Personality (Pa.): a type of personality whose chief love-needs are to be taken care of, described by Freud as the "most typical form of femininity."

Anal Erotism (Pa.): conscious or unconscious wishes associated with pleasurable stimulation of the anus, and with the derivatives of these wishes in conscious thought, act, symptom, or character trait; in theory, those components of the sexual instincts whose primary aim is anal pleasure.

Anal Sadism (Pa.): sadism associated with anal erotism and represented by conscious or unconscious phantasies of beating, exploding, torturing, dirtying, demolishing, etc., and the derivatives of these phantasies in conscious thought, symptom, or behavior.

Analysis (Pa.): colloquial for "psychoanalysis" (*q.v.*).

Anorexia (M.): abnormally diminished or absent appetite for food.

Anus (M.): the external aperture of the intestines.

Anxiety Hysteria (Pa.): a psychoneurosis in which phobias are the most conspicuous symptoms.

Anxiety Neurosis (Pa.): one form of "actual neurosis" (*q.v.*) in which either conscious anxiety without phobia-formation, or the physiological signs of anxiety (palpitation, sweating, etc.), are the most conspicuous symptoms.

Anxiety, Neurotic (Py.): anxiety without, or disproportionate to, realistic justification, contrasted with "fear" of real danger.

Applied Psychoanalysis (Pa.): the non-medical applications of psychoanalytic knowledge and theory to art, literature, biography, sociology, anthropology, public health, etc.

Arthritis (M.): an organic disease of the joints and adjacent tissues; colloquially, "rheumatism."

Asthma (M.): a disease characterized by paroxysmal or continuous inability to breathe air in and out of lungs easily.

Autism (Py.): wishful thoughts, particularly omnipotent, symbolic, delusional, and hallucinatory thoughts, unmodified by rational or realistic processes. Syn., "Primary Process" (*q.v.*).

Autoerotism (Pa.): pleasurable gratification of sexual aims by stimulation of an erotogenic zone, without requiring love of another; unconscious and conscious psychological derivatives of autoerotic needs.

Autonomic Nervous System (M.): that system controlling and co-ordinating those bodily functions which have little mental representation except the experience of moods and emotions.

Bacteriology (M.): the study of microscopic organisms and their relationship to disease.

Bisexuality (Pa.): the fact that the sexual aims and wishes typical of both sexes are present in every individual whether male or female; and those theories of instincts derived from this fact.

Castration Complex (Pa.): a constellation of conscious and unconscious ideas associated with infantile phantasies that a female's penis has been, or a male's penis will be, mutilated, amputated, or destroyed.

Catabolism (M.): those phases of metabolism in which cell and tissue destruction occur.

Catatonic Rage (Py.): very violent, irrational impulses to destroy, occurring in certain types of schizophrenia.

Catharsis: Syn., "Abreaction" (*q.v.*).

Censor (Pa.): in dream psychology, that which compels and effects the disguise of the latent content.

Central Nervous System (M.): that system co-ordinating sensory experience, movement of the muscles of face, trunk, and limbs, and the association of ideas.

Character (Py.): those aspects of a personality (*q.v.*), especially social behavior, which distinguish one from other human beings; what is typical of an individual's ego.

Character Neurosis (Pa.): a psychoneurosis whose most conspicuous feature is the compulsive repetition of characteristic behavior which leads to excessive suffering or failure. Syn., "Neurotic Character."

Child Analysis (Pa.): special techniques developed by psychoanalysts for the treatment of the psychologic and behavior problems of children, fully utilizing play technique and psychoanalytic knowledge and theory.

Child Guidance (Py.): a term nearly synonymous with "child psychiatry" (*q.v.*), which is now rapidly replacing "child guidance" in general usage.

Child Psychiatry (Py.): the study and treatment by psychiatrists of the mental, emotional, and social problems of children.

Clitoris (M.): one of a female's external sexual organs, highly erotogenic and anatomically homologous with the male penis.

Coitus (M.): sexual intercourse.

Coitus Interruptus (M.): voluntary withdrawal of the penis before completion of coitus.

Complex (Pa.): an emotionally charged constellation of closely associated ideas, especially unconscious ideas.

Compulsion (Py.): a psychoneurotic symptom; the need, which cannot easily be controlled by the will, to repeat a rationally purposeless act or ritual, though its futility is intellectually realized.

Compulsion Neurosis (Py.): a psychoneurosis whose most conspicuous symptoms are compulsions (*q.v.*) which seriously impair the fulfillment of mature objectives, closely related to "obsessional neurosis" (*q.v.*).

Compulsive Character (Pa.): a character neurosis, closely related to compulsion neurosis and obsessional neurosis, whose most conspicuous features are the inflexibliity of the character, the inability to abandon or alter a course of action or thought in order to avoid suffering, and often excessive indecisiveness.

Condensation (Pa.): the coincident representation of several unconscious wishes or objects by a single conscious dream-image, thought, act, or symptom.

Confession Compulsion (Pa.): the abnormal compulsion or normal need to confess guilt verbally to another person.

Conflict (Pa.): the opposition of intra-psychic impulses; especially between a repressed wish and a punishment phantasy, between ambivalent instinctual aims, or between different components of the personality structure.

Conscious (1) adjective: being aware, capable of perception or apperception by a voluntary effort of attention.

(2) noun, "the Conscious" (Pa.): an inclusive abstraction of all conscious mental phenomena.

(3) noun, "the System Conscious" (Pa.): in the psychoanalytic theory of personality structure, a dynamic concept implying a functional differentiation of a "region" of the mind, where thoughts are conscious and rationally controlled, from an Unconscious; in early psychoanalytic literature it was used with many of the same implications as "ego" has been later.

Constitution (1) (M.): the hereditary biological endowment.

(2) (Py.): often used with a less precise connotation than "heredity," to include more or less generally what has become either biologically or psychologically fixed, unalterable, and characteristic of the individual.

Control Analysis (Pa.): therapeutic psychoanalysis conducted by a student of a psychoanalytic institute and supervised by a teacher. Syn., "supervised analysis."

Conversion (Pa.): the transformation of an instinctual need mentally represented by a repressed unconscious phantasy into an abnormal physiologic function, often simulating organic nervous disease; according to Freud, the basic mechanism of symptom-formation in hysteria.

Conversion Hysteria (Pa.): a psychoenurosis whose most conspicuous symptoms are localized abnormal functions of sensory or motor nerves, without disease of the tissues, caused by "conversion" (*q.v.*); the same as "hysteria" as used by neurologists and till recently by psychiatrists.

Counter-transference (Pa.): the emotions and phantasies with which the physician reacts to his patient during psychoanalysis or psychotherapy.

Death Instincts (Pa.): a hypothetical group of instincts whose ultimate aim is death, whose biological manifestation is catabolism, and whose psychological derivatives are impulses to destroy or injure oneself or others.

Defense Mechanism (Pa.): an organized psychological reaction, including repression, by which conscious anxiety or guilt associated with an unconscious wish is avoided.

Defloration: rupture of the hymen, usually during the first sexual intercourse of a woman; loss of virginity.

Defusion (Pa.): in later psychoanalytic instinct theory, a process accompanying "regression," characterized by a partial reversal of the "fusion" (*q.v.*) of Eros and the Death Instincts.

Delusion (Py.): an abnormal conscious idea or belief whose logical or realistic absurdity or dubiousness the individual is notably incapable of accepting.

Depression (1) (Py.): melancholia; a psychosis or psychoneurosis whose most conspicuous features are an abnormal degree of melancholy, incapacity for pleasurable experience and useful activity, extensive inhibition and slowing of intellectual activity and behavior, and marked preoccupation with self-abasing ideas, some of which may be delusions.

(2) (Py.): a recurrent phase of "manic-depressive psychosis" (*q.v.*).

(3) (Py.): milder, non-psychotic moods similar to psychotic depressions; "the blues."

Diabetes (M.): a disease caused by deficient secretion of the hormone which normally enables the body to utilize sugars and starches.

Didactic Analysis (Pa.): psychoanalysis of a student at a psychoanalytic institute whose primary purpose is professional education. Syn., "teaching analysis," "training analysis."

Displacement (Pa.): (1) the substitution of the original object of an instinctual impulse by a "surrogate" in act or phantasy.

(2) the substitution of partial aims of the sexual instincts for each other.

Dissociation (Py.): an abnormal process whereby a group of phantasies, which may determine hysterical symptoms and behavior, cannot be controlled or mentally related to the more usual and rational conscious mental systems of the patient.

Dynamic (Py.): based on knowledge of how symptoms, diseases, and normal functions of the personality are affected or determined by ideas, emotions, and psychological development.

Dynamic Psychiatry (Py.): those clinical, theoretical, and therapeutic aspects of modern psychiatry developed by psychoanalysis and other techniques from the premise that the clinical study of psychologic and social data is pre-eminently valuable in learning about psychopathologic processes, personality development and social adaptation, and in therapeutically influencing these processes.

Efferent Nerve (M.): a nerve which carries stimuli away from the brain to muscles and other organs.

Ego (1): the self, that which controls conscious perception, thought, feeling, and behavior, and is experienced as self-awareness.

(2) (Pa.): in the earlier literature Freud considered the ego the seat of the conscious, intellectual, and self-preservative functions, and generally used "ego" interchangeably with "the Conscious," as opposed to "the Unconscious."

(3) (Pa.): in the later concept of personality structure, more exactly described as that organized portion of the personality which enforces repression, other defenses against anxiety and guilt-producing impulses, subserves the Reality Principle, and controls perception, voluntary thought, and the discharge of emotional tensions by behavior.

Ego-defect (Pa.): the absence or insufficiency of a function of the normal ego, predisposing to psychotic or related modes of personality adjustment.

Ego-ideal (Pa.): a narcissistic image of what one aspires to be. (Often confused with "super-ego.")

Ego-instincts (Pa.): instincts which serve the self-preservative functions; in early psychoanalytic theory, those instincts which oppose the sexual instincts and enforce repression; in later theory, that portion of Eros which is utilized by the ego.

Ego-potentiality (Pa.): the potential capacity of an individual, if his psychoneurosis is alleviated, to deal effectively with the emotional and environmentally determined problems of adult life. Syn., "ego-strength."

Ego-psychology (Pa.): those more modern aspects of psychoanalytic investigation and theory which emphasize the organized components of the personality that oppose the gratification of infantile aims, determine defense mechanisms, mediate the normal gratification of instinctual needs, and determine the appraisal of reality, rational thought, and relationship to the environment; especially, the concept of personality structure, the anxiety theory of psychoneurosis, and the psychology of defense mechanisms.

Ego-strength (Pa.): Ego-potentiality (*q.v.*).

Ejaculatio Præcox (M.): a psychoneurotic symptom; that impairment of male genital function characterized by premature discharge of semen with deficient sensual and emotional gratification.

Electra Complex (Pa.): that group of ideas determined by a girl's incestuous phantasies of her father; the synonym, "female Œdipus complex," is much more commonly used.

Endocrine Gland (M.): a gland secreting "hormones," which are transported by the blood to other parts of the body and control many physiologic functions. Syn., "ductless gland."

Endocrinology (M.): the study of hormones, their physiologic effects, and the diseases caused by deficient or excessive secretion of them.

Enuresis (M.), (Py.): involuntary discharge of urine, especially bed-wetting.

Epilepsy, Idiopathic (M.): a group of diseases in which a specific brain damage (except abnormal brain waves in many cases) has not been demonstrated, characterized by generalized convulsions or spells of loss of consciousness of specific types; generally accompanied by marked egocentricity and emotional explosiveness of the general personality, and frequently by progressive mental and social deterioration.

Eros (Pa.): that group of instincts whose aims are sexual pleasure and perpetuation of life, and whose functions are opposed to those of the "Death Instincts"; Syn., the "life instincts."

Erotogenic Zone (Pa.): one of the surface areas of skin or mucous membrane friction of which affords marked voluptuous pleasure; especially the external genitalia, lips, anus, urethra, and skin.

Etiology (M.): the cause of a symptom, disease, or pathologic process.

Exhibitionism (1) (Py.): a sexual perversion in which display of the genitals determines maximal erotic pleasure.

      (2) (Pa.): also, a normal partial aim of infantile and adult sexuality and its derivatives, characterized by the conscious or unconscious wish to be looked at or to be admired; especially the wish to display the genitals. (*See* "Scoptophilia.")

Fixation (Pa.): the persistence of an unconscious wish for an infantile object, or for a specific form of pregenital sexual pleasure normally dominant at an earlier stage of development.

Forepleasure (Pa.): those sensations and actions derived from pregenital aims of the sexual instincts, and used in normal erotic courtship for the intensification of genital desire.

Free Association (Pa.): the fundamental principle of psychoanalytic technique, the reporting by the patient so far as he is able of all thoughts as they become spontaneously conscious, with a minimum of rational or ethical criticism; the thought-processes of spontaneous reverie, contrasted with the intellectual association of ideas.

Frigidity (Py.): any impairment of the female's capacity for genital sensory pleasure, or for any aspect of the emotional experience normally coincident with genital pleasure; it may be of any degree and is usually a psychoneurotic symptom.

Frustration (Pa.): either environmental or intra-psychic prevention of gratification of an instinctual wish.

Functional (M.): in respect to a symptom, etiologically not caused by demonstrable destruction of tissue or primary physiologic abnormality; inexactly but frequently used as a symptom for "hysterical," "psychoneurotic," or "psychogenic."

Fusion (Pa.): in later psychoanalytic theory, an impulse providing gratification of both Eros and Death Instincts; the theoretical origin of sadism, masochism, and normal aggression.

Gastric (M.): pertaining to the stomach.

Genitalia (M.): the sexual and reproductive organs of male and female; especially, the external sexual organs.

Genitality (Pa.): the normal adult organization of the sexual instincts; those aims of psychosexuality which impel to normal adult coitus, and require tenderness and the partner's pleasure as prerequisites of maximal gratification. Roughly synonymous with the non-analytic usage of "sexual instinct."

Grandiosity (Py.): abnormal over-valuation of oneself, expressed in phantasies, delusions, or acts.

Gratification (Pa.): an act or experience which reduces conscious or unconscious emotional tension and yields pleasure; the fulfillment of an instinctual aim; "wish-fulfillment."

Grave's Disease (M.): a disease of the thyroid gland, with over-production of thyroid hormone.

Guilt, Unconscious (Pa.): (1) those mental functions initiated by unconscious punishment phantasies; suffering which results from gratification, or drive toward gratification, of a repressed wish.

(2) theoretically, the tension between ego and super-ego.

Hallucination (Py.): an abnormal perception, conviction in the reality of a sensory experience, such as seeing or hearing, for which no real (external) stimulus exists.

Heredity: those physical and mental components of the organism which are transmitted from parents to child at conception. (Cf. "Constitution.")

Homeostasis (M.): the principle that physiologic processes tend to maintain a state of physico-chemical equilibrium.

Homosexuality (1) (Py.): an abnormal erotic relationship with an individual of one's own sex; or the unusual prominence of psychological traits or behavior usually characteristic of the other sex.

(2) (Pa.): also a "latent" or *unconscious* wish either for "overt" (actual) homosexual experience, or for the characteristics and experiences of the other sex.

(3) (Pa.): "aim-inhibited homosexuality," comprising all conscious and normal affectionate and friendly emotions for members of one's own sex.

(4) (Pa.): theoretically, a normal aim of a portion of the sexual instincts.

Hormone (M.): a chemical substance secreted by an endocrine (ductless) gland (*q.v.*) and carried by the blood to other organs whose function it affects.

Hypnosis (Py.): the induction by psychological suggestion, generally for symptomatic therapy or research, of a special mental state or "trance" somewhat resembling sleep and characterized by unusual responsiveness to suggestions and by the consciousness of memories and ideas repressed at other times. Syn., "mesmerism."

Hypochondria (Py.): a fixated mental attitude, sometimes a psychosis with delusions, involving the erroneous conviction that the body or its organs are diseased.

Hysteria (1) (M.): a psychoneurosis whose most conspicuous features are usually symptoms of abnormal sensations, paralysis, or other functions, without demonstrable abnormality of the nervous system. (Sometimes loosely used in medicine for psychoneurosis in general.)

(2) (Pa.): those closely related psychoneuroses, occurring in people with dominant genital sexual aims and conflicts, referred to as "anxiety hysteria," "conversion hysteria," and "hysterical character" (*q.v.*); in colloquial usage, synonymous with "conversion hysteria," which is symptomatically identical with "hysteria" as used in neurology and general psychiatry.

Hysterical Character (Py.): a character neurosis, most frequent in women and closely related to conversion hysteria, whose most conspicuous features are unpleasant sensations or phantasies when erotically stimulated, excessively volatile, childlike, or theatrical display of emotion, and a pronounced repetitive tendency to sexual relationships which eventuate in quarreling, erotic disappointment, or psychogenic symptoms.

Id (Pa.): in the concept of personality structure, that "region" of the mind characterized by unorganized primitive instinctual wishes.

Identification (Pa.): a complex unconscious process whereby real or imagined characteristics of another person become permanent components of the personality; especially, the typical unconscious solution of an ambivalence (love-hate) conflict, as that of a child reacting to the authority of an adult, resulting in the development and individual features of his super-ego.

Impotence (Py.): partial or complete impairment of the male's capacity for normal erection, orgasm, or erotic pleasure; usually a psychoneurotic symptom.

Infancy (Pa.): technically, in psychoanalysis, the period of life (approximately the first five and a half years) before the Œdipus complex is repressed or resolved and succeeded by the latency period; roughly, the "pre-school" period.

Infantile Sexuality (Pa.): the normal sexuality of infancy, and its unconscious and conscious derivatives in the adult. It includes the phantasies and autoerotism of pregenital sexuality and the Œdipus complex.

Inhibition (Py.): normal or pathological limitation of nerve, muscle, or mental function.

Instinct (Pa.): drive, or impulsion of physiologic origin, producing emotional tension and mentally represented by phantasies or wishes and the need to act in that specific way which yields pleasure by the reduction of tension.

Instinct Representation (Pa.): those components of the mind, especially memories and phantasies, which are accompanied or produced by an emotional need. Syn., a "wish"; "mental-representation."

Insulin (M.): a hormone whose deficiency causes diabetes; sometimes administered for "shock treatment" of psychosis.

Introversion (Pa.): (1) originally used by Freud to designate preoccupation with phantasies of object-love whose actual realization is neurotically inhibited.

(2) used by Jung to designate thoughts, feelings, sensations, and intuitive processes when interest in other people is absent or subsidiary.

(3) later used by Freud for those phantasies in which the self is object of the libido; narcissim; egocentricity.

Iritis (M.): a disease characterized by inflammation and pain of the "iris," the circular, colored portion of the eye whose central aperture is the pupil.

Latency Period (Pa.): the period of psychosexual and personality development between the repression of the Œdipus complex and puberty, lasting approximately from the age of six to thirteen.

Latent Content (Pa.): in dream psychology, those primary unconscious wishes, discovered by analysis of the manifest content (*q.v.*), which have activated a dream.

Lay Analysis (Pa.): therapy by psychoanalysts who have not studied medicine.

Libido (Pa.): the instinctual source of psychosexual needs and their mental representations; in later theory, a derivative of "Eros." Syn.: sexual instincts.

Lumbar Pain (M.): pain in the loins, or lower curvature of the back.

Manic-depressive Psychosis (Py.): a psychosis characterized by "manic" periods of pathological excitement, lack of emotional restraint, incessant heightened mental and physical activity, alternating with periods of depression.

Manifest Content (Pa.): in dream psychology, the conscious waking memory of what has been dreamed in sleep.

Masochism (1) (Py.): a sexual perversion, characterized by the need to experience physical pain in order to attain maximal erotic satisfaction.

(2) (Pa.): also, conscious or unconscious wishes to experience physical or psychological pain, and their derivatives; actual or potential pleasure in pain or suffering.

(3) (Pa.): theoretically, a partial aim of the libido; in later theory, the passive instinctual aims resulting from incomplete fusion of Eros and the Death Instincts.

(4) (Pa.): loosely used in early literature as synonymous with any impulsion toward passive gratification; "passivity."

Megalomania (Py.): a psychotic mental state characterized by delusions that one is a very great personage; psychotic grandiosity.

Melancholia (Py.): a severe psychotic depression *(q.v.)*.

Menopause (M.): the physical and psychological changes accompanying the cessation of menstruation; "change of life" in women.

Mental Status (Py.): a systematic examination whose chief purpose is the determination of abnormalities of the intellectual functions, affects, and behavior of a patient.

Narcissism (Pa.): (1) theoretically, those phenomena which result from a person's body, ego, or mental attributes being the object of his libido; "introversion" of the libido;

(2) conscious or unconscious libidinal wishes which do not require object-love for full gratification; love of self or certain attributes of the self;

(3) in analytic psychopathology, unusual manifestations, or an excessive degree, of self-love.

Narcissism, Primary (Pa.): the original narcissism of normal infancy, before the stage of object-love.

Narcissistic Character (Pa.): an individual many of whose characteristic traits are determined by excessive narcissism and deficient capacity for object-love; colloquially, a "narcissist." Moderate types are closely related to "character neurosis," severe types to "psychosis."

Neonate (M.): a newly born infant.

Neurasthenia (Py.): a non-psychotic syndrome characterized by lassitude, irritability, failure of initiative, mild but often abundant hypochondriacal complaints, excessive worry or fearfulness, constant fatigue, and general psychic incapacity and deficient normal pleasure. (Often misused in general medicine as a diagnosis of almost any psychological difficulty.)

Neurology (M.): the medical study of the organs of the nervous systems and their diseases.

Neurosis (1) (M.): a disease ascribed to abnormal function of the nerves.

(2) (Pa.): in psychoanalysis, the usual colloquial synonym for "psychoneurosis" (*q.v.*).

Neurotic Character (Pa.): a synonym for "character neurosis" (*q.v.*).

Nirvana Principle (Pa.): a phantasy that the ultimate goal of life is peace without tension by death.

Object (Pa.): that person or thing or surrogate which is loved or hated, consciously or unconsciously essential for gratification of a specific instinctual impulse.

Object-love (Pa.): the need to give to, to be tender toward, to provide pleasure for another person, who is consequently subjectively "over-valued," in contrast to autoerotic, narcissistic, and most pregenital love.

Obsession (Py.): a psychoneurotic symptom; an absurd, inconsequential, or irrelevant idea upon which conscious attention must be focused, though it is adequately evaluated by the intellect as futile and opposed by the will.

Obsessional Character (Pa.): a character neurosis closely related to "compulsive character," in which the mind is excessively dominated by elaborate intellectualization without full development of obsessions, recognition of emotional needs is impaired, and a rigidity of personality produces a pattern of repetitive failures to attain reasonable objectives.

Obsessional Neurosis (Py.): a psychoneurosis the most conspicuous feature of which is the occurrence of obsessions which seriously impair normal thought and behavior. Closely related to "compulsion neurosis" (*q.v.*).

Œdipus Complex (Pa.): the conscious or unconscious erotic and tender love of male or female for either parent, with marked jealousy of the other parent; the normal culmination of the infantile period of sexual development. (*See* "Electra Complex.")

Ontogeny (M.): the sequence and relationship of phases of development.

Oral: related to the lips or mouth.

Oral Erotism (Pa.): conscious or unconscious wishes associated with pleasurable sensations of the lips and mouth, and the derivatives of these wishes in thought, act, and symptom; in theory, those components of the sexual instincts whose primary aim is oral pleasure.

Oral Sadism (Pa.): sadism associated with oral erotism and mentally represented by unconscious phantasies of biting or devouring, and the derivates of these phantasies in thought, symptom, or behavior.

Organic Disease (M.): a somatic disease, contrasted with "functional" disease and psychoneurosis (*q.v.*), in which an abnormality of a tissue or organ can be demonstrated or inferred. Syn., "somatic disease."

Ovary (M.): the internal organ of the female which produces ova (eggs).

Overt: direct, actual expression of a wish by conscious behavior. (Cf. "Latent.")

Paranoia (Py.): a paranoid psychosis (*q.v.*) whose delusions are highly systematized, intellectually rationalized, and coherent.

Paranoid Character (Py.): a non-psychotic type of narcissistic character (*q.v.*), whose conspicuous feature is an excessive subjective tendency to suspect others of hostile intentions.

Paranoid Psychosis (Py.): a psychosis whose most conspicuous feature is delusions that certain people are plotting, persecuting, or disloyal.

Parapraxia (Pa.): an unconsciously determined error or mistake, a "symptomatic act."

Partial Aim (Pa.): any one of the various means of gratification of the sexual instincts; especially one of the pregenital aims (oral, anal, phallic, urethral, exhibitionistic, etc.).

Passivity (Pa.): those instinctual aims requiring initiative in the behavior of the object.

Pathological (M.): abnormal.

Pathology (M.): the study of changes in the tissues produced by organic disease.

Personality (Py.): the aggregate of psychological and social reactions which characterize an individual; the aggregate of his subjective, emotional, and organized mental life, his behavior, and his reactions to the environment. Less emphasis on the unique or unalterable traits of a person is connoted by "personality" than by the term "character" (*q.v.*).

Perversion, Sexual (Py.): a dominant conscious preference for attaining maximal erotic gratification by some other sexual act than coitus, or the need to supplement coitus by some unusual voluptuous experience.

Phallic Phase (Pa.): that stage of psychosexual development in which the penis or clitoris is the zone of maximal sensual pleasure, but in which tender object-love and the pleasure of another are not essential for maximal gratification.

Phobia (Py.): a psychoneurotic anxiety experienced when some special object or situation, as a certain animal or street, or the darkness, is encountered or imagined.

Physiology (M.): the study of the functions of tissues and organs.

Pituitary Gland (M.): an endocrine gland within the brain secreting hormones which control the functions of other endocrine glands, often called the "master gland."

Pleasure Principle (Pa.): in instinct theory, the hypothesis that pleasure results from reduction of instinctual tension, that all psychological processes are determined by the desire for maximal pleasure and minimal pain, and that immediate gratification regardless of future consequences is normally characteristic of the instincts when not controlled by an organized and mature ego.

Pleurisy (M.): inflammation of the membranes encasing the lung.

Preconscious (Pa.): in Freud's early theory of personality structure, a portion of the "System Conscious" (*q.v.*), consisting of potentially conscious ideas.

Pregenital Sexuality (Pa.): (1) those phases of infantile psychosexuality which precede maturation of the Œdipus complex and genital object-love and whose maximal gratification is autoerotic.

(2) the wishes of the adult unconscious for autoerotic gratification, and their conscious derivatives.

Primal Horde (Pa.): the hypothetical structure of a primitive human family historically antedating the organization of clans.

Primary Process (Pa.): the laws determining the association of ideas not controlled or altered by such rational and realistic mental processes as logic, recognition of time and spatial relationships, of opposites, of negation, etc.; the "primary process" is considered characteristic of the infantile mind, the adult unconscious, latent dream content, and psychotic thoughts. Syn., "autism."

Prognosis (M.): prediction of the probable outcome of a disease or its treatment.

Projection (Pa.): conscious perception of an imaginary sensation or idea as though it existed in the outer world; especially, the unrealistic ascribing of an unconscious wish, a character trait, or an ideal to another person.

Proteins (M.): complex chemical compounds found in all cells and essential to life.

Pseudo-memory (Pa.): a free association which seems subjectively to be the memory of a real event, though it certainly, or probably, did not actually occur.

Psychiatry (M.): that specialty of medicine which studies and treats mental disease, including psychoses, psychoneuroses, personality and social problems, and the emotional aspects of organic disease.

Psychoanalysis (colloquially, "analysis") (Pa.): the technique of Sigmund Freud based upon free association (*q.v.*); the use of this technique for treatment, and for the study of normal and abnormal *unconscious* psychology; and the data and the theories derived from these studies.

Psychogenic (M.): caused by psychological factors. Syn., "functional."

Psychology: (1) all study of the mind, and all mental phenomena.

(2) specifically, the non-medical science of the mind, including experimental, psychometric, clinical, social, educational, and other branches of psychology, and the practical applications of these.

Psychoneurosis (colloquially, "neurosis") (Py.): a disturbance of psychologic or physiologic functions, of the general personality, or of the social adjustment, without conspicuous evidence of psychosis or emotional indifference to other people, caused by unconscious mental conflict, and productive directly or indirectly of a significant limitation of pleasure or success, or a significant degree of suffering and social failure.

Psychopathic Personality (Py.): a diagnostic term used variously by different psychiatrists. I have used it to designate special types of abnormal personality, with or without definite psychosis, characterized predominantly by a major defect in moral sensitivity, a profound disregard of social institutions, and a marked incapacity to restrain antisocial impulses, though intellectually there is normal awareness of the laws and mores and of the consequences of their violation.

Psychopathology (Py.): the study of abnormalities of mind, personality, and social adjustment.

Psychosexuality (Pa.): (1) psychosexuality, as used in psychoanalysis, comprises all aspects of love and pleasure-seeking; it emphasizes unconscious wishes for sensual gratification and their conscious de-erotized derivatives, normal and abnormal, as well as wishes which culminate in complete and mature heterosexual union. (Colloquially, "sexuality.")

(2) theoretically, the instinctual impulsion of the libido toward acts or thoughts of sensual pleasure, or substitutes for sensual pleasure.

Psychosis (Py.): insanity; medically, one of the forms of mental disease which manifest a striking abnormality of mental function or behavior, usually of a degree incompatible with self-sustained social adjustment, often but not always manifesting delusions or hallucinations.

Psychosomatic (M.): involving the relationships of bodily and mental phenomena, especially psychologic factors in the causation of organic disease.

Psychotherapy (Py.): treatment of disease, psychoneurosis, and personality problems by a psychologic method.

Punishment Phantasy (Pa.): a phantasy, generally unconscious in the adult, of an unpleasant consequence of wish-fulfillment; usually the subjective motive for repression of a wish or of guilt if it is gratified.

Rationalization (Pa.): a simple or philosophical, logically justifiable or fallacious, reasoning process which is unconsciously exploited to explain intellectually an emotionally motivated occurrence.

Reality Principle (Pa.): that normal function of the ego, characteristic of maturity, which governs the temporary denial or postponement of immediate gratification of a wish in order to avoid painful future consequences.

Reality Situation (Pa.): the actual environment of a person, especially the emotional attitudes of other people appraised objectively, and the economic, social, and other practical aspects of the situation. The environment as a person would appraise it if there were no immaturity or neurotic distortion at all.

Reality-testing (Pa.): (1) the discrimination of what has rational validity or actual existence in the person's environment from imaginative or autistic ideas.

(2) theoretically, a conscious mental function organized in the course of development, a normal component of the ego.

Regression (Pa.): unconscious displacement of instinctual aim or object to one whose primacy in normal development is chronologically earlier.

Repetition Compulsion (Pa.): the primitive tendency of instincts to reproduce a typical tension independently of the Pleasure Principle.

Repression (Pa.): (1) the involuntary exclusion from representation in the conscious mind of a sexual or hostile wish, phantasy, memory, or associated emotion; especially the exclusion of wishes associated with infantile sexual objects or aims.

(2) theoretically, one of the defense mechanisms organized by the ego for control of instinctual impulses and avoidance of conscious pain.

Resistance (Pa.): the occurrence during psychoanalysis or psychotherapy of emotional opposition to the method and objective purpose of the treatment.

Reversibility (Py.): the potential capacity of a diseased tissue or organ to return to its healthy state when the original cause of the abnormality is altered.

Sadism (1) (Py.): a sexual perversion, characterized by the need to inflict physical pain in order to attain maximal erotic gratification.

(2) (Pa.): also, conscious and unconscious wishes to cause physical or psychological pain, and their derivatives; pleasure in inflicting pain or injury.

(3) (Pa.): theoretically, active partial aims of the sexual instincts; in later theory considered the result of incomplete fusion of Eros and the Death Instincts.

(4) (Pa.): loosely used in early literature as though synonymous with any aggressive impulse; "activity."

Sado-masochism (Pa.): sadism *and* masochism.

Schizoid Character (Py.): a personality type characterized by marked limitation of self-assertive behavior and object-love, social seclusiveness, and excessive preoccupation with phantasies, which are often of a poetical or symbolic character.

Schizophrenia (Py.): a group of malignant psychoses characterized especially by a profound deficiency of the usual indications of *normal* emotion and capacity for "rapport," and an extreme preoccupation with ideas which are extensively symbolic, neologistic, unreal, and intellectually incomprehensible, often accompanied by bizarre delusions, hallucinations, and behavior. Syn., "dementia præcox."

Scoptophilia (Pa.): conscious or unconscious psychosexual pleasure in looking, especially looking at the genitals, and its derivatives (curiosity); in theory, a partial aim of the libido. (*See* "Exhibitionism.")

Secondary Gains (Pa.): those pleasures which a psychoneurotic person seeks to derive from or attain by his symptoms or immature character traits; they are not the cause, but a consequence of the psychoneurosis.

Secondary Process (Pa.): those laws determining the rational and realistic association of ideas; in the theories of personality structure they are considered functions of the System Conscious or the ego.

Seminal Vesicles (M.): internal organs where semen is stored and from which it is emitted during male orgasm.

Sexual Instincts (Pa.): a group of instincts producing emotional needs for love and sensual pleasures and their substitutes, and for all other manifestations of "psychosexuality" (*q.v.*); each component sexual instinct is distinguished by specificity of its "aim" (*q.v.*). Syn., "libido" (*q.v.*).

Siblings: brothers and sisters.

Structure, Personality (Pa.): (1) originally, in "metapsychology," the description of the mind as composed of three systems, the Unconscious, the Conscious, and the Preconscious (*q.v.*).

(2) later, the theory that all the conscious and unconscious mental components of total personality may be described in three systems, id, ego, and super-ego (*q.v.*).

Sublimation (Pa.): the process by which an unconscious sexual wish is "de-sexualized" and consciously gratified in work, play, or art, without conscious sensual experience, without love of another person, and without contingent suffering. (Cf. "Aim-inhibited Wish.")

Suggestion (Py.): those methods of psychotherapy by which symptoms are cured by direct or implied authoritative reassurance.

Super-ego (Pa.): in the later concept of personality structure, those components of the personality, in the main unconscious, which represent intra-psychically the prohibitions and ideals of adults who had originally imposed external frustrations or punishment; theoretically, the organization of intra-psychic functions which threaten or impose a sense of guilt or psychic suffering.

Supervised Analysis (Pa.): instruction of a student at a psychoanalytic institute in the clinical use of the psychoanalytic method. Syn., "control analysis."

Surrogate (Pa.): a conscious substitute for the unconscious object of a sexual or aggressive wish, the result of object-displacement.

Symbol (Pa.): any mental or behavioral representation of a wish or thing by some simple, poetically toned, and unrealistic substitute; especially those representations of unconscious psychosexual thoughts which are found to be common to many individuals of various cultures, and recur frequently in dreams, art, folklore, and everyday life.

Sympathetic Nervous System (M.): a part of the autonomic nervous system (*q.v.*).

Taboo: the ritualistic or conventional prohibition of certain forms of behavior, especially one of those prohibitions which constitute the ethical codes of primitive societies.

Therapy (M.): treatment of disease or symptoms; (Py.): psychotherapy.

Thyroid Gland (M.): an endocrine gland situated in the neck whose secretion increases physiologic metabolism and psychologic excitability.

Tic (M.): an involuntary, convulsive movement of any muscle-group, usually a psychoneurotic symptom.

Totality Concept (Py.): the concept of psychosomatic medicine that every biologic and mental function, especially emotion and interpersonal experience, is related to the functions of the organism as a whole. Syn., "holistic concept."

Totem: that animal regarded by primitive people as the reincarnation of dead members of their clan, and therefore the object of special taboos and rituals.

Training Analysis (Pa.): synonym for "didactic analysis" (*q.v.*).

Transference (Pa.): a patient's pattern of conscious and unconscious phantasies about the physician, and the emotions and conflicts they represent, developing during psychoanalysis or psychotherapy (and in other professional relationships) in consequence of the patient's repressed needs and earlier object relations.

Transference Neurosis (Pa.): that phase of transference during some psychoanalyses when the most fundamental ambivalence conflicts of the individual are displaced on the therapist and become compulsive.

Trauma (M.): an external event which acts as a primary or precipitating cause of a symptom or disease.

Traumatic Neurosis (Py.): a mental disorder caused by an acute emotional trauma, characterized especially by inhibition of normal functions, intense anxiety, and the marked tendency to repeat the emotions of the trauma, and to reproduce portions of it in hallucinations or catastrophic dreams. "Shell-shock" or "combat neurosis" of soldiers in battle is the most common traumatic neurosis.

Ulcer, Gastric (M.): a medical or psychosomatic disease producing erosions of the inner wall of the stomach.

Umbilical Cord (M.): the cord attaching the unborn fœtus or infant to his mother's womb.

Unconscious: (1) adjective: unaware, inaccessible to consciousness by an effort of voluntary attention.

(2) noun, "the Unconscious" (Pa.): an inclusive abstraction of all unconscious mental phenomena.

(3) noun, the "System Unconscious" (Pa.): in the early theory of personality structure (*q.v.*), a "region" of the mind controlled by the "primary process" (*q.v.*) and differentiated from the System Conscious, or ego.

Urethra (M.): the tube by which urine is excreted from the bladder.

Urethral Erotism (Pa.): (1) conscious or unconscious wishes for sensory pleasure by urination, and associated phantasies.

(2) in theory, a partial aim of the sexual instincts.

Uterus: the female organ in which the infant develops prior to birth; the womb.

Vagina: the female organ which receives the penis in sexual intercourse.

Wild Analysis: therapeutic psychoanalysis by the untrained and unqualified.

Wish (Pa.): a phantasy; the representation of an instinct in the mind, especially unconscious psychosexual and hostile phantasies associated with infantile aims and objects; an "instinct-representation."

INDEX

(Italicized page-references indicate specific discussion of the topic. Most references to published works are indexed under the author.)

IVES HENDRICK was born in New Haven, Connecticut, in 1898. He received his B.A. from Yale in 1921, and his M.D. from the Yale Medical School in 1925. After completing his general internship, he specialized in psychiatry, working at the Boston Psychopathic Hospital and at the Sheppard Enoch Pratt Hospital in Baltimore. He then studied for two years at the Berlin Psycho-analytic Institute, graduating in 1930. Returning to Boston, he began the private practice of psychoanalysis and psychiatry, and was instrumental in the organization of the first professional training program of the Boston Psychoanalytic Institute in 1931.

Dr. Hendrick has been on the faculty of the Harvard Medical School since 1930, becoming Clinical Professor of Psychiatry in 1953; he was also Director of Medical Education at the Boston Psychopathic Hospital from 1949 to 1955. He has been a regular contributor to technical journals, and has served the American Psychoanalytic Association as Councillor, as Chairman of its Board on Professional Standards (1951–3), as President (1953–5), and as a member of the Editorial Board of its *Journal* (1951–5).